Obsessive Compulsive and Related Disorders

Editors

ERIC A. STORCH
WAYNE K. GOODMAN

PSYCHIATRIC CLINICS OF NORTH AMERICA

www.psych.theclinics.com

Consulting Editor
HARSH K. TRIVEDI

March 2023 • Volume 46 • Number 1

ELSEVIER

1600 John F. Kennedy Boulevard • Suite 1800 • Philadelphia, Pennsylvania, 19103-2899

http://www.theclinics.com

PSYCHIATRIC CLINICS OF NORTH AMERICA Volume 46, Number 1
March 2023 ISSN 0193-953X, ISBN-13: 978-0-443-18264-8

Editor: Megan Ashdown
Developmental Editor: Diana Grace Ang

Psychiatric Clinics of North America (ISSN 0193-953X) is published quarterly by Elsevier Inc., 360 Park Avenue South, New York, NY 10010-1710. Months of issue are March, June, September, and December. Business and Editorial Offices: 1600 John F. Kennedy Blvd., Suite 1800, Philadelphia, PA 19103-2899. Periodicals postage paid at New York, NY and additional mailing offices. Subscription prices are $352.00 per year (US individuals), $781.00 per year (US institutions), $100.00 per year (US students/residents), $422.00 per year (Canadian individuals), $519.00 per year (international individuals), $983.00 per year (Canadian & international institutions), and $220.00 per year (international students/residents), $100.00 per year (Canadian & students/residents). Foreign air speed delivery is included in all *Clinics'* subscription prices. All prices are subject to change without notice. **POSTMASTER:** Send address changes to *Psychiatric Clinics of North America*, Elsevier Health Sciences Division, Subscription Customer Service, 3251 Riverport Lane, Maryland Heights, MO 63043. **Customer Service: 1-800-654-2452 (US). From outside the United States, call 1-314-447-8871. Fax: 1-314-447-8029. E-mail: journalscustomerservice-usa@elsevier.com (for print support)** and **journalsonlinesupport-usa@elsevier.com (for online support)**.

Reprints. For copies of 100 or more, of articles in this publication, please contact the Commercial Reprints Department, Elsevier Inc., 360 Park Avenue South, New York, New York 10010-1710. Tel.: 212-633-3874, Fax: 212-633-3820, E-mail: reprints@elsevier.com.

Psychiatric Clinics of North America is covered in *MEDLINE/PubMed (Index Medicus)*, *Current Contents/Social and Behavioral Sciences*, *Social Science Citation Index*, *Embase/Excerpta Medica*, and PsycINFO.

Contributors

CONSULTING EDITOR

HARSH K. TRIVEDI, MD, MBA
President and Chief Executive Officer, Sheppard Pratt, Clinical Professor of Psychiatry, University of Maryland School of Medicine, Baltimore, Maryland, USA

EDITORS

ERIC A. STORCH, PhD
Professor, Vice Chair, and McIngvale Presidential Endowed Chair, Menninger Department of Psychiatry and Behavioral Sciences, Baylor College of Medicine, Houston, Texas, USA

WAYNE K. GOODMAN, MD
D.C. and Irene Ellwood Professor and Chair, Menninger Department of Psychiatry and Behavioral Sciences, Baylor College of Medicine, Houston, Texas, USA

AUTHORS

LINDSAY BACALA, MSW
PhD Student, University of Manitoba, Winnipeg, Manitoba, Canada

LAURA B. BRAGDON, PhD
Clinical Instructor, Department of Psychiatry, New York University School of Medicine, New York, New York, USA; Visiting Scientist, Nathan S. Kline Institute for Psychiatric Research, Orangeburg, New York, USA

CHRISTIANA BRATIOTIS, PhD, MSW
Associate Professor, University of British Columbia, School of Social Work, Vancouver, British Columbia, Canada

MATTI CERVIN, PhD
Department of Clinical Sciences, Lund, Child and Adolescent Psychiatry, Faculty of Medicine, Lund University, Lund, Sweden

KATHERINE A. COLLINS, PhD, LCSW
Research Scientist, Nathan S. Kline Institute for Psychiatric Research, Orangeburg, New York, USA

JAMES J. CROWLEY, PhD
Associate Professor, Departments of Genetics and Psychiatry, The University of North Carolina at Chapel Hill, Chapel Hill, North Carolina, USA

MADELEINE CUNNINGHAM, PhD
Department of Microbiology and Immunology, University of Oklahoma Health Sciences Center, Oklahoma City, Oklahoma, USA

GOI KHIA ENG, PhD
Postdoctoral Fellow, Department of Psychiatry, New York University School of Medicine, New York, New York, USA; Visiting Scientist, Nathan S. Kline Institute for Psychiatric Research, Orangeburg, New York, USA

JOEY K.-Y. ESSOE, PhD
Department of Psychiatry and Behavioral Sciences, Division of Child and Adolescent Psychiatry, Center for OCD, Anxiety, and Related Disorders for Children, Johns Hopkins School of Medicine, Baltimore, Maryland, USA

JENNIFER FRANKOVICH, MD, MS
Stanford Children's Health, PANS Clinic and Research Program, Division of Pediatrics, Department of Allergy, Immunology, Rheumatology, Stanford University School of Medicine, Stanford, California, USA

RON GADOT, BSC
Department of Neurosurgery, Baylor College of Medicine, Houston, Texas, USA

DANIEL A. GELLER, MD
Department of Psychiatry, Massachusetts General Hospital, Harvard Medical School, Boston, Massachusetts, USA

WAYNE K. GOODMAN, MD
D.C. and Irene Ellwood Professor and Chair, Menninger Department of Psychiatry and Behavioral Sciences, Baylor College of Medicine, Houston, Texas, USA

ANDREW G. GUZICK, PhD
Baylor College of Medicine, Houston, Texas, USA

TAL HARMELECH, PhD
BrainsWay Ltd, Jerusalem, Israel

AMITA JASSI, DClinPsy
National and Specialist OCD, BDD, and Related Disorders Service, South London and Maudsley NHS Trust, London, United Kingdom

GEORGINA KREBS, DClinPsy, PhD
National and Specialist OCD, BDD, and Related Disorders Service, South London and Maudsley NHS Trust, Department of Clinical, Educational and Health Psychology, University College London, London, United Kingdom

NANCY LIN, MSW, RSW
PhD Student, University of British Columbia, School of Social Work, Vancouver, British Columbia, Canada

SPENSER MARTIN, BA
Hoarding Wellness Specialist, Canadian Mental Health Association, Winnipeg, Manitoba, Canada

JOSEPH F. McGUIRE, PhD
Department of Psychiatry and Behavioral Sciences, Division of Child and Adolescent Psychiatry, Center for OCD, Anxiety, and Related Disorders for Children, Johns Hopkins School of Medicine, Baltimore, Maryland, USA

JORDANA MUROFF, PhD, MSW
Associate Professor, Boston University, School of Social Work, Boston, Massachusetts, USA

EYAL MUSCAL, MD, MS
Department of Rheumatology, Texas Children's Hospital, Houston, Texas, USA

AINSLEY K. PATRICK, BS
Department of Psychiatry and Behavioral Sciences, Division of Child and Adolescent Psychiatry, Center for OCD, Anxiety, and Related Disorders for Children, Johns Hopkins School of Medicine, Baltimore, Maryland, USA

CHRISTOPHER PITTENGER, MD, PhD
Mears and Jameson Professor of Psychiatry, Departments of Psychiatry, Psychology, and Child Study Center, Center for Brain and Mind Health, Yale University, New Haven, Connecticut, USA

NICOLE PROVENZA, PhD
Department of Neurosurgery, Baylor College of Medicine, Houston, Texas, USA

KESLEY A. RAMSEY, PhD
Department of Psychiatry and Behavioral Sciences, Division of Child and Adolescent Psychiatry, Center for OCD, Anxiety, and Related Disorders for Children, Johns Hopkins School of Medicine, Baltimore, Maryland, USA

NICOLETTE RECCHIA, BS
Research Data Associate, Department of Psychiatry, New York University School of Medicine, New York, New York, USA; Research Assistant, Nathan S. Kline Institute for Psychiatric Research, Orangeburg, New York, USA

YIFTACH ROTH, PhD
BrainsWay Ltd, Jerusalem, Israel; Department of Life Sciences, Ben Gurion University of the Negev, Israel

McKENZIE SCHUYLER, BS
Department of Psychiatry, Massachusetts General Hospital, Boston, Massachusetts, USA

SAMEER A. SHETH, MD, PhD
Department of Neurosurgery, Department of Psychiatry, Baylor College of Medicine, Houston, Texas, USA

BEN SHOFTY, MD, PhD
Department of Neurosurgery, University of Utah, Salt Lake City, Utah, USA

SAMUEL D. SPENCER, MA
Baylor College of Medicine, Houston, Texas, USA

EMILY R. STERN, PhD
Associate Professor, Department of Psychiatry, New York University School of Medicine, New York, New York, USA; Research Scientist, Nathan S. Kline Institute for Psychiatric Research, Orangeburg, New York, USA

JORDAN T. STIEDE, MS
Baylor College of Medicine, Houston, Texas, USA

ERIC A. STORCH, PhD
Professor, Vice Chair, and McIngvale Presidential Endowed Chair, Menninger Department of Psychiatry and Behavioral Sciences, Baylor College of Medicine, Houston, Texas

ARON TENDLER, MD
BrainsWay Ltd, Jerusalem, Israel; Department of Life Sciences, Ben Gurion University of the Negev, Israel

MARGO THIENEMANN, MD
Division of Child and Adolescent Psychiatry and Child Development, Department of Psychiatry, Stanford Children's Health, PANS Clinic and Research Program, Stanford University School of Medicine, Stanford, California, USA

ALLISON VREELAND, PhD
Division of Child and Adolescent Psychiatry and Child Development, Department of Psychiatry, Stanford Children's Health, PANS Clinic and Research Program, Stanford University School of Medicine, Stanford, California, USA

ANDREW D. WIESE, PhD
Baylor College of Medicine, Houston, Texas, USA

Contents

Obsessive-compulsive disorder (OCD) is characterized by time-consuming, distressing, or impairing obsessions and compulsions. Obsessions are recurrent, persistent, and intrusive thoughts, urges, or images. Compulsions are repetitive and often ritualized behaviors or mental acts performed to manage obsession-related distress or prevent harm. OCD affects 1% to 3% of the population, typically begins during adolescence or early adulthood, and can have a chronic or deteriorating course in the absence of effective treatment.

Obsessive-compulsive disorder (OCD) is an impairing mental health disease, generally beginning in childhood, affecting up to ~3% of the population. Using evidence-based assessments (EBAs) is the starting point for the accurate diagnosis and treatment of OCD. EBAs consist of structured and semistructured clinician-administered interviews, parent-report and child-report, and self-report for adults. This article details the practical application, psychometric properties, and limitations of available assessments to determine the presence of OCD and evaluate OCD symptom severity. The following reviews measurement of constructs relevant to OCD (ie, insight, family accommodation, impairment) and details considerations for best clinical interview practices.

A wealth of evidence has shown that genetics plays a major role in susceptibility to obsessive-compulsive disorder (OCD) and all of its related disorders. Several large-scale, collaborative efforts using modern genomic methods are beginning to reveal the genetic architecture of these traits and identify long-sought risk genes. In this article, we summarize current OCD and related disorder genomic knowledge and explain how to communicate this information to patients and their families. The article concludes with a discussion of how genomic discovery in OCD and related disorders can inform our understanding of disease etiology and provide novel targets for therapeutic development.

Cognitive neuroscientific research has the ability to yield important insights into the complex neurobiological processes underlying obsessive-compulsive disorder (OCD). This article provides an updated review of neuroimaging studies in seven neurocognitive domains. Findings from the literature are discussed in the context of obsessive-compulsive phenomenology and treatment. Expanding our knowledge of the neural mechanisms involved in OCD could help optimize treatment outcomes and guide the development of novel interventions.

Sydenham chorea (SC), pediatric autoimmune neuropsychiatric disorders associated with streptococcal infections (PANDAS) and pediatric acute-onset neuropsychiatric syndrome (PANS) are postinfectious neuroinflammatory diseases that involve the basal ganglia and have obsessive-compulsive disorder as a major manifestation. As is true for many childhood rheumatological and neuroinflammatory diseases, SC, PANDAS and PANS lack diagnostic biomarkers and randomized clinical trials. Treatment of these disorders depend on three complementary modes of intervention: treating the symptoms, the source of inflammation, and disturbances of the immune system. Future studies should aim to integrate neuroimaging, inflammation, immunogenetic, and clinical data (noting the stage in clinical course).

Obsessive–compulsive disorder (OCD) frequently affects children and adolescents, with most cases beginning during this time. Symptoms of OCD in youth may present as exaggerated developmental concerns and excessive ritualistic behavior beyond what is part of normal development, yet low levels of insight may prevent recognition. Affected youth commonly have comorbid neurodevelopmental diagnoses, especially males. Early detection and intervention are critical to recovery and remission, as well as family involvement in treatment. Cognitive behavioral therapy and serotonin reuptake inhibitors are first-line treatments.

Pharmacological treatment is a mainstay of the care of individuals with obsessive-compulsive disorder. Robust evidence supports the use of the selective serotonin reuptake inhibitors and the older tricyclic drug clomipramine. Other antidepressants are less effective (or have been insufficiently studied). When first-line treatment with these agents, and with appropriate psychotherapy, is ineffective, several augmentation strategies are available, though their evidentiary support is weaker. A substantial minority of patients have persistent symptoms despite optimal evidence-based treatment. Further work and more treatment options are needed.

Treatment-resistant obsessive-compulsive disorder (trOCD) is a severely disabling, life-threatening psychiatric disorder affecting ~0.5% of the US population. Following the failure of multiple medical and psychotherapeutic treatment lines, patients with trOCD, like others with functional disorders, may benefit from invasive neuromodulation. Cumulative evidence suggests that disrupting abnormal hyperdirect cortico-striato-thalamo-cortical (CSTC) pathway activity offers sustainable, robust symptomatic relief in most patients. Multiple surgical approaches allow for modulation of the CSTC pathway, including stereotactic lesions and electrical stimulation. This review aims to describe the modern neurosurgical approaches for trOCD, recent advances in our understanding of pathophysiology, and future therapeutic directions.

Obsessive-compulsive disorder (OCD) patients need novel therapeutic interventions since most experience residual symptoms despite treatment. Converging evidence suggest that OCD involves dysfunction of limbic cortico-striato-thalamo-cortical loops, including the medial prefrontal cortex (mPFC) and dorsal anterior cingulate cortex (dACC), that tends to normalize with successful treatment. Recently, three repetitive transcranial magnetic stimulation (rTMS) coils were FDA-cleared for treatment-refractory OCD. This review presents on-label and off-label clinical evidence and relevant physical characteristics of the three coils. The Deep TMS™ H7 Coil studies' point to efficacy of mPFC-dACC stimulation, while no clear target stems from the small heterogenous D-B80 and figure-8 coils studies.

Obsessive-compulsive disorder (OCD) is characterized by the presence of debilitating obsessions and compulsions. Cognitive and behavioral models of OCD provide a strong theoretic and empirical foundation for informing effective psychotherapeutic treatment. Cognitive-behavioral therapy (CBT) for OCD, which includes a deliberate emphasis on exposure and response/ritual prevention, has consistently demonstrated robust efficacy for the treatment of pediatric and adult OCD and is the front-line psychotherapeutic treatment for OCD. Two case vignettes describing CBT for OCD in practice as well as recommendations for clinicians are provided.

Hoarding disorder is characterized by difficulty parting with possessions due to strong urges to save the items, leading to the excessive accumulation of items. High clutter levels result in varied personal, social, and legal consequences. Specialized treatments, including individual, virtual, and group cognitive and behavioral therapies, community-based interventions, and peer support approaches have shown preliminary effectiveness. Animal, attachment, and neurobiological models are expanding our understanding of the etiological bases of the disorder. Specialized populations such as children, older adults, and involuntary patients are highlighted as requiring special consideration for intervention and risk mitigation. Directions for future research are identified.

This article summarizes current knowledge of body dysmorphic disorder across the life span. An overview of the epidemiology and phenomenology of this condition is provided, as well as clinical perspectives on assessment and treatment. Barriers to accessing treatment are considered, along with recent developments to improve access. Future directions in research and clinical care for this population are summarized.

PSYCHIATRIC CLINICS OF NORTH AMERICA

FORTHCOMING ISSUES

June 2023
Treatment Resistant Depression
Manish K. Jha and Madhukar H. Trivedi, *Editors*

September 2023
Women's Mental Health
Susan G. Kornstein and Anita H. Clayton, *Editors*

RECENT ISSUES

December 2022
Geriatric Psychiatry
Louis Marino Jr. and George S. Zubenko, *Editors*

September 2022
Addiction Psychiatry: Challenges and Recent Advances
Sunil D. Khushalani, George Kolodner and Christopher Welsh, *Editors*

SERIES OF RELATED INTEREST

Child and Adolescent Psychiatric Clinics of North America
https://www.childpsych.theclinics.com/

Neurologic Clinics
https://www.neurologic.theclinics.com/

Advances in Psychiatry and Behavioral Health
https://www.advancesinpsychiatryandbehavioralhealth.com/

THE CLINICS ARE AVAILABLE ONLINE!
Access your subscription at:
www.theclinics.com

Preface

Obsessive Compulsive and Related Disorders

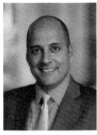 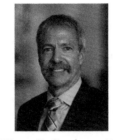

Eric A. Storch, PhD   Wayne K. Goodman, MD
Editors

Obsessive-compulsive disorder (OCD) is a relatively common and impairing condition that runs a chronic course without adequate treatment.[1-3] Characterized by distressing and unwanted obsessions that compel repetitive behaviors and avoidance, OCD is among the most disabling psychiatric conditions[4,5] and confers increased risk of comorbidity as well as early mortality.[6]

As recent as 40 years ago, OCD was considered a difficult-to-treat condition with few available intervention options. Practitioners were stymied in their ability to support their patients. Affected individuals endured lifetimes of sustained illness and impairment with little promise of symptom relief. However, during the 1980s, the outlook began to change. Introduction of targeted psychotherapeutic[7,8] and pharmacologic interventions[9] coupled with validated assessment instruments (eg, Yale-Brown Obsessive-Compulsive Scale)[10] provided hope.

Since then, significant developments have been and continue to be made across multiple frontiers in support of individuals with OCD. Improved appreciation of the phenomenology of the condition has been realized, including appropriate diagnostic classification, patterns of comorbidity, and understanding key clinical characteristics (eg, insight). In addition, the portfolio of validated assessments has dramatically increased such that there are psychometrically sound approaches to capturing obsessive-compulsive severity and cooccurring clinical constructs across the age continuum. Beyond an improved understanding of the clinical presentation of OCD, there have been advances in understanding of the cause of OCD as well as mechanistically informed interventions. For example, building upon models of neurocircuitry, enhancements to existing treatments have taken place as well as development of neuromodulation approaches. Similarly, refining the cognitive-behavioral theory underlying

---

Psychiatr Clin N Am 46 (2023) xiii–xv
https://doi.org/10.1016/j.psc.2022.11.006
0193-953X/23/© 2022 Published by Elsevier Inc.   **psych.theclinics.com**

exposure and response prevention has translated into improved understanding of how this treatment "works" as well as the outcomes of those who receive it.[11]

Despite this progress, more remains to be done. Dissemination of effective therapies is incomplete, particularly to those with fewer resources or in parts of the world where understanding of OCD (and mental health) is limited. Many individuals do not respond sufficiently (or at all) to existing interventions; options for treatment-refractory patients are promising but not sufficiently available yet. Key questions remain on supporting wellness after successful intervention. In the current issue of *Psychiatric Clinics of North America*, we hope to support this continued progress while working to address these remaining issues by compiling a series of articles written by leading scholars. This collection of articles clearly synthesizes information on the clinical phenomenology, assessment, cause, and treatment of OCD across the lifespan. This collection provides "one-stop shopping" for the reader to be updated on the nature and treatment of OCD, and to learn about cutting-edge innovations in intervention, including for those patients who are treatment resistant. It is our hope that this issue (a) disseminates knowledge on how to best support individuals with OCD as well as (b) stimulates continued scientific discovery and innovation.

Eric A. Storch, PhD
Menninger Department of Psychiatry and Behavioral Sciences
Baylor College of Medicine
1977 Butler Boulevard, Suite 4-400
Houston, TX 77030, USA

Wayne K. Goodman, MD
Menninger Department of Psychiatry and Behavioral Sciences
Baylor College of Medicine
1977 Butler Boulevard, Suite 4-400
Houston, TX 77030, USA

E-mail addresses:
Eric.storch@bcm.edu (E.A. Storch)
Wayne.Goodman@bcm.edu (W.K. Goodman)

REFERENCES

1. American Psychiatric Association D-TF: Diagnostic and statistical manual of mental disorders: DSM-5. 5th edition. Washington, DC: American Psychiatric Association; 2013.
2. Rasmussen SA, Eisen JL. The epidemiology and clinical features of obsessive compulsive disorder. Psychiatr Clin North Am 1992;15:743–58.
3. Ruscio AM, Stein DJ, Chiu WT, et al. The epidemiology of obsessive-compulsive disorder in the National Comorbidity Survey Replication. Molecular Psychiatry 2010;15:53–63.
4. Norberg MM, Calamari JE, Cohen RJ, et al. Quality of life in obsessive-compulsive disorder: an evaluation of impairment and a preliminary analysis of the ameliorating effects of treatment. Depress Anxiety 2008;25:248–59.
5. Adam Y, Meinlschmidt G, Gloster AT, et al. Obsessive-compulsive disorder in the community: 12-month prevalence, comorbidity and impairment. Soc Psychiatry Psychiatr Epidemiol 2012;47:339–49.
6. Meier SM, Mattheisen M, Mors O, et al. Mortality among persons with obsessive-compulsive disorder in Denmark. JAMA Psychiatry 2016;73:268–74.

7. Foa EB, Kozak MJ, Steketee GS, et al. Treatment of depressive and obsessive-compulsive symptoms in OCD by imipramine and behaviour therapy. Br J Clin Psychol 1992;31(3). 2792–92.
8. Rachman S, Cobb J, Grey S, et al. The behavioural treatment of obsessional-compulsive disorders, with and without clomipramine. Behav Res Ther 1979; 17(5):4674–8.
9. Goodman WK, Price LH, Delgado PL, et al. Specificity of serotonin reuptake inhibitors in the treatment of obsessive-compulsive disorder. Comparison of fluvoxamine and desipramine. Arch Gen Psychiatry 1990;47:577–85.
10. Goodman WK, Price LH, Rasmussen SA, et al. The Yale-Brown obsessive compulsive scale: I. Development, use, and reliability. Arch Gen Psychiatry 1989;46(11):100610–1.
11. McGuire JF, Storch EA. An inhibitory learning approach to cognitive-behavioral therapy for children and adolescents. Cognit Behav Pract 2019;26(1). 2142–2124.

Obsessive-Compulsive Disorder

Diagnosis, Clinical Features, Nosology, and Epidemiology

Matti Cervin, PhD

KEYWORDS

- Obsessive-compulsive disorder • Obsessions • Compulsions • Diagnosis
- Presentation • Features

KEY POINTS

- Obsessive-compulsive disorder is a disabling mental disorder with a lifetime prevalence of around 2% with similar rates across age groups and countries.
- Diagnosis is made based on a pattern of time-consuming, clinically distressing, or impairing obsessions and compulsions and most cases emerge during puberty or early adulthood.
- Obsessions are recurrent, persistent, and intrusive thoughts, urges, or images, and compulsions are repetitive behaviors or mental acts performed to manage obsession-related distress or prevent harm.
- Symptoms often revolve around intrusive thoughts about harm/scrupulosity and checking or mental rituals, symmetry obsessions and ordering compulsions, and contamination obsessions and cleaning compulsions.
- Obsessive-compulsive disorder is underrecognized, underdiagnosed, and undertreated in all parts of health service, including in psychiatric settings.

INTRODUCTION

Obsessive-compulsive disorder (OCD) is a psychiatric condition characterized by preoccupations with thoughts, objects, sensations, or situations that most individuals experience as neutral or only mildly upsetting. In OCD, these preoccupations are called obsessions and are unwanted, reoccurring, repetitive, and distressing.

Disclosure statement: Dr M. Cervin receives financial compensation from Springer for editorial work outside of the submitted work.
Department of Clinical Sciences, Lund, Child and Adolescent Psychiatry, Faculty of Medicine, Lund University, Sofiavägen 2D, Lund SE-22241, Sweden
E-mail address: matti.cervin@med.lu.se

Obsessions can take on a multitude of forms, but commonly revolve around contamination, possibilities of harm (eg, fires, burglary, accidents, and violence), sex or religion, or asymmetry in one's environment or body. In OCD, obsessions are paired with compulsions, which are repetitive behaviors or mental acts performed to manage or reduce the distress caused by obsessions and/or prevent the risk of unwanted outcomes. An individual with OCD often believes that his or her compulsions are excessive or unnecessary. When a time-consuming, clinically distressing, or impairing pattern of enduring obsessions and compulsions is present, a diagnosis of OCD may be warranted.

DIAGNOSIS
Obsessions

The most up to date and comprehensive diagnostic criteria of OCD are found in the 11th revision of the International Classification of Diseases (ICD-11)[1] and the 5th version of the Diagnostic and Statistical Manual of Mental Disorders (DSM-5).[2,3] Both manuals define obsessions and compulsions separately. ICD-11 states that obsessions are "repetitive and persistent thoughts, images, or impulses/urges that are experienced as intrusive and unwanted, and are commonly associated with anxiety."[1] DSM-5 defines obsessions as "recurrent and persistent thoughts, urges or images that are experienced, at some time during the disturbance, as intrusive, unwanted, and that in most individuals cause marked anxiety or distress."[2,3] Further, both manuals highlight that the thoughts, images, or impulses/urges typically yield attempts to suppress, ignore, or neutralize by performing compulsions.

The diagnostic description of obsessions in the ICD-11 and DSM-5 is largely unchanged from DSM-IV and ICD-10. Both manuals emphasize the heterogeneity of obsessions; they can occur in the form of thoughts, images, or urges, and ICD-11, impulses. They should also be recurrent, repetitive, persistent, and intrusive, meaning that they need to endure over time and in a similar form, setting them apart from everyday worries or concerns. Further, both definitions state that obsessions are unwanted and often experienced as unreasonable or senseless, giving them an "ego dystonic" quality. That is, the obsessive content is not an integrated part of the worldviews of the individual, demarcating them from persecutory delusions and command hallucinations. Anxiety is mentioned in both definitions, and in DSM-5, in combination with distress. Thus, obsessions are unpleasant.

Compulsions

ICD-11 defines compulsions as "repetitive behaviors or rituals, including repetitive mental acts that the individual feels driven to perform in response to an obsession, according to rigid rules, or to achieve a sense of 'completeness.'"[1] The corresponding definition in DSM-5 is "repetitive behaviors or mental acts that the person feels driven to perform in response to an obsession, or according to rules that must be applied rigidly."[2,3] The definitions are very similar and both manuals stress the repetitive nature of compulsions. Both manuals also state that compulsions should be either performed in response to obsessions or according to rigid rules. Further, they should be excessive or not connected in a realistic way to the obsession-related content. In DSM-5, the function of compulsions is described as an effort to prevent or reduce distress or to prevent a dreaded situation or outcome. ICD-11 states that compulsions are attempts to suppress or neutralize obsessions. Thus, according to the ICD-11 and DSM-5 criteria, compulsions are closely related to obsessions and often knowingly performed as a direct response to them.

Additional Criteria

When the presence of clinical obsessions and/or compulsions has been established, an OCD diagnosis mandates that they are either time-consuming, result in significant distress, or yield impairment in important areas of functioning. There is no definitive time limit, but an example of more than 1 hour per day is provided by both manuals. Areas of impairment can be personal, family, social, occupational, or educational. In addition, symptoms should not be better explained by another mental disorder or a general medical condition, or be a direct effect of substances or medication, including withdrawal effects. There is no duration requirement in either manual, but clinicians are cautioned against assigning a diagnosis of OCD when the duration of illness is short, for example, less than 1 month, and in such cases, a careful exploration of other etiologies is warranted.[4]

When OCD has been confirmed, the degree of insight should be specified. In DSM-5, insight is classified into (1) good or fair, (2) poor, or (3) absent/delusional. In ICD-11, insight is classified into (1) fair to good or (2) poor to absent. Insight refers to an acknowledgment that the obsessions and compulsions are (or at least may be) untrue, senseless, or excessive/exaggerated and by a willingness to accept alternative explanations. According to DSM-5, tic-related OCD should be specified when there is a current or past history of a tic disorder. Tic-related OCD has been linked to an earlier onset, a male preponderance, more sensory phenomena in compulsions, and stronger familial patterns.[5] The tic-related specifier is not included in the ICD-11. A synthesis of the diagnostic descriptions of OCD in ICD-11 and DSM-5 is presented in **Box 1**.

Box 1

A synthesis of Diagnostic and Statistical Manual of Mental Disorders-5 and International Classification of Diseases-11 descriptions of obsessive-compulsive disorder

Obsessions

Phenomenology	Recurrent thoughts, images, or urges/impulses
Defining characteristics	Persistent, unwanted, intrusive, and distress-generating
Consequences	Yield attempts to resist, ignore, suppress, or neutralize
Common content	Harm to others or self, violent images, responsibility, making mistakes, sacrilege, sexual concerns, dirt, diseases, germs, contaminants, asymmetry, inexactness, superstition

Compulsions

Phenomenology	Repetitive and often ritualized behaviors or mental acts
Defining characteristics	Excessive or nonlogical and performed in response to obsessions or according to specific rules
Function	Performed to prevent, manage, or ameliorate distress, reach a sense of completeness, or to prevent or lower the probability of harm
Common content	Repeated checking, mental rituals (eg, silently repeating a phrase), handwashing, cleaning of body or items, ordering, arranging, evening out, seeking reassurance from others, counting

Additional criteria

Time-consuming	For example, more than 1 h per day
Or distressing	Clinically significant distress
Or impairing	In occupational, educational, social, personal, or family areas

Rule out other explanations

Other mental disorder	For example, generalized anxiety disorder, body dysmorphic disorder, hoarding disorder, eating disorder, schizophrenia spectrum disorders, autism spectrum disorder
Medical condition	For example, basal ganglia ischemic stroke
Substance, medication	Including withdrawal effects

CLINICAL FEATURES
Symptom Heterogeneity

The heterogeneity of OCD has long been recognized, and a distinction between symptoms characterized by *Folie du doute* (madness of doubt) and *Délire du toucher* (delusion of touch) was proposed already in 1866.[6] Unlike many other mental disorders, where patients often present with similar symptoms, obsessions and compulsions are notoriously idiosyncratic to the point that two patients seldom share the exact same symptoms. Nevertheless, OCD symptoms seem to have commonalities linking them to broader themes or symptom dimensions. The four symptom dimensions with most empirical support are (1) symmetry obsessions and repeating, ordering, and counting compulsions; (2) disturbing thoughts: aggression, sexual, religious, and somatic obsessions and checking compulsions; (3) obsessions and compulsions related to cleanliness, contamination, and germs; and (4) hoarding obsessions and compulsions.[6,7]

These symptom dimensions are temporally stable (with changes from one dimension to another being rare), and they show partly distinct alterations in neurocircuitry and genetic architectures.[8] The multidimensional model of OCD led to a body of work showing that compulsive hoarding was associated with poorer treatment outcome, low co-occurrence of other OCD symptoms, and familial patterns that differed from the other dimensions.[9] This led to the separation of compulsive hoarding from OCD and the introduction of the new diagnostic class of hoarding disorder in DSM-5 and ICD-11 (see Chapter 11). Of note, compulsive hoarding can still be part of OCD, for example, when a patient experiences a strong feeling of incompleteness when discarding an item.

The contamination/cleaning, symmetry/ordering, and disturbing thoughts/checking dimensions have replicated across countries and age groups.[7,10] Recent work, analyzing cross-national data across the lifespan, replicated the three dimensions (and hoarding) but showed that there may be other valid symptom dimensions of OCD.[8,11] Four additional dimensions emerged: obsessions and compulsions related to (1) transformation (ie, fears of turning into somebody or something else), (2) body focus (ie, preoccupations with the body or somatic concerns), (3) superstition (ie, magical thinking), and (4) loss/separation (ie, fear of losing someone). These additional dimensions have been previously recognized in the OCD literature but have not been considered separate dimensions and more work is needed to clarify whether they can yield new insights into OCD. **Fig. 1** provides an overview of the major symptom dimensions of OCD and common symptom within each dimension.

The origin of the symptom dimensions of OCD is unknown, but rigid routines and repetitive behaviors and rituals emerge in normally developing children during the second year of life and are common in other animals.[12] Thus, the clustering of OCD symptoms around broader dimensions may emerge from variation in traits that have been evolutionary conserved.

Avoidance and Insight

Avoidance in OCD refers to the tendency to actively avoid objects, situations, thoughts, or persons to minimize or circumvent triggering obsessions, obsession-related distress, or urges to perform compulsions. Moderate to severe avoidance is found in more than half of all OCD patients irrespective of age,[13,14] contributes to both severity and impairment,[15,16] and predicts poor treatment outcome in youth[14,16] and adults.[13]

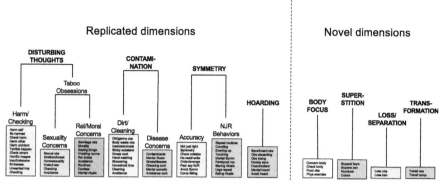

Fig. 1. Symptom structure of OCD with eight broad dimensions: disturbing thoughts (intrusive thoughts about harm or moral failure and checking compulsions), contamination (obsessions about dirt or disease and cleaning compulsions), symmetry (obsessions about accuracy and incompleteness experiences and ordering compulsions), hoarding (excessive saving of and difficulties discarding possessions), body focus (repetitive thoughts and behaviors directed toward the body or somatic concerns), superstition (magical thinking), loss/separation (repetitive thoughts and behaviors related to fears of losing someone), and transformation (fear of turning into someone or something else). The disturbing thoughts, contamination, and symmetry dimensions consist of subdimensions with partly distinct symptom content. The dimensions are based on published empirical work.[8,11]

As stated above, degree of insight should be specified when making an OCD diagnosis. In adults with OCD, 14% to 30% have poor or absent insight[17] and poor insight has been associated with more severe OCD,[17,18] a chronic course,[19] and poorer treatment outcome,[20] although findings for treatment outcome are inconsistent.[14] On average, insight seems to be slightly better in youth: around one in 10 youth with OCD exhibits poor or absent insight, and poor insight does not predict outcome of cognitive-behavioral therapy.[14] In both youth and adults, insight typically improves following treatment.

Co-Occurring Mental and Somatic Conditions

In adults, 60% to 90% of those with lifetime OCD meet lifetime criteria for at least one other mental disorder, with anxiety and depressive disorders being most common.[21,22] In youth, 50% have co-occurring anxiety or depressive disorders and around 15% meet criteria for an externalizing condition (eg, oppositional defiant disorder).[23] Rates of comorbidity varies, with higher rates generally found in clinical samples.[22]

OCD is associated with an increased risk of suicidal thoughts and behaviors and more than 10% of all individuals with OCD attempt suicide at some time during their life.[24] Those with a history of major depression and substance abuse and those struggling with taboo obsessions (ie, obsessions of a religious or sexual nature) seem to be at highest risk.[11]

OCD has been linked to autoimmune diseases, obesity, type 2 diabetes, hypertension, and other metabolic and cardiovascular conditions,[25] with the strongest associations found using register data. It is unclear to which degree these associations reflect the broader OCD population, as only a minority of those with OCD receive a proper diagnosis in registers. In general samples, associations between OCD and somatic health have been weaker or not statistically significant, but findings indicate that

OCD is associated with an increased risk of chronic pain, migraine headaches, respiratory diseases, diabetes, and thyroid disease.[26,27]

Quality of Life and Functional Impairment

Quality of life is generally compromised in OCD. Compared with community samples, adults with OCD show moderately poorer overall quality of life and large differences are found for social, family, and emotional quality of life.[28] In youth with OCD, large differences are found for global quality of life and moderate differences for quality of life in school and in the social arena.[29] It is currently unclear to which degree OCD severity, occurrence of other psychiatric and somatic conditions, and sociodemographic factors each contribute to quality of life in OCD, but some studies indicate pervasiveness, as individuals who achieve remission from OCD still exhibit impaired quality of life.[30]

Most individuals with OCD experience functional impairment in everyday life, and impairment is recognized in the diagnostic criteria of OCD. Impairment relates to all areas of life such as occupational, educational, family, and social areas, and some research indicates that OCD may be particularly strongly linked to functional impairment compared with other mental disorders.[31] Large register-based studies indicate that OCD is associated with poor educational achievement and labor market marginalization,[32,33] but it is currently unclear what contributes to functional impairment and how impairment and interference develop and change over time.

NOSOLOGY
Diagnostic Placement

The newest versions of DSM and ICD include a new group of disorders called *Obsessive-Compulsive and Related Disorders* (OCRDs), with OCD at the center. In DSM-IV, OCD was characterized as an anxiety disorder. The creation of a new diagnostic chapter was based on research showing that OCD may have more in common with conditions revolving around repetitive thoughts and behaviors than with anxiety disorders.[34] Classification in DSM and ICD should reflect and optimize diagnostic validity and relatedness among disorders (eg, shared neurobiology, etiology), and although anxiety is considered common in OCD, it is not necessary. Instead, the new chapter emphasizes repetitive behaviors as the core characteristic of OCD, distinguishing OCD from anxiety disorders, where avoidance is the most prominent behavioral feature.

In DSM-5, the new OCRD chapter includes OCD, body dysmorphic disorder, hoarding disorder, trichotillomania (hair-pulling), and excoriation (skin-picking) disorder. The OCRD chapter in ICD-11 includes the same disorders, but also hypochondriasis (a preoccupation or fear about the possibility of having a serious illness) and olfactory reference disorder (a preoccupation with the belief of omitting an unpleasant body odor).

Removing OCD from the anxiety disorders generated debate, with counterarguments being that the change was based on topographic features of compulsions (i.e., how they appear from the outside) and not functional features (why they are performed).[35] It was further argued that the cognitive-behavioral model of OCD, which applies to both OCD and anxiety disorders, has generated one of the most powerful treatments of the disorder, namely exposure and response prevention, which differs from the indicated treatments for trichotillomania and excoriation disorder.[36]

One goal with the new OCRD chapter was to stimulate research on the related disorders, of which skin-picking and hoarding disorder were new diagnostic classes. **Fig. 2** shows the number of publications related to body dysmorphic disorder, hoarding disorder, trichotillomania, and skin-picking disorder from 1990 to 2021. The year of

2007 is highlighted since by then a consensus about creating a new OCRD chapter in DSM-5 had emerged.[37] Since 2007, there has been an increase in annual publications of 391% for skin-picking disorder, 294% for body dysmorphic disorder, 186% for hoarding disorder, and 127% for trichotillomania; the corresponding increase for OCD is 100%. Thus, although the nosologic placement of OCD is debated, research on other disorders characterized by repetitive thoughts and behaviors has burgeoned.

Placement in the Meta Structure of Psychopathology

DSM and ICD are based on expert consensus and although informed by empirical research, the classifications are not purely data driven. An alternative approach is to examine how OCD as a dimensional trait co-occurs with other psychopathological symptoms and traits. A dimensional approach to psychopathology has been suggested by the Research Domain Criteria initiative[38] and is supported by studies showing that the severity and frequency of obsessions and compulsions are dimensional rather than categorical, with the extreme end representing OCD.[39]

The most influential dimensional structure of psychopathology is provided by the Hierarchical Taxonomy of Psychopathology (HiTOP) framework. In HiTOP, covariance among psychopathological symptoms is parsimoniously represented by variation in three broad dimensions: externalizing, internalizing, and thought disorder symptoms.[40] The extreme end of the externalizing dimension reflects disruptive behaviors, the liability to engage in substance use, and act out with anger and violence in interpersonal contexts. The extreme end of the internalizing dimension reflects vulnerability to depression, stress, and anxiety and this dimension includes two subdimensions: distress (eg, anhedonia, hopelessness, rumination) and fear (eg, panic, phobic avoidance, illness anxiety). The extreme end of the thought disorder dimension reflects psychotic thought processes and unwanted, dysfunctional, and irrational cognitions and perceptions.

At current, most studies indicate that OCD relates to both the fear and thought disorder dimensions, and this shared relationship was confirmed by a recent study that accounted for the heterogeneity of OCD.[41] The placement of OCD in the meta structure of psychopathology is illustrated in **Fig. 3**. Although the "double kinship" of OCD

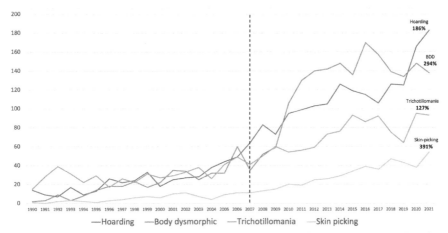

Fig. 2. Increase in number of publications indexed in PubMed from 1990 to 2021 related to hoarding disorder, body dysmorphic disorder, trichotillomania, and skin-picking disorder (defined by the most common keywords).

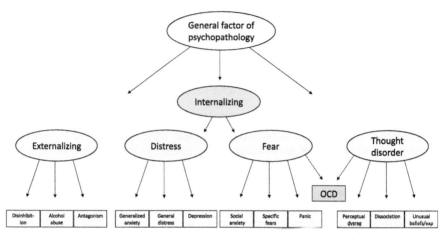

Fig. 3. The placement of OCD in the meta structure of psychopathology.[41]

in this structure should be considered preliminary, it suggests that OCD is related to but also distinct from anxiety disorders, providing some empirical support for the new OCRD chapter. It also supports the decision to place the OCRD chapter directly after the anxiety disorders chapter in DSM-5, which was done to emphasize the relatedness between the two groups of disorders.[2]

Disorders of Compulsivity

The new OCRD chapter centered in on compulsivity. A model of OCD that has been refined during the last decade argues that deficits in goal-directed control, a capacity that protects against the development of rigid maladaptive behaviors, lead to the development of compulsive, non-flexible, and nonadaptive behaviors in OCD.[42] Then, as the individual tries to make sense of these behaviors, intrusive thoughts and anxiety rise as secondary experiences. Deficits in goal-directed behavior relate OCD with other disorders of compulsivity, such as substance use disorders and eating disorders. It is possible that the sense of incompleteness, which is very common in OCD, both as a trigger of compulsive behavior and as a driver of the repetitiveness in compulsions,[43,44] is linked to dysfunction in goal-directed behavior in OCD. However, although deficits in goal-directed behavior could help explain the heterogeneity of compulsions, of which many are not driven by anxiety, and link OCD with other diagnoses characterized by repetitive behaviors, more research is needed to see whether this perspective can aid in the understanding and management of OCD.

EPIDEMIOLOGY
Onset and Natural History

In a large cross-continent study, the mean age of onset in adults with OCD was 16.9 years with most cases onsetting between 12 and 21 years.[45] Similar results were found in a recent meta-analysis showing that the median age of onset of OCD is 19 years and that 60% to 70% onset before age 25.[46] With respect to OCD across the lifespan, these estimates are probably too high as they do not account for childhood-onset cases who reach remission before adulthood. The onset of OCD in youth typically ranges from 8 to 12 years.[47] Thus, the true age of onset of OCD across the lifespan is probably lower than estimates reported using adult samples, and it is reasonable to assume that a majority of lifetime OCD cases onset before adulthood.

Some research indicates that age of onset in OCD has a bimodal distribution, that is, that there may be two distinct peaks in new onsets.[48] The first group is suggested to have a mean age of onset of 11 years with a typical period of onset ranging from 9 to 14 years. The second group has a mean age of onset of 23 years with a much wider typical period of onset. Most cases belong to the early onset group and late-onset OCD remains poorly understood. Early-onset OCD has a male preponderance, more OCD in first-degree relatives, and greater prevalence of tic disorders.[48] A bimodal distribution of age of onset in OCD is intriguing, but large studies with valid age of onset data across age-groups are lacking.

Early research on the natural history of OCD suggested that the disorder may be highly chronic. In 144 individuals with OCD followed-up 40 years after an initial visit, only 20% was in complete recovery and over half had suffered from impairing OCD for at least three decades.[49] Similar findings emerged during shorter time periods and in later adult cohorts, with total remission over 5 years being 17% to 20%.[50,51] Adults receiving adequate treatment may have a better prognosis, with as many as 50% being in remission with an average follow-up time of 5 years.[52] In youth, the prognosis seems to be somewhat better and a recent meta-analysis concluded that 60% of young people whose OCD has been recognized and managed within health care remits.[53] It is reasonable to assume that the risk of chronicity in pediatric OCD increases in the absence of effective treatment, but the natural history of unrecognized OCD in youth is unknown.

How OCD develops over time varies between individuals. In a large Brazilian cohort of 1001 OCD patients, 30% presented with a waxing and waning course, where intensity of symptoms increased and decreased in periods but where periods of minimal symptoms were rare or absent.[54] Twenty-six percent of patients were characterized by a progressive and gradual worsening of symptoms over time. Thirteen percent showed an episodic course, with clearer distinctions between periods of impairing and minimal symptoms, 12% showed a deteriorating course that worsened in plateaus, and only 6% showed a constant, chronic course without much symptom variation over time.

Lifetime and Current Prevalence

OCD was once considered rare, with an early estimation suggesting a prevalence of 0.05% in the general population.[55] Rigorous epidemiologic studies changed this notion. In the Epidemiologic Catchment Area study, conducted in the United States during the 1980s, the lifetime prevalence of OCD in adults was estimated to 2.5% (ie, 50 times greater than the previous estimation of 0.05%) and current prevalence was 1.2%.[55] The investigators concluded that "Although not conclusive, the evidence is strong that OCD is a common mental disorder that, like other stigmatized and hidden disorders in the past, may be ready for discovery and demands for treatment on a large scale."[55] More evidence would emerge as similar lifetime rates for adults were found across continents. In an influential US study, the lifetime prevalence of OCD in a representative sample of adults was 2.3% and the 1-year prevalence 1.3%.[21] A recent systematic review and meta-analysis estimated the lifetime prevalence of OCD in adults to 1.3% and current prevalence to 1.1%.[56]

Similar prevalence rates have been found in children and adolescents. In a US sample of 14 to 19 year olds, the lifetime prevalence of OCD was 1.9% and current prevalence 1.0%.[57] In another US sample of 12 to 16 year olds, lifetime prevalence was 3.0%, with very similar rates across genders, races, and socioeconomic classes.[58] Cross-country similarities have emerged also for OCD in youth, with most work being based on adolescent samples, often finding prevalence rates (lifetime and current) of

1% to 3%,[59–65] with lower current prevalence rates in younger age groups, for example, 0.25% in 5 to 15 year olds in the United Kingdom,[66] indicating that puberty may be a key period of onset. Puberty as a key period of onset is also supported by evidence showing that the frequency and severity of obsessions and compulsions increase from childhood to adolescence among the general population.[67]

The perinatal period is an established risk factor for the onset or exacerbation of OCD. Up to 12% of perinatal women experience clinically significant obsessions and/or compulsions,[68] and perinatal OCD may affect 2.3% of women during pregnancy and 1.7% at postpartum.[69] However, the number of affected women may be higher as prevalence rates increase substantially when women are encouraged to report their obsessions and compulsions, which are often withheld out of shame or fear of negative consequences.[70]

Recognition and Prevalence in Clinical Settings

Most individuals with OCD never seek treatment for their OCD symptoms,[71] making recognition across health services important. Prevalence rates in primary care are on par with prevalence rates of current OCD in the general population and range from 0.6% to 2.2%.[72–75] Rates are substantially higher among psychiatric samples and around 10% of adult psychiatric outpatients meet criteria for OCD, but up to 70% go unrecognized.[76,77] In treatment-seeking youth with mental health problems, 6% to 9% have OCD[78,79]; it is unclear how many are recognized. Among individuals with schizophrenia, 14% meet criteria for current OCD[80] and lifetime prevalence of OCD in individuals with bipolar disorder is 11%.[81] In eating disorders, the lifetime prevalence of OCD is 14% to 18%, with current prevalence being 9% to 15%.[82,83] In youth with autism spectrum disorder as many as 17% meet criteria for OCD[84] and among those with attention-deficit hyperactivity disorder, 3% to 7% have OCD.[85] In addition, up to 40% of youth with tic disorder or Tourette's disorder may meet criteria for OCD.[64] The above estimates show that psychiatric practitioners should expect that around one in 10 of general psychiatric patients meet diagnostic criteria for OCD.

SUMMARY

Individuals with OCD struggle with obsessions and compulsions that are time-consuming and cause distress and impairment. Obsessions can be thoughts, urges, images, or impulses, and compulsions are repetitive and often ritualized behaviors or mental acts performed to reduce distress or prevent harm implicated by obsessions. OCD affects 1% to 3% of the population and seems to be equally common across age groups and counties. The disorder often onsets during adolescence or early adulthood. Around 10% of children and adults in psychiatric settings meet criteria for OCD, but most go unrecognized. The symptom presentation of OCD is heterogenous but revolves around major themes: (1) contamination and cleaning, (2) intrusive and unwanted thoughts about harm/moral failure and checking, and (3) symmetry and ordering. A large majority of those with OCD have co-occurring mental disorders, most often depressive and anxiety disorders. In the newest editions of ICD and DSM, OCD is at the center of a new diagnostic chapter, OCRDs, which also includes other conditions characterized by distressing repetitive thoughts and behaviors. Many patients with OCD engage in avoidance behaviors and 10% to 30% have poor insight, with both factors being associated with more severe OCD and potentially poorer treatment response. OCD can have detrimental effects on quality of life, lead to functional impairment, and follow a chronic course in the absence of effective treatment, making it important for practitioners to recognize the core symptoms of OCD.

CLINICS CARE POINTS

- Obsessive-compulsive disorder is underrecognized in psychiatric settings but can be identified by asking specifically about the most common symptom themes.
- One common theme is intrusive thoughts about harm, responsibility, or moral failure which are often paired with checking compulsions and/or mental rituals.
- Another theme is obsessions about symmetry (that things feel asymmetric, inexact or 'just not right') and ordering, arranging, and evening out compulsions.
- A third major theme revolves around obssessions about contamination or dirt and cleaning compulsions.

REFERENCES

1. World Health Organization. International statistical classification of diseases and related health problems. 11th edition 2019.
2. American Psychiatric Association. Diagnostic and statistical manual of mental disorders. 5th edition 2013.
3. American Psychiatric Association. Diagnostic and statistical manual of mental disorders. 5th edition. American Psychiatric Association; 2022. *text revision.*
4. Stein D, Kogan C, Atmaca M, et al. The classification of obsessive–compulsive and related disorders in the ICD-11. J affective Disord 2016;190:663–74.
5. Brander G, Kuja-Halkola R, Rosenqvist MA, et al. A population-based family clustering study of tic-related obsessive-compulsive disorder. Mol Psychiatry 2021; 26(4):1224–33.
6. Mataix-Cols D, Rosario-Campos MC, Leckman JF. A multidimensional model of obsessive-compulsive disorder. Am J Psychiatry 2005;162(2):228–38. https://doi.org/10.1176/appi.ajp.162.2.228.
7. Bloch MH, Landeros-Weisenberger A, Rosario MC, et al. Meta-analysis of the symptom structure of obsessive-compulsive disorder. Am J Psychiatry 2008; 165(12):1532–42.
8. Cervin M, Miguel EC, Güler AS, et al. Towards a definitive symptom structure of obsessive– compulsive disorder: a factor and network analysis of 87 distinct symptoms in 1366 individuals. Psychol Med 2021;1–13.
9. Mataix-Cols D, Frost RO, Pertusa A, et al. Hoarding disorder: A new diagnosis for DSM-V? Depress anxiety 2010;27(6):556–72.
10. Hojgaard DR, Mortensen EL, Ivarsson T, et al. Structure and clinical correlates of obsessive-compulsive symptoms in a large sample of children and adolescents: a factor analytic study across five nations. Eur Child Adolesc Psychiatry 2016. https://doi.org/10.1007/s00787-016-0887-5.
11. Cervin M, do Rosário MC, Fontenelle LF, et al. Taboo obsessions and their association with suicidality in obsessive-compulsive disorder. J Psychiatr Res 2022; 154:117–22.
12. Evans DW, Leckman JF. Origins of obsessive-compulsive disorder: Developmental and evolutionary perspectives. Developmental Psychopathology: Volume Three: Risk Disord Adaptation 2015;404–35.
13. Wheaton MG, Gershkovich M, Gallagher T, et al. Behavioral avoidance predicts treatment outcome with exposure and response prevention for obsessive–compulsive disorder. Depress anxiety 2018;35(3):256–63.
14. Selles RR, Højgaard DR, Ivarsson T, et al. Avoidance, insight, impairment recognition concordance, and cognitive-behavioral therapy outcomes in pediatric

obsessive-compulsive disorder. J Am Acad Child Adolesc Psychiatry 2020;59(5): 650–9, e2.

15. Storch EA, Rasmussen SA, Price LH, et al. Development and psychometric evaluation of the Yale–Brown Obsessive-Compulsive Scale—Second Edition. Psychol Assess 2010;22(2):223.

16. Nissen JB, Parner E. The importance of insight, avoidance behavior, not-just-right perception and personality traits in pediatric obsessive-compulsive disorder (OCD): a naturalistic clinical study. Nordic J Psychiatry 2018;72(7):489–96.

17. Jacob ML, Larson MJ, Storch EA. Insight in adults with obsessive–compulsive disorder. Compr Psychiatry 2014;55(4):896–903.

18. Fontenelle JM, Harrison BJ, Santana L, et al. Correlates of insight into different symptom dimensions in obsessive-compulsive disorder 2013;25(1):11–6.

19. Bellino S, Patria L, Ziero S, et al. Clinical picture of obsessive-compulsive disorder with poor insight: a regression model. Psychiatry Res 2005;136(2–3):223–31.

20. Gan J, He J, Fu H, et al. Association between obsession, compulsion, depression and insight in obsessive-compulsive disorder: a meta-analysis. Nordic J Psychiatry 2021;1–8.

21. Ruscio AM, Stein DJ, Chiu WT, et al. The epidemiology of obsessive-compulsive disorder in the National Comorbidity Survey Replication. Mol Psychiatry 2010; 15(1):53–63. https://doi.org/10.1038/mp.2008.94.

22. Torres AR, Fontenelle LF, Shavitt RG, et al. Comorbidity variation in patients with obsessive–compulsive disorder according to symptom dimensions: Results from a large multicentre clinical sample. J affective Disord 2016;190:508–16.

23. Peris TS, Rozenman M, Bergman RL, et al. Developmental and clinical predictors of comorbidity for youth with obsessive compulsive disorder. J Psychiatr Res 2017;93:72–8. https://doi.org/10.1016/j.jpsychires.2017.05.002.

24. Pellegrini L, Maietti E, Rucci P, et al. Suicide attempts and suicidal ideation in patients with obsessive-compulsive disorder: a systematic review and meta-analysis. J affective Disord 2020;276.

25. de la Cruz LF, Isomura K, Lichtenstein P, et al. Morbidity and mortality in obsessive-compulsive disorder: A narrative review. Neurosci Biobehavioral Rev 2022;104602.

26. Subramaniam M, Abdin E, Vaingankar J, et al. Obsessive-compulsive disorder in Singapore: prevalence, comorbidity, quality of life and social support. Ann Acad Med Singapore 2020;49(1):15.

27. Witthauer C, T Gloster A, Meyer AH, et al. Physical diseases among persons with obsessive compulsive symptoms and disorder: a general population study. Social Psychiatry Psychiatr Epidemiol 2014;49(12):2013–22.

28. Coluccia A, Fagiolini A, Ferretti F, et al. Adult obsessive–compulsive disorder and quality of life outcomes: a systematic review and meta-analysis. Asian J Psychiatry 2016;22:41–52.

29. Coluccia A, Ferretti F, Fagiolini A, et al. Quality of life in children and adolescents with obsessive–compulsive disorder: a systematic review and meta-analysis. Neuropsychiatr Dis Treat 2017;13:597.

30. Huppert JD, Simpson HB, Nissenson KJ, et al. Quality of life and functional impairment in obsessive–compulsive disorder: a comparison of patients with and without comorbidity, patients in remission, and healthy controls. Depress anxiety 2009;26(1):39–45.

31. Vikas A, Avasthi A, Sharan P. Psychosocial impact of obsessive-compulsive disorder on patients and their caregivers: a comparative study with depressive disorder. Int J Social Psychiatry 2011;57(1):45–56.

32. Perez-Vigil A, Fernandez de la Cruz L, Brander G, et al. Association of Obsessive-Compulsive Disorder With Objective Indicators of Educational Attainment: A Nationwide Register-Based Sibling Control Study. JAMA Psychiatry 2017. https://doi.org/10.1001/jamapsychiatry.2017.3523.

33. Pérez-Vigil A, Mittendorfer-Rutz E, Helgesson M, et al. Labour market marginalisation in obsessive-compulsive disorder: a nationwide register-based sibling control study. Psychol Med 2019;49(6):1015–24. https://doi.org/10.1017/s0033291718001691.

34. Stein DJ, Fineberg NA, Bienvenu OJ, et al. Should OCD be classified as an anxiety disorder in DSM-V? Depress anxiety 2010;27(6):495–506.

35. Abramowitz JS, Jacoby RJ. Obsessive-compulsive disorder in the DSM-5. Clin Psychol Sci Pract 2014;21(3):221.

36. Abramowitz JS, Taylor S, McKay D. Obsessive-compulsive disorder. Lancet 2009;374(9688):491–9. https://doi.org/10.1016/s0140-6736(09)60240-3.

37. Mataix-Cols D, Pertusa A, Leckman JF. Issues for DSM-V: how should obsessive-compulsive and related disorders be classified? Am Psychiatric Assoc; 2007. p. 1313–4.

38. Insel T, Cuthbert B, Garvey M, et al. Research domain criteria (RDoC): toward a new classification framework for research on mental disorders. Am J Psychiatry 2010;167(7):748–51. https://doi.org/10.1176/appi.ajp.2010.09091379.

39. Abramowitz JS, Fabricant LE, Taylor S, et al. The relevance of analogue studies for understanding obsessions and compulsions. Clin Psychol Rev 2014;34(3): 206–17.

40. Kotov R, Krueger RF, Watson D, et al. The Hierarchical Taxonomy of Psychopathology (HiTOP): A dimensional alternative to traditional nosologies. J Abnormal Psychol 2017;126(4):454.

41. Faure K, Forbes MK. Clarifying the placement of obsessive-compulsive disorder in the empirical structure of psychopathology. J Psychopathology Behav Assess 2021;43(3):671–85.

42. Gillan CM, Robbins TW. Goal-directed learning and obsessive-compulsive disorder. Philos Trans R Soc Lond B Biol Sci 2014;(1655):369. https://doi.org/10.1098/rstb.2013.0475.

43. Cervin M, Perrin S, Olsson E, et al. Involvement of fear, incompleteness, and disgust during symptoms of pediatric obsessive-compulsive disorder. Eur Child Adolesc Psychiatry 2020;30(2):271–81. https://doi.org/10.1007/s00787-020-01514-7.

44. da Silva Prado H, do Rosario MC, Lee J, et al. Sensory phenomena in obsessive-compulsive disorder and tic disorders: a review of the literature. CNS spectrums 2008;13(5):425–32.

45. Brakoulias V, Starcevic V, Belloch A, et al. Comorbidity, age of onset and suicidality in obsessive-compulsive disorder (OCD): An international collaboration. Compr Psychiatry 2017;76:79–86. https://doi.org/10.1016/j.comppsych.2017.04.002.

46. Solmi M, Radua J, Olivola M, et al. Age at onset of mental disorders worldwide: large-scale meta-analysis of 192 epidemiological studies. Mol Psychiatry 2021;1–15.

47. Geller DA, Homayoun S, Johnson G. Developmental considerations in obsessive compulsive disorder: comparing pediatric and adult-onset cases. Front Psychiatry 2021;12.

48. Taylor S. Early versus late onset obsessive-compulsive disorder: evidence for distinct subtypes. Clin Psychol Rev 2011;31(7):1083–100. https://doi.org/10.1016/j.cpr.2011.06.007.
49. Skoog G, Skoog I. A 40-year follow-up of patients with obsessive-compulsive disorder. Arch Gen Psychiatry 1999;56(2):121–7.
50. Steketee G, Eisen J, Dyck I, et al. Predictors of course in obsessive compulsive disorder. Psychiatry Res 1999;89(3):229–38.
51. Eisen JL, Sibrava NJ, Boisseau CL, et al. Five-year course of obsessive-compulsive disorder: predictors of remission and relapse. J Clin Psychiatry 2013;74(3):7286.
52. Sharma E, Thennarasu K, Reddy YJ. Long-term outcome of obsessive-compulsive disorder in adults: a meta-analysis. J Clin Psychiatry 2014;75(9):10746.
53. Liu J, Cui Y, Yu L, et al. Long-term outcome of pediatric obsessive-compulsive disorder: A meta-analysis. J Child Adolesc Psychopharmacol 2021;31(2):95–101.
54. Kichuk SA, Torres AR, Fontenelle LF, et al. Symptom dimensions are associated with age of onset and clinical course of obsessive–compulsive disorder. Prog Neuro-Psychopharmacology Biol Psychiatry 2013;44:233–9.
55. Karno M, Golding JM, Sorenson SB, et al. The epidemiology of obsessive-compulsive disorder in five US communities. Arch Gen Psychiatry 1988;45(12):1094–9.
56. Fawcett EJ, Power H, Fawcett JM. Women are at greater risk of OCD than men: a meta-analytic review of OCD prevalence worldwide. J Clin Psychiatry 2020;81(4).
57. Flament MF, Whitaker A, Rapoport JL, et al. Obsessive compulsive disorder in adolescence: an epidemiological study. J Am Acad Child Adolesc Psychiatry 1988;27(6):764–71.
58. Valleni-Basile LA, Garrison CZ, Jackson KL, et al. Frequency of obsessive-compulsive disorder in a community sample of young adolescents. J Am Acad Child Adolesc Psychiatry 1994;33(6):782–91.
59. Apter A, Fallon TJ Jr, King RA, et al. Obsessive-compulsive characteristics: from symptoms to syndrome. J Am Acad Child Adolesc Psychiatry 1996;35(7):907–12.
60. Douglass HM, Moffitt TE, Dar R, et al. Obsessive-compulsive disorder in a birth cohort of 18-year-olds: prevalence and predictors. J Am Acad Child Adolesc Psychiatry 1995;34(11):1424–31.
61. Maina G, Albert U, Bogetto F, et al. Obsessive-compulsive syndromes in older adolescents. Acta Psychiatrica Scand 1999;100(6):447–50.
62. Politis S, Magklara K, Petrikis P, et al. Epidemiology and comorbidity of obsessive–compulsive disorder in late adolescence: a cross-sectional study in senior high schools in Greece. Int J Psychiatry Clin Pract 2017;21(3):188–94.
63. Vivan AdS, Rodrigues L, Wendt G, et al. Obsessive-compulsive symptoms and obsessive-compulsive disorder in adolescents: a population-based study. Braz J Psychiatry 2013;36:111–8.
64. Yan J, Deng H, Wang Y, et al. The Prevalence and Comorbidity of Tic Disorders and Obsessive-Compulsive Disorder in Chinese School Students Aged 6–16: A National Survey. Brain Sci 2022;12(5):650.
65. Barzilay R, Patrick A, Calkins ME, et al. Obsessive-compulsive symptomatology in community youth: typical development or a red flag for psychopathology? J Am Acad Child Adolesc Psychiatry 2019;58(2):277–86, e4.
66. Heyman I, Fombonne E, Simmons H, et al. Prevalence of obsessive–compulsive disorder in the British nationwide survey of child mental health. Br J Psychiatry 2001;179(4):324–9.

67. Luke AK, Ankney R, Wilton EP, et al. Developmental Trajectories of Pediatric Obsessive–Compulsive Symptoms. Res Child Adolesc Psychopathology 2021; 49(12):1635–48.
68. Miller ES, Chu C, Gollan J, et al. Obsessive-compulsive symptoms during the postpartum period. J Reprod Med 2013;58(3–4):115.
69. Fawcett EJ, Fairbrother N, Cox ML, et al. The prevalence of anxiety disorders during pregnancy and the postpartum period: a multivariate Bayesian meta-analysis. J Clin Psychiatry 2019;80(4):1181.
70. Fairbrother N, Collardeau F, Albert AY, et al. High prevalence and incidence of obsessive-compulsive disorder among women across pregnancy and the postpartum. J Clin Psychiatry 2021;82(2):30368.
71. Schwartz C, Schlegl S, Kuelz AK, et al. Treatment-seeking in OCD community cases and psychological treatment actually provided to treatment-seeking patients: A systematic review. J Obsessive-Compulsive Relat Disord 2013;2(4): 448–56.
72. Mergl R, Seidscheck I, Allgaier AK, et al. Depressive, anxiety, and somatoform disorders in primary care: prevalence and recognition. Depress anxiety 2007; 24(3):185–95.
73. Serrano-Blanco A, Palao DJ, Luciano JV, et al. Prevalence of mental disorders in primary care: results from the diagnosis and treatment of mental disorders in primary care study (DASMAP). Social Psychiatry Psychiatr Epidemiol 2010;45(2): 201–10.
74. Gros DF, Magruder KM, Frueh BC. Obsessive compulsive disorder in veterans in primary care: Prevalence and impairment. Gen Hosp Psychiatry 2013; 35(1):71–3.
75. Leon AC, Olfson M, Broadhead WE, et al. Prevalence of mental disorders in primary care: implications for screening. Arch Fam Med 1995;4:857–61.
76. Hantouche E, Bouhassira M, Lancrenon S, et al. Prevalence of obsessive-compulsive disorders in a large French patient population in psychiatric consultation. L'encephale. 1995;21(5):571–80.
77. Wahl K, Kordon A, Kuelz K, et al. Obsessive-Compulsive Disorder (OCD) is still an unrecognised disorder: A study on the recognition of OCD in psychiatric outpatients. Eur Psychiatry 2010;25(7):374–7.
78. Hansen BH, Oerbeck B, Skirbekk B, et al. Non-obsessive–compulsive anxiety disorders in child and adolescent mental health services–Are they underdiagnosed, and how accurate is referral information? Nordic J Psychiatry 2016; 70(2):133–9.
79. Geller D, Biederman J, Faraone SV, et al. Clinical correlates of obsessive compulsive disorder in children and adolescents referred to specialized and non-specialized clinical settings. Depress Anxiety 2000;11(4):163–8.
80. Swets M, Dekker J, van Emmerik-van Oortmerssen K, et al. The obsessive compulsive spectrum in schizophrenia, a meta-analysis and meta-regression exploring prevalence rates. Schizophrenia Res 2014;152(2–3):458–68.
81. Ferentinos P, Preti A, Veroniki AA, et al. Comorbidity of obsessive-compulsive disorder in bipolar spectrum disorders: systematic review and meta-analysis of its prevalence. J affective Disord 2020;263:193–208.
82. Drakes DH, Fawcett EJ, Rose JP, et al. Comorbid obsessive-compulsive disorder in individuals with eating disorders: an epidemiological meta-analysis. J Psychiatr Res 2021;141:176–91.

83. Mandelli L, Draghetti S, Albert U, et al. Rates of comorbid obsessive-compulsive disorder in eating disorders: A meta-analysis of the literature. J Affective Disord 2020;277:927–39.

84. van Steensel FJ, Bögels SM, Perrin S. Anxiety disorders in children and adolescents with autistic spectrum disorders: a meta-analysis. Clin child Fam Psychol Rev 2011;14(3):302.

85. Abramovitch A, Dar R, Mittelman A, et al. Comorbidity between attention deficit/hyperactivity disorder and obsessive-compulsive disorder across the lifespan: A systematic and critical review. Harv Rev Psychiatry 2015;23(4):245–62.

Clinical Considerations for an Evidence-Based Assessment for Obsessive-Compulsive Disorder

Ainsley K. Patrick, BS[a,b], Kesley A. Ramsey, PhD[a,b],
Joey K.-Y. Essoe, PhD[a,b], Joseph F. McGuire, PhD[a,b,*]

KEYWORDS

- Obsessive-compulsive disorder • Evidence-based treatment • Measurement
- Evidence-based assessments • Clinical rating scales

KEY POINTS

- Given the internalizing nature of obsessive-compulsive disorder (OCD) shared phenomenology with other psychiatric illnesses, accurate diagnosis can be challenging for several reasons (eg, lack of reporter insight, social stigma). Evidence-based assessments are the first step in accurately identifying and quantifying OCD symptoms and severity.
- Psychometrically valid scales allow clinicians to track treatment progress over time, tailoring treatment foci to individualize symptom progress for patients.
- Clinicians should administer the most relevant and psychometrically sound assessments for accurate diagnosis and treatment monitoring while considering related constructs (eg, insight, family accommodation).

Introduction

Obsessive-compulsive disorder (OCD) is a debilitating mental health condition, which affects up to ~3% of the population across the lifespan.[1,2] It is characterized by the presence of obsessions—repetitive intrusive *unwanted* thoughts—and compulsions—compensatory behaviors that serve to lessen distress related to obsessions.[3] Although obsessions and compulsions are relatively common in the general

[a] Department of Psychiatry and Behavioral Sciences, Johns Hopkins School of Medicine, 550 North Broadway, Baltimore, MD 21224, USA; [b] Division of Child and Adolescent Psychiatry, Department of Psychiatry & Behavioral Sciences, Center for OCD, Anxiety, and Related Disorders for Children, Johns Hopkins University School of Medicine, 550 North Broadway, Suite 206, Baltimore, MD 21205, USA
* Corresponding author. Division of Child and Adolescent Psychiatry, Department of Psychiatry & Behavioral Sciences, Center for OCD, Anxiety, and Related Disorders for Children, Johns Hopkins University School of Medicine, 550 North Broadway, Suite 206, Baltimore, MD 21205.
E-mail address: jfmcguire@jhmi.edu

Psychiatr Clin N Am 46 (2023) 17–38
https://doi.org/10.1016/j.psc.2022.10.001
0193-953X/23/© 2022 Elsevier Inc. All rights reserved.

population, for a diagnosis of OCD to be conferred, these symptoms must cause significant impairment in social, familial, or academic activities, or be time consuming (ie, present for at least 1 hour per day).[3] Given its internalizing nature and shared phenomenology with other psychiatric conditions (eg, generalized anxiety), it can be challenging for clinicians to accurately diagnose OCD for multiple reasons (eg, lack of reporter insight, social stigma, cultural expectations, and shame).[4–6] However, selecting appropriate rating scales can aid clinicians in arriving at an accurate and reliable OCD diagnosis.

Evidence-based assessment (EBA) is essential for the accurate identification and diagnosis of OCD and related OC spectrum disorders, as well as to appropriately characterize symptom severity. Given that treatments for anxiety, OCD, and OC spectrum disorders differ, an accurate diagnosis is the first step in evidence-based treatment. Moreover, reliable, valid, and treatment-sensitive measures enable clinicians to monitor changes in symptom severity, assess improvement, and inform adjustments to treatment to optimize therapeutic outcomes for each patient. Building on the promising efforts from related conditions (eg, body-focused repetitive behaviors)[7] and prior OCD reviews,[8] this review will provide a summary of OCD measures with psychometric properties to help guide clinicians in conducting an EBA.

The following psychometric properties were considered when describing reliability and validity of measures of OCD listed below.[9,10] Reliability was characterized using interrater reliability, internal consistency, and test–retest reliability. Internal consistency was defined as excellent when α is greater than 0.90, good when α is from 0.80 to 0.89, fair when α is from 0.70 to 0.79, and poor when α is less than 0.70. Interrater reliability was considered excellent with an interclass reliability (ICC) value at 0.75 while lower ICC values were good (0.60–0.74), fair (0.40–0.59), and poor (0.59). Finally, for test–retest reliability, a correlation of greater than 0.80 was considered good, whereas 0.70 to 0.79 represented acceptable, and greater than 0.70 represented poor test–retest reliability.

Validity was evaluated using convergent and discriminant validity. A measure was considered to have good convergent validity when demonstrating r is greater than 0.50 with other measures of OCD severity. Meanwhile, values in which r is from 0.39 to 0.49 were considered fair, and values in which r is less than 0.29 were considered to be poor for convergent validity. Discriminant validity was considered good when correlations of r less than 0.29 were observed between the measure and measures distinct from OCD. When r is from 0.30 to 0.49, discriminant validity was considered fair, and when r greater than 0.50, discriminant validity was considered poor. Measures were described as exhibiting treatment sensitivity when detecting statistically significant reductions in symptom severity after evidence-based treatment.

This article reviews the current EBA tools for OCD. First, it discusses the diagnostic criteria for OCD and accompanying assessment measures. Second, it discusses clinician-rated measures, adult self-report measures, and parent-reported and child-reported measures for youth that can be used to characterize OCD severity. Third, it discusses factors relevant for comprehensive assessment batteries (eg, impairment, family accommodation, insight). Finally, it concludes with recommendations for EBA for OCD across assessment purposes and assessment modalities (eg, telehealth).

Making an Obsessive-Compulsive Disorder Diagnosis

The DSM-5 requires that an individual experiences repetitive, unwanted thoughts (ie, obsessions) and/or repetitive rituals or behaviors to alleviate the distress of obsessions or in response to rigid rules (ie, compulsions) and that these symptoms must cause significant impairment and distress in at least 2 domains (ie, social, familial, and/or academic) to receive an OCD diagnosis.[3] OCD is often diagnosed through informal, unstructured clinical interviews. However, comprehensive assessments with multiple reporters are preferred (eg, family members, self, and others). There are several advantages to evaluating OCD using thorough semistructured or structured clinical interviews including increased reliability and validity of assessments, reduced clinician bias, and a more comprehensive evaluation of symptoms.[11–13] In particular, comprehensive assessments provide differential diagnosis between OCD and related disorders. Although many clinicians are excellent diagnosticians, semistructured and structured interviews are less subject to clinician variability, have stronger interrater reliability,[14] and can help to provide differential diagnoses between OCD and related disorders.

Clinicians should use comprehensive assessments based on DSM criteria instead of using an unstructured clinical interview approach. Such measures include the Mini International Neuropsychiatric Interview (MINI for adults, and MINI-K for youth), the Diagnostic Interview for Anxiety, Mood, and Obsessive-Compulsive Related Disorders (DIAMOND), and the Structured Interview for DSM-IV (SCID-I). The MINI for DSM-IV has been validated with adult and child populations.[15–17] Recently, the MINI 7.0 was revised for use with DSM-5 criteria.[18] The DIAMOND is a semistructured clinical interview based on DSM-5 diagnostic criteria, focusing mainly on anxiety, mood, depression, and obsessive-compulsive–related symptoms in adults.[19] The SCID-I shows good psychometric properties while the new Structured Interview for DSM-5 Disorders-Clinician Version (SCID-5-CV) has shown good validity and reliability for use with DSM-5 criteria.[20–22] Although comprehensive interviews are important for differential diagnosis, clinicians must consider the utility of administering comprehensive assessments because it increases the assessment time burden on patients and families.[23]

Clinician-Rated Measures of Obsessive-Compulsive Disorder Symptom Severity

Yale-Brown Obsessive-Compulsive Scale (Y-BOCS) and Y-BOCS-II. The Y-BOCS is considered the gold-standard measure for OCD. The Y-BOCS comprises a Symptom Checklist and a Severity Scale to evaluate obsessions and compulsions experienced in the past week.[24,25] The Symptom Checklist includes commonly endorsed obsessions and compulsions. On the Severity Scale, clinicians rate the endorsed obsessive-compulsive symptoms on a 4-point scale (0–4) across 5 items including (1) time/frequency, (2) interference, (3) distress, (4) resistance, and (5) degree of control.[8] The severity of obsessions and compulsions are rated separately (range: 0–20) and summed to produce a total score (0–40). Specific ranges on the Y-BOCS Total Score have been found to correspond with mild OCD severity (range: 0–13), moderate OCD severity (range: 14–25), moderate-to-severe severity (range: 25–34), or severe severity (range: 35–40).[26]

The Y-BOCS total score has shown good internal consistency, interrater reliability, and test–retest reliability (**Table 1**).[27] The Y-BOCS total score demonstrates treatment sensitivity across CBT and pharmacotherapy trials and has fair to excellent convergent validity with other measures of OCD.[24,28–32] Although the Y-BOCS total score has shown good divergent validity from anxiety and externalizing symptoms, it has exhibited low divergent validity from depression.[31–33] Additionally, factor analyses of the Y-BOCS have found an inconsistent factor structure. Although some studies support a 2-factor structure, others have found a 3-factor structure.[31,34–36]

Given advancements in the field's understanding of the phenomenology of OCD (eg, the role of avoidance behaviors in OCD),[37] and the concerns identified above, the

Table 1
Clinician-rated measures of obsessive-compulsive disorder symptom severity

Measure	Brief Description	Reliability	Validity	Treatment Sensitivity
The Yale-Brown Obsessive-Compulsive Scale (Y-BOCS)	A semistructured interview to assess the type and severity of obsessive and compulsive symptoms on a symptom checklist. The severity subscales are summed to create a total severity score[1,2]	*Internal consistency:* $\alpha=0.85–0.98$[2,3] *Inter-rater reliability:* $ICC=0.80–0.99$[2-4] *Test-retest reliability:* $r=0.81–0.97$[3,5]	*Convergent validity:* Total score correlates with measures of impairment ($r=0.53$) and obsessive-compulsive symptoms ($r=0.40–0.43$)[6,7] *Discriminant validity:* Large correlations with measures of depression ($r=0.35–0.91$)[6,7]	Yes
The Yale-Brown Obsessive-Compulsive Scale-Second Edition(Y-BOCS-II)	A semistructured interview using a symptom checklist and severity scale to rate 54 common obsessive-compulsive symptoms. A total score is created by adding the 5-item Obsession Severity and Compulsion scales[8]	*Internal consistency:* $\alpha=0.83–0.96$[8-10] *Interrater reliability:* $ICC=0.96–0.99$[8,10] *Test-retest reliability:* $ICC=0.81–0.95$[8-10]	*Convergent validity:* Correlations with measures of OCD symptom severity ($r=0.84–0.85$)[8,10] *Discriminant validity:* Small-to-moderate correlations with depression ($r=0.35–0.41$), and anxiety ($r=0.22–0.24$)[8,10]	Yes
The Children's Yale-Brown Obsessive-Compulsive Scale (CY-BOCS)	A 10-item semistructured interview using a symptom checklist to assess obsessions and compulsions across the past week with parents and children. Obsessions and compulsions are rated for 5 items each on a 4-point Likert scale. A total score (range: 0–40) is created by summing the scores of the 10 items	*Internal consistency:* Severity scales $\alpha=0.80–0.82$ Total score $\alpha=0.72–0.95$[11,12] *Interrater reliability:* $ICC=0.70–0.84$[11,12(p200)] *Test-retest reliability:* $ICC=0.79$[12]	*Convergent validity:* Significant correlations with measures of OCD ($r=0.63–0.75$)[12,13] *Discriminant validity:* Moderate associations with externalizing ($r=0.53–0.56$), small-to-moderate correlations with anxiety and depression ($r=0.12–0.44$)[12,13]	Yes

Measure	Description	Reliability	Validity	
Children's Yale-Brown Obsessive-Compulsive Scale-II (CY-BOCS-II)	Semistructured interview with a symptom checklist measuring symptoms and severity of OCD in the past 30 days for children. The 10 items are rated on a 6-point Likert scale	Internal consistency: α=0.75–0.88[14] Interrater reliability: ICC=0.86–0.92[14] Test–retest reliability: ICC=0.95–0.98[14]	Convergent validity: Moderate-to-large correlations with other measures of OCD symptoms and severity (r=0.35–0.79)[14] Discriminant validity: Small-to-moderate correlations with measures of anxiety (r=0.25–0.34), mood (r=0.24–0.36), and externalizing symptoms (r=0.24)[14]	Yes
The Dimensional Yale-Brown Obsessive-Compulsive Scale (DY-BOCS)	Respondents rate symptoms across 6 obsessive-compulsive dimensions. Clinicians review endorsed symptoms. Each dimension is rated for severity, distress, and impairment (range: 0–5). Global frequency, impairment, and distress are rated (range: 05, max score: 15). The global severity score (max score: 30) is created by summing the global ratings (max score: 15) and a global impairment rating (range:0–15)[15]	Internal consistency: α=0.70–0.97[16,17] Interrater reliability: ICC=0.98[15]	Convergent validity: Large correlations with other measures of OCD severity (r=0.48–0.85)[18] Discriminant validity: Significant correlations with depression (r=0.57) and functional impairment (r=0.67)[18]	Yes
National Institute of Mental Health-Global Obsessive-Compulsive Scale (NIMH-GOCS)	A single-item rating of OCD symptom severity, rated from 0 to 15, with a higher score indicating higher severity[19]	Interrater reliability: ICC=0.77–0.95[20] Test–retest reliability: ICC=0.87–0.98[20]	Convergent validity: Associations with measures of OCD severity (r=0.43–0.80)[20]	Yes

Y-BOCS-II was developed. The Y-BOCS-II has the same overall structure as the Y-BOCS (ie, Symptom Checklist and Severity Scale) but has incorporated several key changes.[38] The Y-BOCS-II updated the Symptom Checklist by removing the sub-headings, including language relevant for "just right" feelings and active avoidance symptoms commonly experienced by adults with OCD.[38] The Severity Scale was updated by replacing the "resistance to obsessions" item with an "obsession-free interval," and also increasing to a 6-point Likert scale (range: 0–50) in order to increase the sensitivity of the measure.[38] The Y-BOCS-II has shown fair to excellent internal consistency, good to excellent interrater reliability, fair to excellent test–retest reliability, and is sensitive to treatment (see **Table 1**).[38–41] It also maintains good convergent validity with other measures of OCD symptoms and shows good discriminant validity from symptoms of anxiety and depression.[40–42]

Children's Obsessive-Compulsive Scale (CY-BOCS) and CY-BOCS-II. Although the Y-BOCS and Y-BOCS-II are specific for adults, the CY-BOCS and CY-BOCS-II are parallel versions for children and adolescents. Similar to the Y-BOCS, the CY-BOCS comprises a Symptom Checklist and Severity Scale to evaluate obsessions and compulsions. On the severity scale, clinicians rate the endorsed obsessive-compulsive symptoms across 5 items including (1) time/frequency, (2) interference, (3) distress, (4) resistance, and (5) degree of control. The severity score of obsessions and compulsions is calculated separately (range: 0–20) and the total score is created by adding all items together (range: 0–40).[29] Specific ranges on the CY-BOCS Total Score have been shown to correspond with mild OCD severity (range: 0–4), moderate OCD severity (range: 14–24), moderate-to-severe severity (range: 25–30), or severe severity (range: 30–40).[29]

The CY-BOCS has demonstrated good internal consistency for the Obsession and Compulsion severity scales, excellent internal consistency for the Total Severity scale, and good test–retest reliability (see **Table 1**).[43–45] The CY-BOCS has demonstrated good to excellent interrater reliability across several studies, and has demonstrated good convergent and divergent validity.[42–44]

Given advances in the field's understanding of the phenomenology of childhood OCD, the CY-BOCS-II was created.[38] These changes paralleled the revision of the Y-BOCS-II to allow consistent examinations across the lifespan. The CY-BOCS-II is reported to have good internal consistency for Obsession and Total Severity Scales while the Compulsion Severity Scale was fair (see **Table 1**).[46] The interrater reliability and test–retest reliability for the Total Severity scores were excellent.[46] The CY-BOCS-II has strong convergent validity with expected measures while maintaining divergent validity from unrelated measures (ie, impulsiveness) and moderate correlations with depression.[46]

Dimensional Yale-Brown Obsessive-Compulsive Scale (DY-BOCS). The DY-BOCS is an 88-item self-report measure, which can then be used in clinical interviews to assess the presence and severity of OCD symptoms. The DY-BOCS assesses individual severity levels of 6 dimensions of obsessions and related compulsions. Then, the dimensions are summed to rate total severity and to inform a global impairment score. The DY-BOCS has been shown to have good internal consistency and interrater reliability and has demonstrated sensitivity to treatment outcomes (see **Table 1**).[47–49] The DY-BOCS has not been evaluated for test–retest reliability. The DY-BOCS has good convergent validity with other measures of OCD severity (ie, Y-BOCS) but poor divergent validity from depression.[48–50]

National Institute of Mental Health-Global Obsessive Compulsive Scale (NIMH-GOCS). The NIMH-GOCS is a clinician-rated single-item, Likert scale (range: 1–15) that measures overall OCD symptom severity, with higher scores representing greater overall OCD severity. The NIMH-GOCS has shown excellent interrater reliability, good test–retest reliability, and sensitivity to treatment while maintaining good convergent validity with other measures of OCD (see **Table 1**).[51–56]

Self-Report Measures of Obsessive-Compulsive Disorder Symptom Severity

Yale-Brown Obsessive Compulsive Scale-Self-Report (Y-BOCS-SR). The Y-BOCS-SR is a self-report version of the clinician-administered Y-BOCS. The self-report structure is similar to the Y-BOCS, with a Symptom Checklist and a Severity Scale.[57] The Y-BOCS-SR has shown good internal consistency and test–retest reliability with moderate-to-high correlations with the clinician-administered Y-BOCS (**Table 2**).[58–60] The Y-BOCS has shown good convergent validity; however, divergent validity has been reported as low for depression measures.[60] A self-report version of the Y-BOCS-II is under evaluation.

Obsessive Compulsive Inventory-Revised (OCI-R). The OCI-R is the updated version of the Obsessive Compulsive Inventory (OCI) that offers several advantages to the original OCI (eg, reduced administration time, simplified scoring).[61] The OCI-R is an 18-item self-report measure that assesses the type and severity of OCD symptoms. Items are rated on the 5-point Likert scale and divided evenly into 6 subscales of symptoms (ie, 3-items per subscale). An early evaluation shows good internal consistency with the exception of the neutralizing domain, fair-to-excellent test–retest reliability, good convergent and divergent validity, and treatment sensitivity (see **Table 2**).[61–63] Further psychometric examination has attempted to reduce the items on the OCI to develop a screening measure. These investigations have produced the OCI-4, which have been developed to screen for OCD symptoms for adults.[64]

Obsessive Compulsive Inventory-12 (OCI-12). The OCI-12 is a new 12-item self-report measure derived from OCI-R that removes the hoarding and neutralizing subscales.[65] The measure has shown good internal consistency, good test–retest reliability, treatment sensitivity, and fair to good convergent and good divergent validity (see **Table 2**).[65]

Florida Obsessive-Compulsive Inventory (FOCI). The FOCI is a 25-item self-report measure for assessing the number and severity of obsessions and compulsions.[66] The measure inquires about the presence of common obsessions (10 items) and compulsions (10 items) on the Symptom Checklist. Afterward, patients use these symptoms to guide ratings on the 5-item severity scale. The FOCI has good internal consistency, high interrater reliability, and is sensitive to treatment (see **Table 2**).[67,68] The FOCI has strong convergent validity with the Y-BOCS and the Y-BOCS-II.[66] The FOCI has shown fair discrimination from anxiety but fair to poor divergent validity from depression.[66,67]

Dimensional Obsessive-Compulsive Scale (DOCS). The DOCS is a 20-item measure with 4 subscales: (1) contamination, (2) responsibility for harm, (3) unacceptable thoughts, and (4) symmetry. Each of these scales consists of 5 items that are rated on a 0 to 4 Likert scale, assessing the severity of specific symptom dimensions derived from the Y-BOCS.[69] The DOCS has excellent internal consistency, good test–retest reliability, and is sensitive to treatment (see **Table 2**).[70,71] The DOCS also shows good convergent validity with OCD-related measures and good divergent validity from anxiety and depression measures.[69]

Dimensional Obsessive-Compulsive-Short Form (DOCS-SF). The DOCS-SF is a 5-item measure of OCD symptoms, in which items are rated on a 9-pointt Likert Scale (range: 0-8). The DOCS-SF is based off of the DOCS and Y-BOCS, and is only available in Norwegian at present.[72,73] The measure has fair to excellent internal consistency and is treatment sensitive.[72,73] However, the DOCS-SF does not have

Table 2
Self-report measures of obsessive-compulsive disorder symptom severity

Measure	Brief Description	Reliability	Validity	Treatment Sensitivity
The Yale-Brown Obsessive-Compulsive Scale-Self-Report (Y-BOCS-SR)	A self-report measure with a symptom checklist and severity scale assessing obsessions and compulsions over the past week. Respondents also rank their current top 3 OCD symptoms[21]	Internal consistency: α=0.78–0.89[22,23] Test–retest reliability: r=0.88[23]	Convergent validity: Strong correlations with clinician-rated measures of OCD (r=0.75)[23] Discriminant validity: Moderate-to-strong correlations with anxiety symptoms (r=0.44–0.77)[24,25]	Not reported
Obsessive-Compulsive Inventory-Revised (OCI-R)	An 18-item self-report measure rated on a 5-point Likert scale from 0 (not at all) to 4 (very much) with 6 subscales, which are summed for a total score. The subscales are washing, obsessing, hoarding, ordering, checking, and neutralizing[26]	Internal consistency: Total score α=0.83–0.90[26–29] Test–retest reliability: r=0.70–0.96[26,28,30]	Convergent validity: Strong associations with other measures of OCD (r=0.41–0.85)[26,27] Discriminant validity: Moderate-to-large correlations with depression (r=0.39–0.70) and anxiety (r=0.42)[26–28]	Yes
Obsessive-Compulsive Inventory-12 (OCI-12)	Derived from the OCI-R, this 12-item measure has 4 subscales: washing, checking, ordering, and obsessing which are summed for a total score[31]	Internal consistency: α=0.79[31] Test–retest reliability: ICC=0.85[31]	Convergent validity: Significant correlations with other measures of OCD symptoms (r=0.30–0.67)[31] Discriminant validity: Small-to-moderate correlations with depression (r=0.28) and anxiety (r=0.27–0.33)[31] symptoms	Yes

Measure	Description	Reliability	Validity	
Florida Obsessive-Compulsive Inventory (FOCI)	A 25-item measure, assessing obsessions (10 items) and compulsions (10 items) experienced during the past month. A 5-item severity scale is included, with a maximum severity score of 0–25[32]	Internal consistency: α=0.89[32] Test-retest reliability: r=0.57[33]	Convergent validity: Correlations between symptom checklist and self-report OCD (r=0.68–0.76) and between severity scale and YBOCS (r=0.61–0.78)[32–34] Discriminant validity: Significant correlations with anxiety (r=0.33–0.46) and depression (r=0.25–0.73)[32–34]	Yes
Dimensional Obsessive-Compulsive Scale (DOCS)	A 20-item measure across four subscales: contamination, responsibility for harm, unacceptable thoughts, and symmetry. Each item is rated on a 0–4 scale with total subscale scores summing to make a total score[35]	Internal consistency: α=0.89–0.93[17,35,36] Test-retest reliability: r = 0.66–0.79[17,35]	Convergent validity: Significant correlations with measures of OCD (r=0.54–0.70)[35,36] Discriminant validity: Significant correlations with measures of anxiety (r=0.33–0.52) and depression (r=0.37–0.38)[35]	Yes
Brief Obsessive-Compulsive Scale (BOCS)	Respondents rate experiences of OCD symptoms on 15 items. Severity is measured by 6 items, rated on a 0–4 Likert scale, focused on any symptoms endorsed in the preceding 15 items	Internal consistency: Symptom checklist: α=0.84 Severity scale, α=0.94[37] Interrater reliability: r=0.67[37]	Convergent validity: Significant negative associations with global functioning (r = −0.28)[37]	Yes

significant correlations with other OCD measures and has mixed correlations with measures of anxiety and depression, lending to questions about its convergent and divergent validity.[72]

The Brief Obsessive-Compulsive Scale (BOCS). Informed by the Y-BOCS, the BOCS consists of 15 items and a separate 6-item severity scale combining obsessions and compulsions.[74] The BOCS shows strong internal consistency and is sensitive to treatment (see **Table 2**). To our knowledge, test–retest reliability has not been evaluated. The BOCS showed convergent validity with the Y-BOCS but divergent validity has not been evaluated.[74,75]

Child and Parent Reports of Obsessive-Compulsive Disorder Severity

Children's Yale-Brown Obsessive-Compulsive Scale (CY-BOCS) Child Report (CR)/ Parent Report (PR). The CY-BOCS-CR/PR contain 10 items for each reporter (10 for child-patient and 10 for parent/caregiver) to assess the severity of common obsessive and compulsive symptoms. These self-report items were adapted from the CY-BOCS and aim to capture input from youth and parent respondents.[76] The CY-BOCS self-report has shown good internal consistency (**Table 3**). To our knowledge, the CY-BOCS-CR/PR has not been evaluated for test–retest reliability or treatment sensitivity. Good convergent validity for the CR and PR was evidenced by strong correlations with other measures of OCD, and good to fair divergent validity from low correlations of externalizing problems.[76,77]

Obsessive-Compulsive Inventory-Child Version (OCI-CV). The OCI-CV is a child and adolescent self-report that measures the frequency and presence of common obsessions and compulsions based on the DSM-IV criteria.[78] There are 21 items across 6 subscales parallel to the adult OCI: (1) doubting/checking, (2) obsessions, (3) hoarding, (4) washing, (5) ordering, and (6) neutralizing. A total score is produced by summing all subscales. The OCI-CV has shown fair to good internal consistency, fair to adequate test–retest reliability, and sensitivity to treatment (see **Table 3**).[78–80] However, convergent validity was poor to fair across similar measures of OCD and discriminant validity was poor to good across depression and anxiety measures.[81]

Obsessive-Compulsive Inventory-Child Version-Revised (OCI-CV-R). Based on further psychometric evaluations, the 18-item OCI-CV-R was modified from the 21-item OCI-CV to exclude items assessing hoarding based on our advanced phenomenological understanding of OCD and to investigate the possible factorial invariance between younger (aged 7–11 years) and older children (aged 12–17 years).[82] Internal consistency was good, except for neutralizing, which was poor (see **Table 3**).[82] To our knowledge, the OCI-CV-R has not been evaluated for test–retest reliability or treatment sensitivity, likely due to the novelty of the measure. Convergent validity was fair with the OCI-CV and discriminant validity was fair with measures of depression.[82] In addition to the OCI-CV-R, the OCI-CV-5 is an ultrabrief screener version of the OCI-CV-R for common pediatric OCD symptoms.[83]

Children's Florida Obsessive-Compulsive Inventory (C-FOCI). The C-FOCI is the parallel child-version of the FOCI. It includes a symptom checklist of 20 common obsessions and compulsions rated during the past month and a severity scale. Endorsed symptoms are rated across 5 items on a 0 to 5 Likert scale to characterize OCD severity (range: 0–20). The C-FOCI demonstrates fair-to-excellent internal consistency, treatment sensitivity, and correlations between the C-FOCI and other measures of OCD are strong, indicating good convergent validity (see **Table 3**).[84,85] However, correlations with measures of anxiety and depression were also significant indicating poor discriminant validity.[84] The C-FOCI was not related to externalizing disorders.[84,85]

Table 3
Parent-report and child-report measures of obsessive-compulsive disorder symptom severity

Measure	Brief Description	Reliability	Validity	Treatment Sensitivity
Children's Yale-Brown Obsessive-Compulsive Scale-Child and Parent Report Form (CY-BOCS-CR and CY-BOCS-PR)	10-item self-report measures for children and for parents. Items are rated on a Likert-scale and correspond with items from the clinician-administered CY-BOCS	Internal consistency: Child report, α=0.87; parent report, α=0.86[38]	Convergent validity: Associations of clinician-rated OCD severity with parent (r=0.72) and child (r=0.58) ratings[38] Discriminant validity: Externalizing symptoms (r=0.14–0.40) and aggression (r=0.32–0.46) showed small-to-moderate correlations[38]	Yes
Obsessive-Compulsive Inventory-Child Version (OCI-CV)	21-items are rated across 6 subscales: doubting/checking, obsessions, hoarding, washing, ordering, and neutralizing. A total score is produced by summing each subscale	Internal consistency: α=0.85–0.96[39,40] Test–retest reliability: r=0.77[39]	Convergent validity: Significant correlations with measures of OCD symptoms (r=0.59–0.61) and OCD impairment (r=0.50–0.55)[39] Discriminant validity: No correlations with measures of global functioning (r=−0.14–0.07) or irritability (r=−0.02)[41]	Yes
Obsessive-Compulsive Inventory-Child Version-Revised (OCI-CV-R)	18 items rated on a 0–2 Likert scale across 5 subscales: doubting/checking, obsessing, washing, ordering, and neutralizing. Subscales are summed to create a total score[42]	Internal consistency: α=0.86[42]	Convergent validity: Total score correlates with CYBOCS total score (r=0.32)[42] Discriminant validity: Total score correlates with measures of depression and anxiety (r=0.38–0.49) (Güler et al., 2016; Pertusa et al., 2012; Rosario-Campos et al., 2006)[42]	Not reported

(continued on next page)

Table 3
(continued)

Measure	Brief Description	Reliability	Validity	Treatment Sensitivity
The Children's Florida Obsessive-Compulsive Inventory (C-FOCI)	Consists of a symptom checklist of 17 common obsession and compulsions assessed during the past month. 5 items, rated on a scale of 0–4 creates a total severity score out of 20[44]	Internal consistency: Severity Scale α=0.79–0.89; Symptom checklist KR-20=0.73–0.76[43,44] Test–retest reliability: r=0.55[44]	Convergent validity: Severity scale correlates with CYBOCS total score (r=0.27–0498) and COIS-P/C (r=0.417–0.485)[43,44] Discriminant validity: Nonsignificant correlations of total score with externalizing symptoms (r=0.11) and small correlations with anxiety and depression symptoms (r=0.25–0.62)[43,44]	Yes
Children's Obsessive-Compulsive Inventory-Revised (ChOCI-R)	Obsessions and compulsions are rated on 16 items each. The first 10 items on each scale measure the presence of symptoms while the last 6 items of each section measure the severity of symptoms	Internal consistency: Total impairment α, child and parent-report= 0.86–0.87[45]	Convergent validity: Significant correlations of the Total score with CYBOCS Total impairment score (r=0.45–0.55)[45] Discriminant validity: Small-to-large correlations with SDQ emotional problems (r=0.30–0.51) and hyperactivity (r=0.26–0.32)[45]	Not reported

Children's Obsessive-Compulsive Inventory-Revised (ChOCI-R). The ChOCI-R is a 32-item measure assessing the presence and severity of obsessive and compulsive symptoms in youth aged 7 to 17 years.[86] The measure is divided into 2 sections: obsessions, and compulsions, with 16 items each. Each section begins with 10 questions (range: 0–3) evaluating the presence of symptoms, followed by 6 items (range:0–4) measuring the severity of the symptoms. The ChOCI-R demonstrated fair-to-good internal consistency for subscales (see **Table 3**).[86] Test–retest reliability and treatment sensitivity have not been examined for this measure. There are both parent and child report versions of the ChOCI-R, which show fair to good convergent validity with other OCD measures.[86] Both the child and parent report show fair to poor divergent validity with emotional problems and have good divergent validity from conduct or hyperactivity concerns on the Strengths and Difficulties Questionnaire.[86]

Important Related Factors

In addition to characterizing symptom severity, several factors should be considered when evaluating OCD. Here, impairment, family accommodation, and limited insight are discussed. First, impairment is a main diagnostic criterion for OCD. Functional impairment and perceived distress affect patients' quality of life and thus are key treatment targets to lessen the overall burden of OCD.[1,87,88] Second, family accommodation can present as overreassurance, participating in rituals, assisting with avoidance, or any other reaction to a person's OCD behaviors.[89] Family accommodation is among the top negative predictors of treatment response and is associated with increased symptom severity and functional impairment, by means of reducing engagement with evidence-based therapy.[90] Finally, limited insight is associated with delayed treatment seeking behaviors, worse prognosis, and poor treatment outcomes.[8,91] Thus, assessing these 3 factors is important for a comprehensive EBA in OCD.

Impairment. Several rating scales are useful for assessing impairment. For children, a commonly used measure of OCD-specific impairment is the Child Obsessive-Compulsive Impact Scale-Revised (COIS-R).[92] The 33-item measure assesses functional impairment of OCD symptoms across several domains (home, school, social), through parallel parent and child report options.[92,93] The parent and child versions of the COIS-R have demonstrated treatment sensitivity, as demonstrated in several OCD treatment studies including medication and cognitive-behavioral therapy, with one study using the COIS-R to predict treatment outcomes.[93–96] Meanwhile, for adults, the 48-item Adult OCD Impact Scale was adapted from the COIS-R to assess OCD impairment across work/school, home, social, and intimate domains.[97] Items are rated on a 5-point Likert scale with higher scores indicating greater impairment.[97]

For more general ratings of impairment, the 5-item Sheehan Disability Scale (SDS) is a measure that can be used to assess OCD symptom interference in work, family, and social life in adult patients. The SDS maintains good psychometric properties and is sensitive to treatment.[98,99] The SDS has been modified to assess youth-the Child Sheehan Disability Scale-Parent Report and Child Report (CSDS-P/C). The CSDS-P/C has a parallel format to the adult self-report, measuring functional impairment across 3 domains: school, home, and social life.[100,101]

Family Accommodation. Several studies have shown that family accommodation is common for children and adults with OCD, and it is associated with poorer treatment outcomes and more severe psychopathology because accommodation can serve the same function as a compulsion.[90,102,103] There are several measures to capture family accommodation. First, the Family Accommodation Scale (FAS) is a clinician-administered, semistructured interview capturing level of family accommodation for individuals with OCD.[104,105] Adult patients with OCD have a self-report version of the FAS, the Family Accommodation Scale-Patient Version (FAS-PV), which asks about their perceived familial accommodation activities.[106] The Family Accommodation Scale Self-Report is appropriate for use with adult OCD patients' family members to assess the level of accommodation family members individually contribute.[107] Finally, the FAS-PV can be administered to parents of youth with OCD.[104,108,109]

Insight. Limited insight is associated with worse clinical outcomes for both adults and youth with OCD.[1,91,94,110] The Y-BOCS and Y-BOCS-II both have a single item of insight, whereas the CY-BOCS and CY-BOCS-II have a single item of insight for youth. Although clinician ratings are preferred over self-report measures, single items may not capture all facets of patient insight. The Brown Assessment of Beliefs Scale is a clinician-rated, semistructured interview assessing insight.[111] The clinician inquires about the patient's beliefs related to their symptoms during the past week across 7 items. Multiple beliefs about the same disorder are scored compositely, with higher scores indicating less insight into their psychological symptoms.[111]

DISCUSSION

This article reviewed EBAs for use by clinicians as a resource for building EBA batteries. The following recommendations are of note in the assessment process.

Screening Assessment. Brief evidence-based self-reports are useful in assessing symptoms and severity in time-constrained situations. Self-reports are cost and time effective and do not require substantial training to administer. Quick screening measures, including the OCI-CV-5 for children and OCI-4 for adults are useful for brief administration during intake procedures. If OCD symptoms are endorsed, clinicians could administer the self-report ratings to adults (eg, OCI-R, OCI-12, FOCI) and/or youth (eg, OCI-CV, OCI-CV-R) to obtain greater detail regarding OCD symptoms.

Differential Diagnosis Assessment. Structured and semistructured interviews can assist in determining an OCD diagnosis and potential comorbidities, which is useful for clinical presentations with overlapping symptoms. Clinicians can choose developmentally appropriate interviews for determining diagnoses and can supplement these with self-report measures when needed. There are several semistructured interviews with strong psychometric properties and discriminant validity across diagnoses including the DIAMOND, SCID-5-CV, MINI, and MINI-K. Structured clinical interviews can be supplemented other rating scales to further inform an accurate differential diagnosis and discriminate between common comorbidities. For instance, the FOCI (for adults) and C-FOCI (for youth) show fair discriminant validity from anxiety and may be informative to administer in such cases.

Initial assessment. Initial assessments should be conducted with psychometrically sound clinician-rated measures to characterize symptoms and their symptom severity.[8] Assessment batteries should include reports from multiple informants (eg, patient, family members), as well as clinician judgements and observations. Indeed, multifaceted information is particularly helpful when assessing individuals with limited insight.[112]

The gold standard for clinician-administered, semistructured OCD severity assessment is the Y-BOCS/Y-BOCS-II for adults and CY-BOCS/CY-BOCS-II for children. There are guidelines for characterizing OCD severity based on the Y-BOCS and CY-BOCS Total Scores. Alongside identifying OCD symptoms and characterizing their severity, it is important to obtain information about impairment, familial accommodation, and insight. Impairment, accommodation behaviors, and insight are important clinical features that can inform patients' prognosis and treatment targets.

Treatment monitoring. Clinicians need to monitor therapeutic progress to help guide clinical decisions. Although it is optimal to use clinician-administer scales such as the Y-BOCS/Y-BOCS-II for adults and the CY-BOCS/CY-BOCS-II for children, the full administration of these semistructured interviews can be somewhat time intensive for patients and clinicians. Thus, validated brief self-report measures with treatment sensitivity can serve as useful alternative when administered regularly to monitor patients' therapeutic progress.

Virtual assessments. The COVID-19 pandemic challenged the norm of some in-person clinical assessments, and lead to increased usage of telehealth and mHealth appointments worldwide.[113,114] Clinicians must consider external factors related to virtual assessments that may affect the validity of diagnostic evaluations. Brief measures should be chosen, and supplemental self-reports should be used to lessen "zoom fatigue" from lengthy assessments conducted remotely.[115] Additionally, clinicians should encourage the use of stable Internet and limited distractions for optimal remote assessments.

Future directions. Finally, using technology may enhance OCD assessment through increased engagement and data points. Ecological momentary assessment in OCD, using prompts on smart devices to assess mood in the moment and to track mood over time, has been shown to be treatment sensitive.[116] Technological advances allow the possibility to move from clinician-based scales to other game-like tasks for assessment, potentially increasing engagement in the assessment process.

CLINICS CARE POINTS

- Clinicians should use psychometrically validated rating scales and interviews to evaluate the presence and severity of OCD psychopathology. Though some rating scales are time intensive, the accurate understanding of symptoms is essential to provide proper care.

- When assessing an individual for the presence and severity of OCD, clinicians should consider and measure outside factors including family accommodation and level of insight. These considerations may impact prognosis and treatment targets.

- Psychometrically valid tools for OCD diagnosis are constantly evolving. Clinicians should stay current on the literature to maintain knowledge about relevant, useful diagnostic measures for OCD and related constructs.

SUMMARY

This article reviewed current assessments for youth and adults with OCD across self-report, parent-report, and clinician-administered measures. Recommendations for an EBA were made based on clinical and research goals. Importantly, EBAs for OCD should include measures from multiple informants and clinicians should use judgment when evaluating information across several sources. Because assessments are increasingly administered over telehealth platforms, clinicians must stay cognizant of best telehealth administration practices.

REFERENCES

1. Ruscio AM, Stein DJ, Chiu WT, et al. The Epidemiology of Obsessive-Compulsive Disorder in the National Comorbidity Survey Replication. Mol Psychiatry 2010;15(1):53–63.

2. Wadsworth LP, Potluri S, Schreck M, et al. Measurement and impacts of intersectionality on obsessive-compulsive disorder symptoms across intensive treatment. Am J Orthop 2020;90(4):445.

3. APA. Diagnostic and statistical Manual of mental disorders: DSM-5. American Psychological Association; 2013.

4. Fernández de la Cruz L, Kolvenbach S, Vidal-Ribas P, et al. Illness perception, help-seeking attitudes, and knowledge related to obsessive-compulsive disorder across different ethnic groups: a community survey. Soc Psychiatry Psychiatr Epidemiol 2016;51(3):455–64.

5. Fineberg NA, Krishnaiah RB, Moberg J, et al. Clinical Screening for Obsessive-Compulsive and Related Disorders. Isr J Psychiatry Relat Sci 2008;45(3):13.

6. Jakubovski E, Pittenger C, Torres AR, et al. Correlates of Insight Level in Obsessive-Compulsive Disorder with Dimensions of Symptomology. Prog Neuropsychopharmacol Biol Psychiatry 2011;35(7):1677–81.

7. McGuire JF, Kugler BB, Park JM, et al. Evidence-based assessment of compulsive skin picking, chronic tlc disorders and trichotillomania in children. Child Psychiatry Hum Dev 2012;43(6):855–83.

8. Rapp AM, Bergman RL, Piacentini J, et al. Evidence-Based Assessment of Obsessive–Compulsive Disorder. J Cent Nerv Syst Dis 2016;8:13–29.

9. Cicchetti DV. Guidelines, criteria, and rules of thumb for evaluating normed and standardized assessment instruments in psychology. Psychol Assess 1994; 6(4):284–90.

10. Nunnally J. Psychometric theory. 2nd edition. McGraw-Hill; 1978.

11. Calinoiu I, McClellan J. Diagnostic interviews 2004;8. Published online.

12. Hughes CW, Rintelmann J, Mayes T, et al. Structured Interview and Uniform Assessment Improves Diagnostic Reliability. J Child Adolesc Psychopharmacol 2000;10(2):119–31.

13. Lewin AB. Evidence-Based Assessment of Child Obsessive-Compulsive Disorder (OCD): Recommendations for Clinical Practice and Treatment Research. In: Farrell LJ, Ollendick TH, Muris P, editors. Innovations in CBT for childhood anxiety, OCD, and PTSD. 1st edition. Cambridge University Press; 2019. p. 313–31.

14. Mueller AE, Segal DL. Structured versus Semistructured versus Unstructured Interviews. In: The Encyclopedia of clinical Psychology. John Wiley & Sons, Ltd; 2015. p. 1–7.

15. Sheehan DV, Lecrubier Y, Sheehan KH, et al. The Mini-International Neuropsychiatric Interview (M.I.N.I.): the development and validation of a structured diagnostic psychiatric interview for DSM-IV and ICD-10. J Clin Psychiatry 1998; 59(Suppl 20):22–33 [quiz: 34-57].

16. Sheehan DV, Sheehan KH, Shytle RD, et al. Reliability and Validity of the Mini International Neuropsychiatric Interview for Children and Adolescents (MINI-KID). J Clin Psychiatry 2010;71(3):17393.

17. Whiteside SPH, Riemann BC, McCarthy DM. Using the Child Sheehan Disability Scale to Differentiate Severity Level in Youth With Anxiety Disorders and Obsessive Compulsive Disorder. Assess Published Online February 2022;21. 107319112210772.

18. Sheehan DV. The Mini-International Neuropsychiatric interview, version 7.0 for DSM-5 (MINI 7.0). Medical Outcomes Systems; 2014.

19. Tolin DF, Gilliam CM, Davis E, et al. Psychometric properties of the Hoarding Rating Scale-Interview. J Obsessive-compuls Relat Disord 2018;16:76–80.

20. First MB, Williams JBW, Karg RS, et al. Structured Clinical Interview for DSM-5 Disorders-Clinician Version SCID-5-CV. 2016. Available at: https://www.appi.

org/Products/Interviewing/Structured-Clinical-Interview-for-DSM-5-Disorders. Accessed July 25, 2022.

21. Osório FL, Loureiro SR, Hallak JEC, et al. Clinical validity and intrarater and test-retest reliability of the Structured Clinical Interview for DSM-5 - Clinician Version (SCID-5-CV). Psychiatry Clin Neurosci 2019;73(12):754–60.

22. Shabani A, Masoumian S, Zamirinejad S, et al. Psychometric properties of Structured Clinical Interview for DSM-5 Disorders-Clinician Version (SCID-5-CV). Brain Behav 2021;11(5). https://doi.org/10.1002/brb3.1894.

23. Ford-Paz RE, Gouze KR, Kerns CE, et al. Evidence-based assessment in clinical settings: Reducing assessment burden for a structured measure of child and adolescent anxiety. Psychol Serv 2019;17(3):343.

24. Goodman WK, Price LH, Rasmussen SA, et al. The Yale-Brown Obsessive Compulsive Scale. II. Validity. Arch Gen Psychiatry 1989;46(11):1012–6.

25. Goodman WK, Price LH, Rasmussen SA, et al. The Yale-Brown Obsessive Compulsive Scale. I. Development, use, and reliability. Arch Gen Psychiatry 1989;46(11):1006–11.

26. Storch EA, De Nadai AS, Conceição do Rosário M, et al. Defining clinical severity in adults with obsessive–compulsive disorder. Compr Psychiatry 2015;63:30–5.

27. López-Pina JA, Sánchez-Meca J, López-López JA, et al. The Yale–Brown Obsessive Compulsive Scale: A Reliability Generalization Meta-Analysis. Assessment 2015;22(5):619–28.

28. Farris SG, McLean CP, Van Meter PE, et al. Treatment response, symptom remission, and wellness in obsessive-compulsive disorder. J Clin Psychiatry 2013;74(7):685–90.

29. Lewin A, Piacentini J, De Nadai A, et al. Defining Clinical Severity in Pediatric Obsessive-Compulsive Disorder. Psychol Assess 2013;26. https://doi.org/10.1037/a0035174.

30. Tolin DF, Abramowitz JS, Diefenbach GJ. Defining Response in Clinical Trials for Obsessive-Compulsive Disorder: A Signal Detection Analysis of the Yale-Brown Obsessive Compulsive Scale. J Clin Psychiatry 2005;66(12):4081.

31. Storch EA, Shapira NA, Dimoulas E, et al. Yale-Brown Obsessive Compulsive Scale: the dimensional structure revisited. Depress Anxiety 2005;22(1):28–35.

32. Taylor S. Assessment of obsessions and compulsions: Reliability, validity, and sensitivity to treatment effects. Clin Psychol Rev 1995;15(4):261–96.

33. Woody SR, Steketee G, Chambless DL. Reliability and validity of the Yale-Brown Obsessive-Compulsive Scale. Behav Res Ther 1995;33(5):597–605.

34. Anholt GE, van Oppen P, Cath DC, et al. The Yale-Brown Obsessive-Compulsive Scale: Factor Structure of a Large Sample. Front Psychiatry 2010;1:18.

35. Deacon BJ, Abramowitz JS. The Yale-Brown Obsessive Compulsive Scale: factor analysis, construct validity, and suggestions for refinement. J Anxiety Disord 2005;19(5):573–85.

36. Moritz S, Meier B, Kloss M, et al. Dimensional structure of the Yale-Brown Obsessive-Compulsive Scale (Y-BOCS). Psychiatry Res 2002;109(2):193–9.

37. McGuire JF, Storch EA, Lewin AB, et al. The role of avoidance in the phenomenology of obsessive-compulsive disorder. Compr Psychiatry 2012;53(2):187–94.

38. Storch EA, Rasmussen SA, Price LH, et al. Development and psychometric evaluation of the Yale–Brown Obsessive-Compulsive Scale—Second Edition. Psychol Assess 2010;22(2):223–32.

39. Alić M, de Leeuw A, Selier J, et al. Responsiveness and other psychometric properties of the Yale-Brown Obsessive-Compulsive Scale Severity Scale-Second Edition in a Dutch clinical sample. Clin Psychol Psychother 2022. https://doi.org/10.1002/cpp.2715.

40. Castro-Rodrigues P, Camacho M, Almeida S, et al. Criterion Validity of the Yale-Brown Obsessive-Compulsive Scale Second Edition for Diagnosis of Obsessive-Compulsive Disorder in Adults. Front Psychiatry 2018;9:431.

41. Wu MS, McGuire JF, Horng B, et al. Further psychometric properties of the Yale-Brown Obsessive Compulsive Scale - Second Edition. Compr Psychiatry 2016; 66:96–103.

42. Zhang CC, Gong H, Zhang Y, et al. Development and psychometric evaluation of the Mandarin Chinese version of the Yale-Brown Obsessive-Compulsive Scale – Second Edition. Braz J Psychiatry 2019;41(6):494–8.

43. Scahill L, Riddle MA, McSWIGGIN-HARDIN M, et al. Children's Yale-Brown Obsessive Compulsive Scale: Reliablllty and Validity. J Am Acad Child Adolesc Psychiatry 1997;36(6):844–52.

44. Storch EA, Murphy TK, Geffken GR, et al. Psychometric evaluation of the Children's Yale-Brown Obsessive-Compulsive Scale. Psychiatry Res 2004; 129(1):91–8.

45. Yucelen AG, Rodopman-Arman A, Topcuoglu V, et al. Interrater reliability and clinical efficacy of Children's Yale-Brown Obsessive-Compulsive Scale in an outpatient setting. Compr Psychiatry 2006;47(1):48–53.

46. Storch EA, McGuire JF, Wu MS, et al. Development and Psychometric Evaluation of the Children's Yale-Brown Obsessive-Compulsive Scale Second Edition. J Am Acad Child Adolesc Psychiatry 2019;58(1):92–8.

47. Cervin M, Perrin S, Olsson E, et al. Validation of an interview-only version of the Dimensional Yale-Brown Obsessive-Compulsive Scale (DY-BOCS) in treatment-seeking youth with obsessive-compulsive disorder. Psychiatry Res 2019;271: 171–7.

48. Pertusa A, Fernández de la Cruz L, Alonso P, et al. Independent validation of the Dimensional Yale-Brown Obsessive-Compulsive Scale (DY-BOCS). Eur Psychiatry 2012;27(8):598–604.

49. Rosario-Campos MC, Miguel EC, Quatrano S, et al. The Dimensional Yale–Brown Obsessive–Compulsive Scale (DY-BOCS): an instrument for assessing obsessive–compulsive symptom dimensions. Mol Psychiatry 2006;11(5): 495–504.

50. Güler AS, do Rosário MC, Ayaz AB, et al. Psychometric properties of the DY-BOCS in a Turkish sample of children and adolescents. Compr Psychiatry 2016;65:15–23.

51. Insel TR, Murphy DL, Cohen RM, et al. Obsessive-compulsive disorder. A double-blind trial of clomipramine and clorgyline. Arch Gen Psychiatry 1983; 40(6):605–12.

52. Kim S, Dysken M, Kuskowski M, et al. The Yale-Brown Obsessive-Compulsive Scale and the NIMH Global Obsessive-Compulsive Scale: a reliability and validity study. 1993. Available at: https://scholar.google.com/scholar_lookup?hl=en&volume=3&publication_year=1993&pages=37-44&author=S.W.+Kimauthor=M.W.+Dyskenauthor=M.+Kuskowskiauthor=K.M.+Hoover&title=The+Yale-Brown+Obsessive-Compulsive+Scale+and+the+NIMH+Global+Obsessive-Compulsive+Scale%3A+a+reliability+and+validity+study. Accessed July 26, 2022.

53. Kim SW, Dysken MW, Kuskowski M. The symptom checklist-90: Obsessive-compulsive subscale: A reliability and validity study. Psychiatry Res 1992; 41(1):37–44.
54. March JS, Biederman J, Wolkow R, et al. Sertraline in children and adolescents with obsessive-compulsive disorder: a multicenter randomized controlled trial. JAMA 1998;280(20):1752–6.
55. Tek C, Uluğ B, Rezaki BG, et al. Yale-Brown Obsessive Compulsive Scale and US National Institute of Mental Health Global Obsessive Compulsive Scale in Turkish: reliability and validity. Acta Psychiatr Scand 1995;91(6):410–3.
56. Yaryura-Tobias JA, Grunes MS, Walz J, et al. Parental obsessive-compulsive disorder as a prognostic factor in a year long fluvoxamine treatment in childhood and adolescent obsessive-compulsive disorder. Int Clin Psychopharmacol 2000;15(3):163–8.
57. Baer L, Brown-Beasley MW, Sorce J, et al. Computer-assisted telephone administration of a structured interview for obsessive-compulsive disorder. Am J Psychiatry 1993;150(11):1737–8.
58. Federici A, Summerfeldt LJ, Harrington JL, et al. Consistency between self-report and clinician-administered versions of the Yale-Brown Obsessive-Compulsive Scale. J Anxiety Disord 2010;24(7):729–33.
59. Rosenfeld R, Dar R, Anderson D, et al. A computer-administered version of the Yale-Brown Obsessive-Compulsive Scale. Psychol Assess 1993;4(3):329.
60. Steketee G, Frost R, Bogart K. The Yale-Brown Obsessive Compulsive Scale: Interview versus self-report. Behav Res Ther 1996;34(8):675–84.
61. Foa EB, Huppert JD, Leiberg S, et al. The Obsessive-Compulsive Inventory: Development and validation of a short version. Psychol Assess 2002;14(4): 485–96.
62. Huppert JD, Walther MR, Hajcak G, et al. The OCI-R: Validation of the subscales in a clinical sampe. J Anxiety Disord 2007. https://doi.org/10.1016/j.janxdis.2006.05.006.
63. wen PZ, han YW, dong MG, et al. The Chinese version of the Obsessive-Compulsive Inventory-Revised scale: Replication and extension to non-clinical and clinical individuals with OCD symptoms. BMC Psychiatry 2011;11:129.
64. Abramovitch A, Abramowitz JS, McKay D. The OCI-4: An ultra-brief screening scale for obsessive-compulsive disorder. J Anxiety Disord 2021;78:102354.
65. Abramovitch A, Abramowitz JS, McKay D. The OCI-12: A syndromally valid modification of the obsessive-compulsive inventory-revised. Psychiatry Res 2021;298:113808.
66. Storch EA, Bagner D, Merlo LJ, et al. Florida obsessive-compulsive inventory: Development, reliability, and validity. J Clin Psychol 2007;63(9):851–9.
67. Aldea MA, Geffken GR, Jacob ML, et al. Further psychometric analysis of the Florida Obsessive-Compulsive Inventory. J Anxiety Disord 2009;23(1):124–9.
68. Saipanish R, Hiranyatheb T, Lotrakul M. Reliability and Validity of the Thai Version of the Florida Obsessive-Compulsive Inventory. Sci World J 2015; 2015:240787.
69. Abramowitz JS, Deacon BJ, Olatunji BO, et al. Assessment of obsessive-compulsive symptom dimensions: Development and evaluation of the Dimensional Obsessive-Compulsive Scale. Psychol Assess 2010;22(1):180.
70. López-Nicolás R, Rubio-Aparicio M, López-Ibáñez C, et al. A Reliability Generalization Meta-analysis of the Dimensional Obsessive-Compulsive Scale. Psicothema 2021;33(3):481–9.

71. Ong ML, Reuman L, Youngstrom EA, et al. Discriminative Validity of the Dimensional Obsessive–Compulsive Scale for Separating Obsessive–Compulsive Disorder From Anxiety Disorders. Assessment 2020;27(4):810–21.

72. Eilertsen T, Hansen B, Kvale G, et al. The Dimensional Obsessive-Compulsive Scale: Development and Validation of a Short Form (DOCS-SF). Front Psychol 2017;8. Available at: https://www.frontiersin.org/articles/10.3389/fpsyg.2017.01503. Accessed July 18, 2022.

73. Wetterneck CT, Rouleau TM, Williams MT, et al. A New Scrupulosity Scale for the Dimensional Obsessive-Compulsive Scale (DOCS): Validation With Clinical and Nonclinical Samples. Behav Ther 2021;52(6):1449–63.

74. Bejerot S, Edman G, Anckarsäter H, et al. The Brief Obsessive-Compulsive Scale (BOCS): a self-report scale for OCD and obsessive-compulsive related disorders. Nord J Psychiatry 2014;68(8):549–59.

75. Patel SR, Basaraba C, Rose S, et al. The brief obsessive-compulsive scale: Development and validation of a self-report (BOCS-SR). J Obsessive-compuls Relat Disord 2022;33:100730.

76. Storch EA, Murphy TK, Adkins JW, et al. The children's Yale-Brown obsessive–compulsive scale: Psychometric properties of child- and parent-report formats. J Anxiety Disord 2006;20(8):1055–70.

77. Conelea CA, Schmidt ER, Leonard RC, et al. The Children's Yale–Brown Obsessive Compulsive Scale: Clinician versus self-report format in adolescents in a residential treatment facility. J Obsessive-compuls Relat Disord 2012;1(2):69–72.

78. Foa EB, Coles M, Huppert JD, et al. Development and Validation of a Child Version of the Obsessive Compulsive Inventory. Behav Ther 2010;41(1):121–32.

79. McGuire JF, Geller DA, Murphy TK, et al. Defining Treatment Outcomes in Pediatric Obsessive-Compulsive Disorder Using a Self-Report Scale. Behav Ther 2019;50(2):314–24.

80. Opakunle T, Aloba O, Akinsulore A. Obsessive Compulsive Inventory - Child Version (OCI-CV): Confirmatory factor analysis, reliability, validity and correlates among Nigerian adolescents. Malawi Med J J Med Assoc Malawi 2018;30(4):262–9.

81. Jones AM, De Nadai AS, Arnold EB, et al. Psychometric Properties of the Obsessive Compulsive Inventory: Child Version in Children and Adolescents with Obsessive–Compulsive Disorder. Child Psychiatry Hum Dev 2013;44(1):137–51.

82. Abramovitch A, Abramowitz JS, McKay D, et al. The OCI-CV-R: A Revision of the Obsessive-Compulsive Inventory - Child Version. J Anxiety Disord 2022;86:102532.

83. Abramovitch A, Abramowitz JS, McKay D, et al. An ultra-brief screening scale for pediatric obsessive-compulsive disorder: The OCI-CV-5. J Affect Disord 2022;312:208–16.

84. Piqueras JA, Rodríguez-Jiménez T, Ortiz AG, et al. Factor Structure, Reliability, and Validity of the Spanish Version of the Children's Florida Obsessive Compulsive Inventory (C-FOCI). Child Psychiatry Hum Dev 2017;48(1):166–79.

85. Storch EA, Khanna M, Merlo LJ, et al. Children's Florida Obsessive Compulsive Inventory: Psychometric Properties and Feasibility of a Self-Report Measure of Obsessive–Compulsive Symptoms in Youth. Child Psychiatry Hum Dev 2009;40(3):467–83.

86. Uher R, Heyman I, Turner CM, et al. Self-, parent-report and interview measures of obsessive–compulsive disorder in children and adolescents. J Anxiety Disord 2008;22(6):979–90.

87. Asnaani A, Kaczkurkin AN, Alpert E, et al. The effect of treatment on quality of life and functioning in OCD. Compr Psychiatry 2017;73:7–14.

88. Storch EA, Small BJ, McGuire JF, et al. Quality of Life in Children and Youth with Obsessive-Compulsive Disorder. J Child Adolesc Psychopharmacol 2018;28(2):104–10.

89. La Buissonnière-Ariza V, Guzik AG, Schneider SC, et al. Family Accommodation of Symptoms in Adults With Obsessive-Compulsive Disorder: Factor Structure and Usefulness of the Family Accommodation Scale for OCD–Patient Version. J Psychiatr Pract 2022;28(1):36–47.

90. Lebowitz ER, Panza KE, Bloch MH. Family accommodation in obsessive-compulsive and anxiety disorders: a five-year update. Expert Rev Neurother 2016;16(1):45–53.

91. Stein DJ, Costa DLC, Lochner C, et al. Obsessive–compulsive disorder. Nat Rev Dis Primer 2019;5(1):52.

92. Piacentini J, Peris TS, Bergman RL, et al. Functional impairment in childhood OCD: development and psychometrics properties of the Child Obsessive-Compulsive Impact Scale-Revised (COIS-R). J Clin Child Adolesc Psychol Off J Soc Clin Child Adolesc Psychol Am Psychol Assoc Div 2007;36(4):645–53.

93. Skarphedinsson G, Melin KH, Valderhaug R, et al. Evaluation of the factor structure of the Child Obsessive–Compulsive Impact Scale – Revised (COIS-R) in Scandinavia with confirmatory factor analysis. J Obsessive-compuls Relat Disord 2015;7:65–72.

94. Garcia AM, Sapyta JJ, Moore PS, et al. Predictors and Moderators of Treatment Outcome in the Pediatric Obsessive Compulsive Treatment Study (POTS I). J Am Acad Child Adolesc Psychiatry 2010;49(10):1024–33.

95. Piacentini J, Bergman RL, Chang S, et al. Controlled comparison of family cognitive behavioral therapy and psychoeducation/relaxation training for child obsessive-compulsive disorder. J Am Acad Child Adolesc Psychiatry 2011;50(11):1149–61.

96. Storch EA, Caporino NE, Morgan JR, et al. Preliminary investigation of web-camera delivered cognitive-behavioral therapy for youth with obsessive-compulsive disorder. Psychiatry Res 2011;189(3):407–12.

97. Wetterneck CT, Pinciotti CM, Knott L, et al. Development and validation of the Adult OCD Impact Scale (AOIS): A measure of psychosocial functioning for adults with obsessive-compulsive disorder. J Context Behav Sci 2020;18:287–93.

98. Leon AC, Olfson M, Portera L, et al. Assessing Psychiatric Impairment in Primary Care with the Sheehan Disability Scale. Int J Psychiatry Med 1997;27(2):93–105.

99. Sheehan KH, Sheehan DV. Assessing treatment effects in clinical trials with the discan metric of the Sheehan Disability Scale. Int Clin Psychopharmacol 2008;23(2):70–83.

100. Soler CT, Vadlin S, Olofsdotter S, et al. Psychometric evaluation of the Swedish Child Sheehan Disability Scale in adolescent psychiatric patients. Scand J Child Adolesc Psychiatry Psychol 2021;9:137–46.

101. Whiteside SP. Adapting the Sheehan Disability Scale to Assess Child and Parent Impairment Related to Childhood Anxiety Disorders. J Clin Child Adolesc Psychol 2009;38(5):721–30.

102. Stewart KE, Sumantry D, Malivoire BL. Family and couple integrated cognitive-behavioural therapy for adults with OCD: A meta-analysis. J Affect Disord 2020; 277:159–68.
103. Strauss C, Hale L, Stobie B. A meta-analytic review of the relationship between family accommodation and OCD symptom severity. J Anxiety Disord 2015;33: 95–102.
104. Calvocoressi L, Lewis B, Harris M, et al. Family accommodation in obsessive-compulsive disorder. Am J Psychiatry 1995;152(3):441–3.
105. Calvocoressi L, Mazure CM, Kasl SV, et al. Family accommodation of obsessive-compulsive symptoms: instrument development and assessment of family behavior. J Nerv Ment Dis 1999;187(10):636–42.
106. Wu MS, Pinto A, Horng B, et al. Psychometric properties of the Family Accommodation Scale for Obsessive-Compulsive Disorder-Patient Version. Psychol Assess 2016;28(3):251–62.
107. Pinto A, Van Noppen B, Calvocoressi L. Development and preliminary psychometric evaluation of a self-rated version of the Family Accommodation Scale for Obsessive-Compulsive Disorder. J Obsessive-compuls Relat Disord 2013;2(4): 457–65.
108. Flessner CA, Sapyta J, Garcia A, et al. Examining the Psychometric Properties of the Family Accommodation Scale-Parent-Report (FAS-PR). J Psychopathol Behav Assess 2009;31(1):38–46.
109. Monzani B, Vidal-Ribas P, Turner C, et al. The Role of Paternal Accommodation of Paediatric OCD Symptoms: Patterns and Implications for Treatment Outcomes. J Abnorm Child Psychol 2020;48(10):1313–23.
110. Selles RR, Højgaard DRMA, Ivarsson T, et al. Symptom Insight in Pediatric Obsessive-Compulsive Disorder: Outcomes of an International Aggregated Cross-Sectional Sample. J Am Acad Child Adolesc Psychiatry 2018;57(8): 615–9, e5.
111. Eisen JL, Phillips KA, Baer L, et al. The Brown Assessment of Beliefs Scale: reliability and validity. Am J Psychiatry 1998;155(1):102–8.
112. Gan J, He J, Fu H, et al. Association between obsession, compulsion, depression and insight in obsessive-compulsive disorder: a meta-analysis. Nord J Psychiatry 2021;0(0):1–8.
113. Hong JS, Sheriff R, Smith K, et al. Impact of COVID-19 on telepsychiatry at the service and individual patient level across two UK NHS mental health Trusts. Evid Based Ment Health 2021;24(4):161–6.
114. Reay RE, Looi JC, Keightley P. Telehealth mental health services during COVID-19: summary of evidence and clinical practice. Australas Psychiatry 2020;28(5): 514–6.
115. Deniz ME, Satici SA, Doenyas C, et al. Zoom Fatigue, Psychological Distress, Life Satisfaction, and Academic Well-Being. Cyberpsychology Behav Soc Netw 2022;25(5):270–7.
116. Rupp C, Falke C, Gühne D, et al. A study on treatment sensitivity of ecological momentary assessment in obsessive–compulsive disorder. Clin Psychol Psychother 2019;26(6):695–706.

Genomics of Obsessive-Compulsive Disorder and Related Disorders

What the Clinician Needs to Know

James J. Crowley, PhD[a,b],*

KEYWORDS

- Obsessive-compulsive disorder • Trichotillomania • Excoriation disorder
- Hoarding disorder • Body dysmorphic disorder • Genetic • Genomic • Twin

KEY POINTS

- Obsessive-compulsive disorder (OCD) and its related disorders are all complex traits that result from genetic and environmental factors in roughly equal proportions.
- Genomic studies of OCD and its related disorders are just beginning to yield replicable results and long-sought risk genes.
- Most genomic findings for OCD and its related disorders are not yet clinically actionable, but pharmacogenetic data may be one exception.

OVERVIEW

Despite their high prevalence and disabling effects, obsessive-compulsive disorder (OCD) and related disorders (OCD-RDs) have traditionally been under-represented in psychiatric genomics research. Thankfully, however, several large-scale, collaborative efforts using modern genomic methods have begun to reveal the genetic architecture of these traits and identify long-sought risk genes. The purpose of this article is to summarize what we know now and how this information can be useful for clinicians and their patients. We first detail the latest genetic epidemiology and molecular genetic findings for OCD and all four related disorders defined by the DSM-5 (trichotillomania, skin picking disorder, hoarding disorder, and body dysmorphic disorder). Next, we describe the current state of knowledge on the pharmacogenetics of serotonin reuptake inhibitors in OCD. The article concludes with several clinical implications of

[a] Department of Genetics, University of North Carolina at Chapel Hill, 120 Mason Farm Road, Chapel Hill, NC 27599, USA; [b] Department of Psychiatry, University of North Carolina at Chapel Hill, 120 Mason Farm Road, Chapel Hill, NC 27599, USA
* Department of Genetics, University of North Carolina at Chapel Hill, 120 Mason Farm Road, Chapel Hill, NC 27599.
E-mail address: crowley@unc.edu

Psychiatr Clin N Am 46 (2023) 39–51
https://doi.org/10.1016/j.psc.2022.11.003
0193-953X/23/© 2022 Elsevier Inc. All rights reserved.

genetic findings in OCD-RDs. Specifically, we provide guidance for using pharmaco-genetics information in pharmacotherapy for OCD-RDs, suggest answers to questions commonly asked by patients and families about OCD-RD genetics and outline the implications of genetic findings for understanding the etiology of OCD-RDs and novel therapeutic development.

Heritability and Molecular Genetics of Obsessive-Compulsive Disorder and Related Disorders

Obsessive-compulsive disorder

tTwin and family studies consistently show that OCD is roughly 50% heritable.[1-5] Early OCD twin studies (summarized by van Grootheest and colleagues[4]) revealed a greater concordance in OCD diagnoses between monozygotic than dizygotic twin pairs, indicating a role for genetics in OCD risk. More contemporary twin studies have focused on obsessive-compulsive symptoms, rather than clinical OCD, in large twin cohorts. For example, Mataix-Cols and colleagues[1] examined 16,383 twin pairs from Sweden and found that additive genetic factors accounted for 47% (95% confidence interval [CI], 42% to 52%) of the variation in liability for obsessive-compulsive symptoms. In the same paper from Sweden, Mataix-Cols and colleagues[1] examined the risk for OCD among the relatives of 24,768 individuals with OCD and found that the risk for OCD increased proportionally to genetic relatedness. For example, first-degree relatives of individuals diagnosed with OCD showed a four- to eightfold increased risk of OCD. In sum, these twin and family studies have provided unequivocal evidence that genetics explains about half of the risk of OCD, which has motivated hundreds of molecular genetic studies of OCD over the past 30+ years. The other half of OCD risk is of course due to environmental factors and the field is beginning to identify robust risk factors, such as perinatal complications and maternal smoking during pregnancy.[6-8]

Until roughly 10 years ago, molecular genetic studies of OCD suffered from the same limitations as other traits that show complex patterns of inheritance, including reliance on an unproven approach and small sample sizes. For example, OCD linkage studies (reviewed by Pauls and colleagues[9]) and >100 "candidate gene" studies (meta-analyzed by Taylor and colleagues[10]) produced inconsistent results. OCD genomics took a major step forward in 2013 when Stewart and colleagues[11] published the first genome-wide association study (GWAS) of OCD. GWAS is a modern approach in which the genomes of many different people are scanned in an agnostic fashion to find genetic markers associated with a trait or disease. In Stewart and colleagues, the authors collected DNA from 1,465 OCD cases, 5,557 controls, and 400 families and genotyped all samples for ~1 million single-nucleotide polymorphisms (SNPs) spread throughout the genome. As with other complex traits, this sample proved to be underpowered as no genome-wide significant loci were identified. However, polygenic risk analysis revealed that common genetic variation indeed contributed to risk for OCD and that increased sample size would lead to the discovery of significant loci. Two subsequent OCD GWAS[12,13] were published that also advanced the field but were still underpowered.

The first well-powered OCD GWAS was assembled by the Psychiatric Genomics Consortium (PGC) OCD Working Group and posted as a preprint in October 2021.[14] This study was limited to European ancestry individuals ($N = 14,140$ OCD cases and $N = 562,117$ controls), but it did identify the first genome-wide significant locus for OCD and strengthened previous literature suggesting genetic correlations with disorders often comorbid with OCD (eg, Tourette syndrome and anorexia nervosa). The PGC OCD Working Group is currently working on publishing a much larger OCD GWAS with >50,000 cases and >1 million controls. This marked increase in sample size has led to a tremendous step forward in OCD genomics, in the form of 30 genome-wide significant loci where common genetic variation is associated with OCD (results presented at the 2022 World Congress of Psychiatric Genetics, Florence, Italy). This study is an important advance and has facilitated many informative "post-GWAS" analyses, such as polygenic risk score (PRS) analysis. PRS estimates an individual's genetic risk for a disease or trait (calculated by summing the effect of many common variants) and has the potential to be clinically useful.

One major limitation, however, of the forthcoming OCD GWAS is that it is far from diverse. More than 95% of the OCD cases included are of European ancestry since there has been no large-scale collection of non-European OCD cases. This Eurocentric bias makes it such that OCD genetic findings are more accurate for individuals of European ancestry than other ancestries, thereby contributing to health disparities in potential future applications of genomics in precision medicine. Thankfully, however, the US NIMH has recently funded an effort to collect DNA and comprehensive phenotypic data from 5000 Latin American OCD cases in a study called the Latin American Trans-ancestry INitiative for OCD genomics (LATINO). We expect that LATINO and similar studies of OCD in diverse populations such as those from Asia and Africa will help to accelerate gene discovery for this understudied condition.

There is no question that GWAS is a powerful method to associate commonly occurring genetic variation with OCD, but it is blind to rare variation. Thresholds vary, but in general, common genetic variants are found in 1% or more of the population while rare variants are found in <1% and sometimes so rare that they have never been observed before in hundreds of thousands of samples. In isolation, common genetic risk variants generally have a modest effect on risk (eg, a relative risk ~ 1.1), but can have large effects in aggregate. Rare risk variants, on the other hand, generally have a larger effect on risk (eg, relative risks of 2 to >20), and are often more clinically actionable. The first modern genomic method used to interrogate rare variation in OCD risk was copy number variant (CNV) analysis, which involves the identification of stretches of DNA where the number of copies differs from the expectation of two (one maternal copy and one paternal copy). CNV deletions refer to the loss of a copy and CNV duplications refer to the gain of a copy. Two OCD CNV studies have been published thus far. McGrath and colleagues[15] examined 1,613 OCD cases and 1,789 controls and found no global CNV burden in cases, but did observe a trend toward an increased burden of large deletions previously associated with neurodevelopmental disorders, particularly deletions located at chromosome 16p13.11 (5 in cases, 0 in controls). Mahjani and colleagues[16] recently published a CNV analysis of 993 OCD cases and, like McGrath and colleagues, also found the 16p13.11 region to harbor the most potentially damaging CNVs (one deletion and two duplications in cases). Thus, genes within the 16p13.11 region are potential OCD risk genes.

Another powerful method that has been used to identify rare genetic risk factors for OCD is whole exome sequencing (WES). WES involves sequencing the protein-coding regions (exons) of all genes (the "exome") in an individual's genome. The exome represents just $\sim 1\%$ of the genome but is known to be highly enriched for disease-relevant rare variants. A particularly powerful application of WES is to sequence an affected proband as well as their parents. This is termed a "trio" analysis and has the advantage of being able to assign variants as *de novo* in origin (a new mutation not found in either parental genome). Thus far, two OCD WES studies have been published. The first, from Cappi and colleagues,[17] included WES data from 222 OCD trios and found that *de novo* mutations predicted to damage gene function are enriched in OCD probands (rate ratio, 1.52; $P = .0005$). They further identified two high-confidence risk genes, each containing two damaging mutations in unrelated probands: *CHD8* and *SCUBE1*. The second study, from Halvorsen and colleagues,[18] reported WES results from the largest OCD cohort to date. This study included WES data from a total of 1313 OCD cases, consisting of 587 trios, 644 "singletons" (probands without parent data) and 41 quartets (two siblings with OCD and their parent data). Overall, relative to healthy controls, OCD cases carried an excess of rare variants that are expected to damage gene function ("loss of function" variants) in genes that are generally intolerant to such variation ("loss of function intolerant" genes). This was also true of *de novo* variants found in trios. In case-control analyses, the most significant single-gene result was *SLITRK5* (odds ratio = 8.8, $P = 2.3 \times 10^{-6}$), which is known to influence synapse formation. Taken together, these data support the contribution of rare coding variants to OCD genetic risk. Like other psychiatric disorders, sequencing larger OCD cohorts will power the discovery of novel risk genes and provide greater insight into disease biology.

Trichotillomania

Trichotillomania (TTM) is a psychiatric disorder where patients recurrently pull out their own hair, leading to hair loss and impaired functioning.[19,20] It affects ~1 to 2% of the population and is often comorbid with OCD, anxiety/depressive disorders, and attention-deficit/hyperactivity syndrome (ADHD).[21] TTM typically begins in childhood and affects males and females equally, though fewer males seek treatment.[21] The evidence suggests that TTM has a genetic component. Several case reports,[22–24] five family studies[25–29] and two twin studies[30,31] all support a role for genetics in the etiology of TTM. For example, Keuthen and colleagues[26] found that first-degree relatives of individuals with TTM were roughly 8 times more likely to meet the criteria for TTM than relatives of healthy controls.

As mentioned above, selecting candidate genes based on unproven biological hypotheses has not been a successful approach in psychiatry. Currently, only a handful of such candidate gene studies have been reported for TTM. For example, Zuchner and colleagues[32,33] provided evidence that rare coding variants in *SLITRK1* and *SAPAP3* may be associated with TTM, but replication of these findings is needed. Thus far, there have been no GWAS, CNV, or WES studies focused on TTM, so the literature lacks an agnostic genome-wide analysis of TTM using modern genomic methods. One of the unique aspects of TTM is that it is considerably easier to model in non-human organisms as compared with other psychiatric disorders. For example, compulsive grooming in mice is quantifiable and thought to have relatively high face validity for human TTM. Thus far, single-gene knockouts of multiple genes in mice have been shown to induce compulsive grooming, including *Sapap3*,[34] *Slitrk5*[35] and *Hoxb8*.[36] Overall, for gene discovery in TTM to advance, there is a need for large, modern genomic studies such as those described above for OCD.

Excoriation (skin picking) disorder

Skin picking disorder (SPD) is defined as recurrent skin picking that results in skin lesions despite repeated attempts to stop the behavior, resulting in clinically significant distress or impairment.[19,37,38] Research on SPD is in the early stages and only one twin study has been published. Monzani and colleagues[39] examined the prevalence and heritability of SPD in 2518 adult twin pairs from a community sample in the UK. The prevalence of SPD was 1.2% and genetic factors accounted for ~40% of the variance in SPD risk. Therefore, SPD appears to be a relatively common problem with a genetic component similar in magnitude to OCD and TTM. In fact, SPD is clinically very similar to TTM and they seem to be genetically correlated, according to multivariate twin modeling.[30]

To our knowledge, there have been no molecular genetic studies focused on SPD. Thankfully, at least two ongoing, large-scale OCD genomics efforts are collecting data on SPD in OCD patients: the LATINO study mentioned above and the Nordic OCD and Related Disorders Consortium (NORDiC),[40] but the need exists for SPD-specific genetic studies.

Hoarding disorder

Hoarding disorder (HD) is defined as persistent difficulty discarding or parting with possessions, regardless of their actual value, resulting in cluttered living spaces.[19,41] The hoarding causes clinically significant distress or impairment in social, occupational, or other important areas of functioning (including maintaining a safe environment for oneself or others). HD is present in 1% to 3% of the population[42,43] and hoarding symptoms (HS) are found in 5% to 10% of the population.[44,45] As HD is a relatively new diagnosis, most genetic studies thus far have focused on HS. Twin studies have estimated the heritability of HS to be between 30% and 60%, with variation attributed to study differences in sex, age and ascertainment methods.[44–49] Family studies also support the role of genetics in HS.[50–54]

Few molecular genetic studies of HS have been performed and many were performed in patients who were ascertained for OCD. As with other OCD-RDs, candidate gene[55–59] and linkage studies[53,60,61] have been unrevealing. There have been two relatively small GWAS of HS,[62,63] with the results indicating that, like OCD, larger samples are likely to yield significant loci.

Body dysmorphic disorder

Body dysmorphic disorder (BDD) is defined as a preoccupation with one or more perceived defects or flaws in physical appearance that are not observable or appear slight to others.[19,64] At some point during the course of the disorder, the individual has performed repetitive behaviors or mental acts in response to the appearance concerns and the preoccupation causes clinically significant distress or impaired functioning. The prevalence of BDD is approximately 1% to 2%, with a significantly higher prevalence in females than males.[65] BDD is associated with high levels of psychiatric comorbidity, self-harm, suicide attempts, desire for cosmetic procedures, and school dropout.[66,67] BDD twin studies[65,68,69] all indicate a heritability of ~40 to 50% and one family study[70] found that first-degree relatives of BDD cases were 4 to 8 times more likely to meet criteria for BDD than the general population.

Just two small candidate genes studies[71,72] have been published on BDD. No genome-wide studies have been performed. As with SPD mentioned above, at least two ongoing, large-scale OCD genomics efforts are collecting data on BDD in OCD patients (LATINO and NORDiC), but the need exists for BDD-specific genetic studies.

Pharmacogenetics

The two primary treatment options for OCD are cognitive behavioral therapy (CBT) and serotonin reuptake inhibitors (SRIs). Access to evidence-based CBT for OCD is limited, so many patients rely on SRIs for symptom relief. Unfortunately, however, roughly 50% of OCD patients do not improve with SRI treatment.[73,74] This leaves a large number of patients without adequate treatment, which increases the risk of chronic disability,[75] quality of life impairment,[76] and suicide.[77] The goals of precision medicine are to deliver the right treatment to the right patient at the right time. If clinicians were able to predict which OCD patients were likely to fail SRI treatment, experience undesirable side effects or need dosing adjustments, they could tailor SRI treatments to the individual and hopefully increase response rates. This is the basic idea of pharmacogenetics (PGx), which is defined as the study of variability in drug response due to heritable factors.

PGx has recently shown clinical utility in psychiatry, after many years of promise. For example, Brown and colleagues[78] systematically reviewed and meta-analyzed clinical trials for PGx-guided antidepressant therapy in patients with major depressive disorder (MDD). In total, 13 trials comprising 4767 patients were analyzed. Patients who received PGx-guided antidepressant therapy (N = 2395) showed a 40% increase in remission compared with treatment as usual (odds ratio of 1.41, P = .001). Likewise, Greden and colleagues[79] showed that PGx-guided treatment modifications in MDD led to a greater symptom improvement (33.5% vs 21.1% reduction, P = .002), response rate (28.5% vs 16.7%, odds ratio 1.96, P = .036), and remission rate (21.5% vs 8.5%, OR 2.9, P = .007) compared with those without such modifications. This was replicated by Perlis and colleagues[80] where PGx-guided treatment modifications in MDD led to higher remission rates (33.7% vs 18.5%, OR 2.23, P = .005). In sum, PGx-guided antidepressant therapy causes a modest but significant increase in MDD remission. The effect size may seem small, but there are currently ~25 million Americans taking SRIs, so even a modest improvement in remission rates can benefit a large number of people. Furthermore, the effect size will improve as PGx moves away from a candidate gene approach based mostly on common metabolic polymorphisms (eg, poor and rapid metabolizers defined by $CYP2C19$ genotypes) and toward a genomic approach that incorporates common and rare variation for all genes.

OCD PGx studies have been vastly underpowered compared with MDD. Zai[81] provides a comprehensive review of ~25 relevant publications, most of which are small, retrospective candidate gene studies. These publications fall into two categories: those examining pharmacodynamic genes (eg, the serotonin transporter $SLC6A4$) and those examining pharmacokinetic genes (eg, the liver enzyme $CYP2D6$). Although most of these studies were unrevealing, some encouraging results were found in $CYP2D6$ and $CYP2C19$. This is consistent with MDD PGx, where pharmacokinetic variants are the most informative. To date, there are no large-scale OCD PGx studies, even though OCD has several advantages over MDD for PGx studies. Specifically, compared with MDD, OCD has a stronger SRI dose–response relationship,[82–84] a two-fold higher diagnostic inter-rater reliability,[85–87] a two-fold lower placebo response rate,[88] higher heritability[89] and a tenfold lower rate of spontaneous remission.[78,90] Therefore, we anticipate that PGx-guided treatment modifications in OCD may have a greater effect on response and remission rates than that found in MDD.

Clinical Implications

PGx-guided pharmacotherapy for obsessive-compulsive disorder and related disorders

PGx data is currently the most immediately actionable form of genetic data for OCD-RDs but is rarely used due to the uncertainty of how beneficial it is (see Zai and colleagues[81]). There are several companies that market commercial PGx tests that provide specific treatment recommendations to the clinician. As noted above, more research is needed to validate these treatment recommendations and therefore PGx is not widely used in OCD. There have been recommendations published by the FDA,[91] the Clinical Pharmacogenetics Implementation Consortium (CPIC)[92] and the International Society of Psychiatric Genetics (ISPG).[93] Overall, there is agreement that PGx data are one of many clinical variables worth considering before starting a patient on drug therapy. It is important to note that the recommendations are drug-specific, not disorder-specific. The ISPG statement[93] reads "Evidence to support widespread use of pharmacogenetic tests at this time is still inconclusive, but when pharmacogenetic testing results are already available, providers are encouraged to integrate this information into their medication selection and dosing decisions. Genetic information for CYP2C19 and CYP2D6 would likely be most beneficial for individuals who have experienced an inadequate response or adverse reaction to a previous antidepressant or antipsychotic trial."

Zai and colleagues[81] provided some practical advice for clinicians interested in using PGx to guide drug treatment for OCD. First, if a patient's CYP2D6 profile indicates that they are likely an unusually rapid or slow metabolizer, one could prescribe an SSRI that is not metabolized by CYP2D6 such as escitalopram, citalopram, or sertraline. Second, if a CYP2D6 poor metabolizer requires clomipramine, it would be prudent to measure serum clomipramine levels at a low initial dose to reduce the risk of adverse effects. Third, if a patient is a CYP2C19 ultra-rapid metabolizer, the clinician may want to avoid citalopram and escitalopram as very high doses may be needed for a therapeutic effect. High doses of citalopram and escitalopram are contraindicated by many regulatory authorities due to dose-dependent QT interval prolongation, which can cause serious cardiovascular complications (namely Torsades de Pointes, ventricular tachycardia, and sudden death). Fourth, if a patient is a CYP2C19 poor metabolizer, a low starting dose may be warranted. As the field of OCD PGx advances, there are likely to be additional and perhaps more specific recommendations. As recently shown in MDD, these advances will likely require large-scale randomized trials to show clinical utility.

Answers to common questions from patients about obsessive-compulsive disorder and related disorder genetics
Patients and families often have practical questions about what genetic research findings mean for them. **Table 1** lists several such questions and suggested answers based on our current knowledge of OCD-RD genetics.

Understanding etiology and novel therapeutic development
A major goal of genetics research in OCD-RDs is to help provide a deeper understanding of the etiology of these conditions to guide the development of more effective treatments. In terms of etiology, the genetic results thus far support a model where complex interactions between environmental and genetic risk factors predispose individuals to OCD-RDs, though the details are only beginning to be revealed, as

Table 1 Answers to common questions from patients about obsessive-compulsive disorder and related disorder genetics	
Question	**Suggested Answer**
I have OCD. What are the chances my relatives will develop it too?	Your closest relatives (siblings, children, and parents) are at moderate risk (around 10% chance).
My child has trichotillomania. Did I give it to them?	No. Most cases involve the chance inheritance of hundreds of gene variants from mom and dad. In some cases, brand-new variants not found in mom or dad occur by chance.
I have OCD, but my brother has ADHD. Why don't we have the same diagnosis?	OCD risk genes partially overlap with risk genes for other psychiatric disorders.
Can you predict skin picking disorder from genetic data alone?	No. Even identical twins of patients with skin picking disorder only have it half the time, so genes aren't everything.
Why should I participate in a genetic study?	In time, large genetic studies of OCD-RDs can help lead to new and improved treatment approaches.

described above. In terms of novel therapeutic development, there is currently only limited drug development in OCD-RDs,[94] due in part to a lack of novel targets for rational drug design or repurposing (identifying a novel therapeutic indication for an FDA-approved drug). In other psychiatric disorders, such as schizophrenia, the discovery of risk genes and biological pathways through genomic research has nominated several novel targets for rational drug design and repurposing.[95] For example, multiple voltage-gated calcium channel genes (eg, *CACNA1C* and *CACNA1D*) were among the first genes to be reliably linked to schizophrenia through both common and rare genetic variation.[96,97] As several FDA-approved calcium channel blockers and modulators are in use for cardiovascular indications (eg, verapamil for high blood pressure), a logical approach is to see if repurposing these agents for schizophrenia could improve outcomes. Based on this approach, there are five calcium channel blockers currently being tested for efficacy in schizophrenia.[98]

Some drug repurposing trials are also underway in OCD and, in some cases, genetic data were informative in the selection of targets for repurposing agents.[94] For example, the literature suggests a role for genetic variation in glutamatergic genes in OCD.[99] Motivated by these findings, Biohaven Pharmaceuticals is currently performing a phase three trial evaluating the efficacy and safety of adjunctive troriluzole in OCD.[100] Troriluzole is a prodrug of the glutamate-modulating agent riluzole, which is FDA-approved for amyotrophic lateral sclerosis. Troriluzole reduces synaptic glutamate levels and increases synaptic glutamate absorption. The Biohaven phase three trial was designed to enroll 700 participants and is expected to be completed in 2023. Overall, as we learn more about the genomics of OCD-RDs, we expect to nominate more novel targets for rational drug design and repurposing.

CLINICS CARE POINTS

- Genetic factors play a major role in the risk for OCD and its related disorders
- Patients and families often have questions for clinicians about what genetic findings mean for them and communicating this information requires great care
- Genomic studies are just beginning to identify specific genetic risk loci and genes and, in time, this information is likely to inform novel therapeutic development
- Most genomic findings for OCD and its related disorders are not yet clinically actionable, but pharmacogenetic data could potentially become the first exception with further research

DISCLOSURE

Dr J.J. Crowley has no commercial or financial conflicts of interest and acknowledges funding from the National Institutes of Health, United States.

REFERENCES

1. Mataix-Cols D, Boman M, Monzani B, et al. Population-based, multigenerational family clustering study of obsessive-compulsive disorder. JAMA Psychiatry 2013;70:709–17.
2. Pauls DL. The genetics of obsessive-compulsive disorder: a review. Dialogues Clin Neurosci 2010;12:149–63.
3. Bolton D, Rijsdijk F, O'Connor TG, et al. Obsessive-compulsive disorder, tics and anxiety in 6-year-old twins. Psychol Med 2007;37:39–48.

4. van Grootheest DS, Cath DC, Beekman AT, et al. Twin studies on obsessive-compulsive disorder: a review. Twin Res Hum Genet 2005;8:450–8.
5. Iervolino AC, Rijsdijk FV, Cherkas L, et al. A multivariate twin study of obsessive-compulsive symptom dimensions. Arch Gen Psychiatry 2011;68:637–44.
6. Brander G, Pérez-Vigil A, Larsson H, et al. Systematic review of environmental risk factors for Obsessive-Compulsive Disorder: A proposed roadmap from association to causation. Review Neurosci Biobehav Rev 2016;65:36–62.
7. Brander G, Rydell M, Kuja-Halkola R, et al. Association of perinatal risk factors with obsessive-compulsive disorder: a population-based birth cohort, sibling control study. JAMA Psychiatry 2016;73(11):1135–44.
8. Yilmaz Z, Larsen JT, Nissen JB, et al. The role of early-life family composition and parental socio-economic status as risk factors for obsessive-compulsive disorder in a Danish national cohort. J Psychiatr Res 2022;149:18–27.
9. Pauls DL, Abramovitch A, Rauch SL, et al. Obsessive-compulsive disorder: an integrative genetic and neurobiological perspective. Nat Rev Neurosci 2014;15:410–24.
10. Taylor S. Molecular genetics of obsessive-compulsive disorder: a comprehensive meta-analysis of genetic association studies. Mol Psychiatry 2013;18:799–805.
11. Stewart SE, Yu D, Scharf JM, et al. Genome-wide association study of obsessive-compulsive disorder. Mol Psychiatry 2013;18:788–98.
12. Mattheisen M, Samuels JF, Wang Y, et al. Genome-wide association study in obsessive-compulsive disorder: results from the OCGAS. Mol Psychiatry 2015;20:337–44.
13. International Obsessive Compulsive Disorder Foundation Genetics Collaborative (IOCDF-GC) and OCD Collaborative Genetics Association Studies (OCGAS). Revealing the complex genetic architecture of obsessive-compulsive disorder using meta-analysis. Mol Psychiatry 2018;23:1181–8.
14. Strom NI, Yu D, Gerring ZF, et al. Genome-wide association study identifies new locus associated with OCD. medRxiv 2021;2021. 10.13.21261078.
15. McGrath LM, Yu D, Marshall C, et al. Copy number variation in obsessive-compulsive disorder and tourette syndrome: a cross-disorder study. J Am Acad Child Adolesc Psychiatry 2014;53:910–9.
16. Mahjani B, Birnbaum R, Buxbaum Grice A, et al. Phenotypic Impact of Rare Potentially Damaging Copy Number Variation in Obsessive-Compulsive Disorder and Chronic Tic Disorders. Genes 2022;13(10):1796.
17. Cappi C, Oliphant ME, Péter Z, et al. De Novo Damaging DNA Coding Mutations Are Associated With Obsessive-Compulsive Disorder and Overlap With Tourette's Disorder and Autism. Biol Psychiatry 2020;87:1035–44.
18. Halvorsen M, Samuels J, Wang Y, et al. Exome sequencing in obsessive-compulsive disorder reveals a burden of rare damaging coding variants. Nat Neurosci 2021;24:1071–6.
19. American Psychiatric Association. Diagnostic and Statistical Manual of Mental Disorders. DSM Library. Available at: https://dsm.psychiatryonline.org/doi/book/10.1176/appi.books.9780890425596. Accessed November 4, 2022.
20. Grant JE, Chamberlain SR. Trichotillomania Am J Psychiatry 2016;173:868–74.
21. Grant JE, Dougherty DD, Chamberlain SR. Prevalence, gender correlates, and co-morbidity of trichotillomania. Psychiatry Res 2020;288:112948.
22. Sanderson KV, Hall-Smith P. Tonsure trichotillomania. Br J Dermatol 1970;82:343–50.
23. Kerbeshian J, Burd L. Familial trichotillomania. Am J Psychiatry 1991;148:684–5.

24. Galski T. Hair pulling (trichotillomania). Psychoanal Rev 1983;70:331–46.
25. Schlosser S, Black DW, Blum N, et al. The demography, phenomenology, and family history of 22 persons with compulsive hair pulling. Ann Clin Psychiatry 1994;6:147–52.
26. Keuthen NJ, Altenburger EM, Pauls D. A family study of trichotillomania and chronic hair pulling. Am J Med Genet B Neuropsychiatr Genet 2014;165B: 167–74.
27. Lenane MC, Swedo SE, Rapoport JL, et al. Rates of Obsessive Compulsive Disorder in first degree relatives of patients with trichotillomania: a research note. J Child Psychol Psychiatry 1992;33:925–33.
28. Swedo SE, Rapoport JL. Annotation: trichotillomania. J Child Psychol Psychiatry 1991;32:401–9.
29. Christenson GA, Mackenzie TB, Reeve EA. Familial trichotillomania. Am J Psychiatry 1992;149(2):283.
30. Monzani B, Rijsdijk F, Harris J, et al. The structure of genetic and environmental risk factors for dimensional representations of DSM-5 obsessive-compulsive spectrum disorders. JAMA Psychiatry 2014;71(2):182–9.
31. Novak CE, Keuthen NJ, Stewart SE, et al. A twin concordance study of trichotillomania. Am J Med Genet B Neuropsychiatr Genet 2009;150B:944–9.
32. Zuchner S, Cuccaro ML, Tran-Viet KN, et al. SLITRK1 mutations in trichotillomania. Mol Psychiatry 2006;11:887–9.
33. Züchner S, Wendland JR, Ashley-Koch AE, et al. Multiple rare SAPAP3 missense variants in trichotillomania and OCD. Mol Psychiatry 2009;14:6–9.
34. Welch JM, Lu J, Rodriguiz RM, et al. Cortico-striatal synaptic defects and OCD-like behaviours in Sapap3-mutant mice. Nature 2007;448:894–900.
35. Shmelkov SV, Hormigo A, Jing D, et al. Slitrk5 deficiency impairs corticostriatal circuitry and leads to obsessive-compulsive-like behaviors in mice. Nat Med 2010;16:598–602, 1p following 602.
36. Greer JM, Capecchi MR. Hoxb8 is required for normal grooming behavior in mice. Neuron 2002;33:23–34.
37. Grant JE, Redden SA, Leppink EW. Trichotillomania and skin picking disorder. New York, NY: Oxford Medicine Online; 2017.
38. Silva B, Canas-Simião H, Cavanna AE. Neuropsychiatric aspects of impulse control disorders. Psychiatr Clin North Am 2020;43:249–62.
39. Monzani B, Rijsdijk F, Cherkas L, et al. Prevalence and heritability of skin picking in an adult community sample: a twin study. Am J Med Genet B Neuropsychiatr Genet 2012;159B:605–10.
40. Mataix-Cols D, Hansen B, Mattheisen M, et al. Nordic OCD & Related Disorders Consortium: Rationale, design, and methods. Am J Med Genet B Neuropsychiatr Genet 2020;183:38–50.
41. Steketee G, Frost RO. Introduction to hoarding disorder. Treat Hoarding Disord 2013;1–12. https://doi.org/10.1093/med:psych/9780199334964.003.0001.
42. Nordsletten AE, Reichenberg A, Hatch SL, et al. Epidemiology of hoarding disorder. Br J Psychiatry 2013;203:445–52.
43. Postlethwaite A, Kellett S, Mataix-Cols D. Prevalence of hoarding disorder: a systematic review and meta-analysis. J Affect Disord 2019;256:309–16.
44. Mathews CA, Delucchi K, Cath DC, et al. Partitioning the etiology of hoarding and obsessive-compulsive symptoms. Psychol Med 2014;44:2867–76.
45. Burton CL, Park LS, Corfield EC, et al. Heritability of obsessive-compulsive trait dimensions in youth from the general population. Transl Psychiatry 2018;8:191.

46. Iervolino AC, Perroud N, Fullana MA, et al. Prevalence and heritability of compulsive hoarding: a twin study. Am J Psychiatry 2009;166:1156–61.
47. Ivanov VZ, Mataix-Cols D, Serlachius E, et al. Prevalence, comorbidity and heritability of hoarding symptoms in adolescence: a population based twin study in 15-year olds. PLoS One 2013;8:e69140.
48. López-Solà C, Fontenelle LF, Alonso P, et al. Prevalence and heritability of obsessive-compulsive spectrum and anxiety disorder symptoms: A survey of the Australian Twin Registry. Am J Med Genet B Neuropsychiatr Genet 2014; 165B:314–25.
49. Taylor S, Jang KL, Asmundson GJG. Etiology of obsessions and compulsions: a behavioral-genetic analysis. J Abnorm Psychol 2010;119:672–82.
50. Frost RO, Gross RC. The hoarding of possessions. Behav Res Ther 1993;31: 367–81.
51. Pertusa A, Fullana MA, Singh S, et al. Compulsive hoarding: OCD symptom, distinct clinical syndrome, or both? Am J Psychiatry 2008;165:1289–98.
52. Samuels J, Bienvenu OJ 3rd, Riddle MA, et al. Hoarding in obsessive compulsive disorder: results from a case-control study. Behav Res Ther 2002;40: 517–28.
53. Samuels J, Shugart YY, Grados MA, et al. Significant linkage to compulsive hoarding on chromosome 14 in families with obsessive-compulsive disorder: results from the OCD Collaborative Genetics Study. Am J Psychiatry 2007;164: 493–9.
54. Steketee G, Kelley AA, Wernick JA, et al. Familial patterns of hoarding symptoms. Depress Anxiety 2015;32:728–36.
55. Alonso P, Gratacòs M, Menchón JM, et al. Genetic susceptibility to obsessive-compulsive hoarding: the contribution of neurotrophic tyrosine kinase receptor type 3 gene. Genes Brain Behav 2008;7:778–85.
56. Lochner C, Kinnear CJ, Hemmings SMJ, et al. Hoarding in obsessive-compulsive disorder: clinical and genetic correlates. J Clin Psychiatry 2005; 66:1155–60.
57. Sinopoli VM, Erdman L, Burton CL, et al. Serotonin system genes and hoarding with and without other obsessive-compulsive traits in a population-based, pediatric sample: A genetic association study. Depress Anxiety 2020;37:760–70.
58. Timpano KR, Schmidt NB, Wheaton MG, et al. Consideration of the BDNF gene in relation to two phenotypes: hoarding and obesity. J Abnorm Psychol 2011; 120:700–7.
59. Wendland JR, Moya PR, Timpano KR, et al. A haplotype containing quantitative trait loci for SLC1A1 gene expression and its association with obsessive-compulsive disorder. Arch Gen Psychiatry 2009;66:408–16.
60. Liang K-Y, Wang Y, Shugart YY, et al. Evidence for potential relationship between SLC1A1 and a putative genetic linkage region on chromosome 14q to obsessive-compulsive disorder with compulsive hoarding. Am J Med Genet B Neuropsychiatr Genet 2008;147B:1000–2.
61. Zhang H, Leckman JF, Pauls DL, et al. Genomewide scan of hoarding in sib pairs in which both sibs have Gilles de la Tourette syndrome. Am J Hum Genet 2002;70:896–904.
62. Alemany-Navarro M, Cruz R, Real E, et al. Looking into the genetic bases of OCD dimensions: a pilot genome-wide association study. Transl Psychiatry 2020;10:151.
63. Perroud N, Guipponi M, Pertusa A, et al. Genome-wide association study of hoarding traits. Am J Med Genet B Neuropsychiatr Genet 2011;156:240–2.

64. Phillips K. Body dysmorphic disorder: advances in research and clinical practice. New York, NY: Oxford University Press; 2017.
65. Enander J, Ivanov VZ, Mataix-Cols D, et al. Prevalence and heritability of body dysmorphic symptoms in adolescents and young adults: a population-based nationwide twin study. Psychol Med 2018;48:2740–7.
66. Rautio D, Jassi A, Krebs G, et al. Clinical characteristics of 172 children and adolescents with body dysmorphic disorder. Eur Child Adolesc Psychiatry 2022; 31:133–44.
67. Krebs G, Fernández de la Cruz L, Rijsdijk FV, et al. The association between body dysmorphic symptoms and suicidality among adolescents and young adults: a genetically informative study. Psychol Med 2022;52:1268–76.
68. Monzani B, Rijsdijk F, Harris J, et al. The structure of genetic and environmental risk factors for dimensional representations of DSM-5 obsessive-compulsive spectrum disorders. JAMA Psychiatry 2014;71:182–9.
69. Monzani B, Rijsdijk F, Iervolino AC, et al. Evidence for a genetic overlap between body dysmorphic concerns and obsessive-compulsive symptoms in an adult female community twin sample. Am J Med Genet B Neuropsychiatr Genet 2012; 159B:376–82.
70. Bienvenu OJ, Samuels JF, Riddle MA, et al. The relationship of obsessive-compulsive disorder to possible spectrum disorders: results from a family study. Biol Psychiatry 2000;48:287–93.
71. Wang S-K, Lee Y-H, Kim J-L, et al. No effect on body dissatisfaction of an interaction between 5-httlpr genotype and neuroticism in a young adult korean population. Clin Psychopharmacol Neurosci 2014;12:229–34.
72. Phillips KA, Zai G, King NA, et al. A preliminary candidate gene study in body dysmorphic disorder. J Obsessive-Compulsive Relat Disord 2015;40(10):72–6.
73. Stein DJ, Costa DLC, Lochner C, et al. Obsessive-compulsive disorder. Nat Rev Dis Primers 2019;5:52.
74. Goodman WK, Storch EA, Sheth SA. Harmonizing the neurobiology and treatment of obsessive-compulsive disorder. Am J Psychiatry 2021;178:17–29.
75. Storch EA, Abramowitz JS, Keeley M. Correlates and mediators of functional disability in obsessive-compulsive disorder. Depress Anxiety 2009;26:806–13.
76. Norberg MM, Calamari JE, Cohen RJ, et al. Quality of life in obsessive-compulsive disorder: an evaluation of impairment and a preliminary analysis of the ameliorating effects of treatment. Depress Anxiety 2008;25(3):248–59.
77. Albert U, De Ronchi D, Maina G, et al. Suicide risk in obsessive-compulsive disorder and exploration of risk factors: a systematic review. Curr Neuropharmacol 2019;17:681–96.
78. Brown LC, Stanton JD, Bharthi K, et al. Pharmacogenomic testing and depressive symptom remission: a systematic review and meta-analysis of prospective, controlled clinical trials. Clin Pharmacol Ther 2022. https://doi.org/10.1002/cpt.2748.
79. Greden JF, Parikh SV, Rothschild AJ, et al. Impact of pharmacogenomics on clinical outcomes in major depressive disorder in the GUIDED trial: A large, patient- and rater-blinded, randomized, controlled study. J Psychiatr Res 2019; 111:59–67.
80. Perlis RH, Dowd D, Fava M, et al. Randomized, controlled, participant- and rater-blind trial of pharmacogenomic test-guided treatment versus treatment as usual for major depressive disorder. Depress Anxiety 2020;37:834–41.
81. Zai G. Pharmacogenetics of Obsessive-compulsive disorder: an evidence-update. Curr Top Behav Neurosci 2021;49:385–98.

82. Rabinowitz I, Baruch Y, Barak Y. High-dose escitalopram for the treatment of obsessive-compulsive disorder. Int Clin Psychopharmacol 2008;23:49–53.
83. Ninan PT, Koran LM, Kiev A, et al. High-dose sertraline strategy for nonresponders to acute treatment for obsessive-compulsive disorder: a multicenter double-blind trial. J Clin Psychiatry 2006;67:15–22.
84. Koran LM, Hanna GL, Hollander E, et al. Practice guideline for the treatment of patients with obsessive-compulsive disorder. Am J Psychiatry 2007;164:5–53.
85. Regier DA, Narrow WE, Clarke DE, et al. DSM-5 field trials in the United States and Canada, Part II: test-retest reliability of selected categorical diagnoses. Am J Psychiatry 2013;170(1):59–70.
86. Goodman WK, Price LH, Rasmussen SA, et al. The yale-brown obsessive compulsive scale. I. development, use, and reliability. Arch Gen Psychiatry 1989;46:1006–11.
87. DSM-IV field trial: obsessive-compulsive disorder. Am J Psychiatry 1995;152(1): 90–6 [published erratum appears in Am J Psychiatry 1995;152(4):654].
88. Li F, Nasir M, Olten B, et al. Meta-analysis of placebo response in adult antidepressant trials. CNS Drugs 2019;33(10):971–80.
89. Brainstorm Consortium, Anttila V, Bulik-Sullivan B, et al. Analysis of shared heritability in common disorders of the brain. Science 2018;360.
90. Pallanti S, Hollander E, Bienstock C, et al. Treatment non-response in OCD: methodological issues and operational definitions. Int J Neuropsychopharmacol 2002;5:181–91.
91. Center for Drug Evaluation. Research. Table of pharmacogenomic biomarkers in drug labeling. U.S. food and drug administration. Available at: https://www.fda. gov/drugs/science-and-research-drugs/table-pharmacogenomic-biomarkers-drug-labeling. Accessed November 4, 2022.
92. Hicks JK, Sangkuhl K, Swen JJ, et al. Clinical pharmacogenetics implementation consortium guideline (CPIC) for CYP2D6 and CYP2C19 genotypes and dosing of tricyclic antidepressants: 2016 update. Clin Pharmacol Ther 2017; 102:37–44.
93. Genetic Testing Statement. Available at: https://ispg.net/genetic-testing-statement. Accessed November 4, 2022.
94. Grassi G, Cecchelli C, Vignozzi L, et al. Investigational and experimental drugs to treat obsessive-compulsive disorder. J Exp Pharmacol 2020;12:695–706.
95. Lago SG, Bahn S. The druggable schizophrenia genome: from repurposing opportunities to unexplored drug targets. NPJ Genom Med 2022;7:25.
96. Schizophrenia psychiatric genome-wide association study (GWAS) consortium. genome-wide association study identifies five new schizophrenia loci. Nat Genet 2011;43:969–76.
97. Purcell SM, Moran JL, Fromer M, et al. A polygenic burden of rare disruptive mutations in schizophrenia. Nature 2014;506:185–90.
98. Lago SG, Bahn S. Clinical trials and therapeutic rationale for drug repurposing in schizophrenia. ACS Chem Neurosci 2019;10:58–78.
99. Rajendram R, Kronenberg S, Burton CL, et al. Glutamate genetics in obsessive-compulsive disorder: a review. J Can Acad Child Adolesc Psychiatry 2017;26: 205–13.
100. Efficacy and safety study of adjunctive troriluzole in obsessive compulsive disorder. Available at: https://clinicaltrials.gov/ct2/show/NCT04641143. Accessed November 4, 2022.

Cognitive Neuroscience of Obsessive-Compulsive Disorder

Laura B. Bragdon, PhD[a,b,*], Goi Khia Eng, PhD[a,b],
Nicolette Recchia, BS[a,b], Katherine A. Collins, PhD, LCSW[b],
Emily R. Stern, PhD[a,b]

KEYWORDS

- Error monitoring • Response inhibition • Cognitive flexibility • Reward
- Decision-making • Threat conditioning • Habit • Goal-directed

KEY POINTS

- Paradigms used in the cognitive neuroscientific study of obsessive-compulsive disorder (OCD) can elucidate the underlying mechanisms of the disorder.
- Prefrontal hyperactivation in response to errors and hypoactivation during switching tasks are the most consistent neuroimaging findings in OCD.
- Accumulating evidence points to dysfunction in fronto-limbic areas during decision-making involving uncertainty and risk.
- No single model is likely to fully explain OCD, and interactions between domains are likely.
- Continuing to study the cognitive neuroscience of OCD can contribute to treatment optimization and identification of novel interventional targets.

INTRODUCTION

The advancement in neuroimaging techniques over the past decades has enabled the examination of the neurocircuitry underlying obsessive-compulsive disorder (OCD). These advances, alongside a growing emphasis on examining neural mechanisms independent of symptom provocation, have allowed for a better understanding of the neurobiological underpinnings of cognitive-affective dysfunction in OCD. However, despite an increasing understanding of the pathophysiology of OCD, current treatments have remained largely unchanged over the past 30 years, and further, as

The authors have nothing to disclose.
[a] Department of Psychiatry, New York University School of Medicine, One Park Avenue, 8th floor, New York, NY 10016, USA; [b] Nathan S. Kline Institute for Psychiatric Research, 140 Old Orangeburg Road, Orangeburg, NY 10962, USA
* Corresponding author. Department of Psychiatry, New York University School of Medicine, One Park Avenue, 8th floor, New York, NY 10016.
E-mail address: Laura.Bragdon@NYULangone.org

many as 50%–70% of patients remain symptomatic following either psychotherapy or pharmacotherapy.[1] Further elucidation of the cognitive neuroscience underlying OCD can provide insights for enhancing treatment outcomes by improving treatment-matching (ie, personalizing treatment to match the impairment), optimization of strategies for combining or augmenting therapies, and identification of novel targets for intervention.

In this review, we provide an updated[2] discussion of the neuroscientific literature examining the cognitive-affective constructs that may underlie OCD phenomenology. We summarize the state of the literature in seven key domains: error detection, response inhibition, cognitive flexibility (task switching and reversal), reward processing, decision-making, threat conditioning and extinction, and the balance between goal-directed and habitual behavior. Each domain is discussed in the context of obsessive-compulsive phenomenology and implications for research and treatment are considered.

Error Monitoring

Much research into neuroimaging correlates of OCD has taken place in the field of error detection. The "cybernetic" model of OCD proposed that symptoms of the disorder could be due to abnormality in a control system that compares perceptual input signals with an internal reference.[3] Typically, this system generates an "error signal" when a mismatch is detected, which drives behavioral adjustment to reduce the error. In the case of OCD, this theory proposes that the error or mismatch signal is persistently high and resistant to reduction through behavioral adjustments, leading to OCD symptoms including incompleteness and "not-just-right-experiences" (NJREs) (ie, obsessions) along with repetitive attempts at behavioral adjustments (ie, compulsions).[3]

Functional neuroimaging studies in healthy controls (HCs) consistently point to the involvement of dorsal medial frontal cortex (MFC) including dorsal anterior cingulate cortex (dACC), supplementary motor area (SMA), and pre-SMA, which are linked to the general detection of mismatch or cognitive conflict even in the absence of an error.[4,5] In addition to dorsal MFC regions, errors often activate a broader range of brain areas including bilateral anterior insula/frontal operculum (aI/fO) as well as more rostral areas of ACC (rACC), dorsolateral and ventrolateral prefrontal cortex (vlPFC), and inferior lateral parietal cortex.[6] Broadly speaking, neural regions linked to error detection overlap with those ascribed to the "salience network" (also called cingulo-opercular network), primarily, as well as "frontoparietal network" (FPN).[7,8] Electrophysiologically, errors elicit a large negative-going event-related potential (ERP) waveform that peaks approximately 100 ms after an error is made, called the "error-related negativity" (ERN). The ERN is largest over frontal midline electrodes (Cz and FCz) and has a major generator in dorsal MFC.[9]

Over two decades ago, the first publication of the ERN in OCD reported a significantly increased amplitude of the waveform in patients compared with HCs.[10] Since then, the association between OCD or OC symptoms and a larger ERN has been replicated and extended in over 30 additional studies in both adults and children/adolescents,[11] making the ERN arguably one of the most replicated biomarkers of OCD.[12,13] In a recent meta-analysis of functional magnetic resonance imaging (fMRI) studies of error processing in adults with OCD, patients showed significantly greater activation of dorsal MFC regions (dACC, SMA, and pre-SMA), right aI/fO, and anterior lateral prefrontal cortex in response to errors compared with HCs.[14] Although not found in the meta-analytic results, two earlier studies found greater activation (or reduced deactivation) of the ventromedial prefrontal cortex (vmPFC) in response to errors in OCD children[15] and adults[16] compared with control subjects. The vmPFC is a key area of the default mode network (DMN) that typically deactivates during externally focused cognitive tasks,[17,18] including the detection of errors,[16] but activates more (or deactivates less) during tasks of internally focused cognition such as event imagination, episodic memory, and self-processing.[17,19] The vmPFC node of DMN in particular appears to be involved in mental processes with affective components.[17] Given this context, the above-described findings of increased error-related vmPFC activity in OCD were interpreted as potentially reflecting excessive intrusion of internally focused thought processes or negative emotions when detecting a mistake.

Though imaging studies comparing OCD patients with HCs have considerably advanced the understanding of neurocircuit mechanisms of error processing in the disorder, it is well recognized that OCD is phenotypically heterogeneous, which is likely underpinned by heterogeneity in neurocircuit functioning. Addressing this question, De Nadai and colleagues[20] conducted an innovative latent profile analysis examining neural variability of error-related activations within a large OCD sample. Three OCD subgroups were revealed: one subgroup showed a neural response to errors that were similar to a separate HC group; another group showed hyperactive responses compared with HCs in the dorsal ACC, SMA, and aI/fO as well as reduced deactivation (ie, increased activity) of putamen and vmPFC; and the last subgroup had larger deactivations (ie, reduced activity) compared with HCs in the putamen, vmPFC, and posterior cingulate cortex (PCC). Intriguingly, the second subgroup, compared with the first, showed a trend toward a poorer response to 12 weeks of cognitive-behavioral therapy. Although this initial study warrants further research, it illuminates the important issue of variability in OCD brain function and highlights the need for future work to consider heterogeneity of neural responses within patient samples.

Overall, the literature on OCD is remarkably consistent in identifying an increased neural response to errors among patients, thus providing support for the "overactive mismatch detector" (cybernetic) theory of OCD.[3] However, the majority of studies examined responses to actual (real) errors, whereas the OCD phenotype is more consistent with the detection of errors or mismatches where there are none (or their presence is uncertain). Thus, although hyperactive error responses in OCD may reflect an important characteristic of the disorder related to sensitivity to mistakes, these studies do not directly probe the neural mechanisms associated with the feeling that something is wrong in the absence of overt errors. ERP studies have attempted to address this issue by examining the "correct related negativity" (CRN), a small negative deflection that is the analog to the ERN on correct trials. Results from these investigations have been inconsistent, with only a portion of those studies examining the CRN finding it to be significantly enhanced in OCD.[12] Although CRN studies make up only a small subset of the research on error-related processing in OCD, they represent an important complement to prior work.

Owing to the strong empirical evidence of altered dorsal MFC activation in OCD, two recent clinical trials tested the effects of modulating this region using deep transcranial magnetic resonance imaging (TMS). The first study was an open-label pilot trial of 10 OCD patients using low-frequency 1 Hz stimulation, which is thought to be inhibitory, for 10 sessions conducted over 2 weeks.[21] Patients showed significantly reduced OCD symptom severity both at the end of the 2-week period and at 1-month follow-up.[21] The second study was a multisite, sham-controlled trial of 94 OCD patients using high-frequency stimulation at 20 Hz, which is thought to be excitatory, for 6 weeks of almost-daily treatment.[22] This study also found reduced symptom severity in the high-frequency stimulation group compared with the sham group at the end of the trial and follow-up.[22] In a pilot study using a subsample from this larger trial, high-frequency deep-TMS-related reductions in severity scores among 16 OCD patients were associated with an increase in ERN amplitude from pre- to posttreatment,[23] suggesting that *increasing* activity of the dorsal MFC and associated neurophysiological responses to errors lead to symptom improvement. Results from these two studies provide essentially opposite findings; the high-frequency TMS study was larger and sham-controlled, but provides results that are difficult to reconcile with the cybernetic or "enhanced mismatch detector" model of OCD and extant literature. Indeed, the researchers conducting the high-frequency TMS trial themselves acknowledge the counterintuitive nature of their results, and point out that their pilot testing included a low-frequency arm that was halted early for futility.[23] It has been recently suggested that greater error-related dorsal MFC responses in OCD, rather than being a primary dysfunction driving obsessions and compulsions, may reflect a compensatory over-activation aiming to correct deficient cognitive control processes that are unable to sufficiently regulate anxiety.[14] Within this framework, interventions that increase dorsal MFC would allow for more recruitment of cognitive control and regulation of OCD symptoms, which would be consistent with the findings from the high-frequency trial.[22] Overall, abnormal neural responses to errors are reliably associated with OCD and should be taken into consideration when devising treatments. However, given the conflicting findings in the literature, further work is needed to disentangle these or other possible interpretations of error hyperactivity in OCD.

Response Inhibition

Obsessions and compulsions may reflect, in part, a deficit in the ability to inhibit highly practiced thoughts and actions when a rapid change in thinking or response is required.[24] Experimenters studying response inhibition commonly use tasks where participants are trained to make rapid motor responses to a more frequent "go" stimulus but also asked to either suppress (go/no-go task) or cancel (stop-signal task) the same motor response when cued by an occasional "no-go" or "stop-signal" cue. The stop-signal task, in which a "stop" cue is given only after the prepotent behavior has been initiated, is the most direct probe of inhibitory motor control.[25]

Because successful performance on tasks of response inhibition requires both conflict monitoring (frequent "go" versus infrequent "no-go" trials) as well as motor suppression or cancelation, it is not surprising that "no-go" trials elicit activity in many of the same brain regions as conflict monitoring such as the dACC, SMA, and pre-SMA.[26,27] No-go trials, however, have also been linked to activation of lateral frontal and inferior parietal regions, predominantly in the right hemisphere, as well subcortical structures such as the basal ganglia and thalamus.[26,27] Of these, the right interior frontal gyrus (IFG) is the most common neural landmark linked to response inhibition.[27] Disruption of right IFG signaling by both lesions[28] and experimental deactivation[29] has also been observed to impair it.

OCD diagnosis has been linked to both relative deficits in activation of the right IFG, SMA, ACC, inferior parietal cortex, and orbitofrontal cortex (OFC) and relative excesses of activation in medial and lateral frontal regions, insula, premotor cortex, middle temporal cortex, PCC, and cerebellum during response inhibition.[14,30–35] Both hypo-[14,30–35] and hyper-activity[33] in the striatum and thalamus during effective inhibition have been linked to OCD pathology as well. Shephard and colleagues[36] describe a "ventral cognitive circuit" including the thalamus, ventral caudate, IFG, and vlPFC as hubs, as a key mediator of "self-regulatory" behaviors in general, and response inhibition in particular, in OCD patients.[36]

Meta-analyses suggest that impairment in response inhibition is likely characteristic of OCD,[14,37]. Interestingly, Hagland and colleagues[38] observed a significant reduction of OCD symptoms but no changes in stop signal behavior or brain activation after a course of brief but intensive exposure and response-prevention psychotherapy, suggesting that response inhibition deficits could be a trait characteristic. However, the literature includes studies showing no impairment in response inhibition in OCD[39,40] or deficits that are linked only to certain types of symptoms. Berlin and Lee,[41] for instance, report that stop-signal task performance is a significant predictor of compulsions, but not obsessions or overall OCD severity.[41] Other studies link response inhibition deficits to checking, in contrast to washing, compulsions.[42] Additional investigations exploring how symptom heterogeneity interacts with both neural and behavioral measures of response inhibition are warranted.

Cognitive Flexibility

The ability to shift attention between competing stimuli, tasks, or reinforcement contingencies allows for flexibility in adopting new goals or objectives.[43] OCD is marked by patterns of inflexible thinking and behavior, which may relate to difficulty shifting attention in response to changing environmental demands. Indeed, deficits in a variety of cognitive flexibility measures such as task switching and reversal learning have been found.[44] Task-switching paradigms require switching between two or more discrete tasks following an explicit instruction or cue. Neural correlates of task switching are distributed in a network of frontal and parietal regions including the dorsolateral prefrontal cortex (DLPFC), dACC, inferior and superior parietal lobe, and subcortical areas such as the striatum and thalamus.[45] Unsurprisingly, these regions appear very similar to those of a "FPN," or executive control network, which is thought to be involved in higher level executive functions.[46] Previous work investigating neural correlates of task switching reports widespread hypoactivation of frontoparietal regions extending into the OFC in OCD patients compared with HCs.[47–49] In addition to insufficient recruitment of the FPN, one study also found hyperactivation of the putamen and dACC in patients during task switching.[49] Further, hypoactivation of FPN regions such as the anterior PFC and hyperactivation of the putamen and ACC during task switching was associated with increased symptom severity within patients.[49] In a naturalistic follow-up of this study, symptom reduction over time was correlated with increased activity in the anterior PFC, DLPFC, and thalamus, and decreased activity of the ACC, during task switching,[50] which suggests dysfunctional FPN activity in patients may be state-dependent.

Reversal learning (ie, affective switching) paradigms are also commonly used as measures of cognitive flexibility and involve changing reinforcement contingencies. Affective switching occurs when a stimulus-response (S-R) association is reversed, such that a previously rewarded S-R association is punished and/or a previously punished S-R association is rewarded. Although task switching is thought to involve lateral prefrontal regions, affective switching may rely primarily on the OFC.[51] Studies investigating the neural underpinnings of reversal learning often isolate activity related to affective switching by comparing neural activations during failed reversal trials (ie, errors that do not lead to the acquisition of a new S-R association) and successful reversal trials (ie, errors that do lead to the acquisition of a new S-R association). For these comparisons, insufficient recruitment of the OFC has been implicated in OCD, but hypoactivation of FPN regions such as the DLPFC, bilateral insula, and putamen has also been found.[52–54] A naturalistic follow-up to one of these studies found that hypoactivation of the ACC and DLPFC during affective switching normalized at follow-up and was related to decreased symptom severity.[55] Interestingly, recruitment of the OFC remained stable over time and did not relate to symptom severity[55]

Overall, these findings suggest hypoactivation of a variety of cortical regions in OCD patients during task and affective switching. Although previous work suggests a dissociation in orbital and lateral frontal cortex involvement in these processes, hypo-activation amongst patients does not seem to be localized to either region. Indeed, reduced recruitment of the DLPFC and OFC is seen in both the reversal of reward contingencies and switching of cognitive sets in OCD. Continuing to examine the shared and unique brain networks involved in task switching and reversal learning will help elucidate our understanding of the role of cognitive inflexibility in OCD.

Reward Processing

A hallmark of OCD involves difficulty terminating maladaptive, repetitive behaviors which may relate to deficits in satiety (subjective experience of goal attainment),[56] and its neural representation in the reward system following task completion.[57] In healthy samples, a neural network with hubs in the ventral tegmental area (VTA), ventral pallidum, striatum (including the nucleus accumbens [NAc], caudate, and putamen), thalamus, ACC, and OFC encodes the experience of reward.[58] There is evidence of signaling abnormalities throughout the reward network in OCD with some investigations linking OCD to relative deficits in neural activity in reward structures during reward anticipation[59,60] or receipt.[52,53,61–63] OCD patients, in addition, report anhedonia[64] and, in at least some investigations, underperform on reward-based learning and decision-making tasks.[65,66] Together, these findings support hypotheses proposing that reward hyposensitivity drive OCD pathology.

There is also research supporting an alternative theory: OCD patients may repeat compulsions not because they fail to elicit sufficient relief, but because they are excessively (in magnitude and/or persistence over time) rewarding. OCD has been associated with relatively robust functional connectivity between reward network subregions including the NAc and OFC at rest,[67,68] and during task-induced reward anticipation.[67] Some patients, in addition, directly report that compulsion completion is rewarding and associated with positive emotion.[69] It may make more sense, however, to interpret this work by conceptualizing compulsions primarily as a strategy to proactively prevent (imagined) aversive consequences. Hence, the avoidance of aversive affect rather than the repetitive thoughts or behaviors themselves would be rewarding. Studies investigating punishment or reward omission have linked OCD to improved learning from punishment,[70] less frequent risk taking in gambling paradigms,[71] more robust ACC signaling in response to the omission of an expected reward,[72] and enhanced activation in the reward circuit during the anticipation of punishment, but not reward.[61,65]

It seems likely that neither a generalized reward hypo- nor hyper-sensitivity is characteristic of OCD. Findings linking brain activation during reward paradigms to specific symptom clusters suggest that a focus on heterogeneity could be productive in future investigations of reward and punishment in OCD.[59,60] Beyond symptom-specific heterogeneity, examining individual differences in reward processing may have important implications for the treatment of OCD. For example, Norman and colleagues[73] found that greater pretreatment activation in the vmPFC/OFC during an incentive flanker task predicted better response to exposure and response preventions (Ex/RP), possibly reflecting, in part, motivational processes necessary for engaging in the treatment. Thus, continuing to examine reward processing in OCD may also contribute to a greater understanding of treatment-matching strategies.

Decision-Making Under Uncertainty

Impaired decision-making is a prominent feature in OCD[74,75] which can manifest as intolerance of uncertainty (IU)[76] and an aversion to risk-taking.[62] Uncertainty can be manipulated in experimental tasks by varying the amount of ambiguity and/or risk associated with a decision. Ambiguity exists when the outcome probabilities associated with a decision are unknown (eg, the outcome of a decision can be either A or B), whereas risk occurs when probabilities are explicit but the outcome is still uncertain (eg 60% chance for outcome A, 40% chance for outcome B). A recent meta-analysis in healthy samples suggests that although both conditions engage the anterior insula, ambiguity specifically engages cognitive control and probability calculation regions (DLPFC, inferior parietal) whereas risk specifically recruits areas involved in reward and conflict detection (ventral striatum/NAc and dorsal MFC, respectively).[77]

Studies in OCD have documented the involvement of additional brain regions not typically seen in risk and ambiguity processing in HCs; compared with controls, OCD samples show both amygdala hyper- and hypo-activation in relation to uncertainty.[62,78,79] Functional alterations in other emotional processing areas such as the insula,[78,80] posterior cingulate,[79] and lingual gyrus[79] have also been documented during both risk and ambiguity. In addition, activation of reward-related areas such as the ventral ACC and OFC has been shown in OCD during both types of decision-making.[79,81] Not surprisingly, there is evidence that clinical heterogeneity relates to different neural patterns. Naaz and colleagues[82] found increased bilateral inferior parietal activation during decision-making under ambiguity in OCD patients with high doubting versus low doubting symptoms. This could suggest that when faced with an ambiguous or uncertain choice, higher doubting symptoms led to engagement in cognitive control areas involved in evidence accumulation.[82]

Overall, decision-making under risk and ambiguity in OCD appears to relate to altered functioning in areas involved in reward[78,79,81] and emotional processing.[78,80] The involvement of areas not typically seen in healthy populations, such as the amygdala, may suggest greater emotional involvement when processing uncertainty during decision-making.[62,78,79] Despite the dissociation of brain regions involved in decision-making under risk versus ambiguity in healthy samples,[77] results in OCD are less clear. Differences between paradigms and relatively few studies investigating these behaviors in OCD suggest the need for additional study.

Threat Conditioning and Extinction

Cognitive-behavioral models emphasize the role of threat acquisition and extinction in the etiology, maintenance, and treatment of OCD. These models have formed the foundation for evidence-based psychotherapies such as Ex/RP.[83] Pavlovian threat conditioning involves the pairing of a neutral, conditioned stimulus ("CS," eg a blue light) with an inherently aversive, or unconditioned, stimulus ("US," eg shock) until the CS elicits a conditioned response ("CR") that mirrors reaction to the US. This acquisition or conditioning phase is followed by extinction trials, where the CS is repeatedly presented without the US until the CR decreases. Laboratory research in OCD samples has provided some, albeit mixed results for the abnormal acquisition of conditioned threat responses, and stronger evidence for deficient extinction learning, compared with HCs.[84]

In healthy samples, a neural network including the ACC, vmPFC, insula, amygdala, and hippocampus is involved in the acquisition and expression of conditioned threat responses.[85] Despite the centrality of threat conditioning and extinction to behavioral models and treatments for OCD, few studies have investigated the neurobiological correlates. Both hypo-[86] and hyperactivity[87] in the vmPFC during acquisition have been found in OCD samples compared with controls. Milad and colleagues[86] also found decreased activation in the hippocampus and caudate during threat conditioning, potentially representing dysfunctional encoding of the fear memory. Cano and colleagues[88] identified decreased activation in the right insulo-opercular region and dACC, regions involved in the processing of interoceptive information, threat detection, and appraisal.[89,90] Interestingly, these authors also found that less pretreatment activation in the right insula predicted greater symptom reduction following a course of Ex/RP.[88] These findings complement a growing body of research demonstrating disrupted interoceptive processes in OCD.[91]

Extinction learning in OCD has been linked to decreased activation in the vmPFC, as well as the putamen, PCC, and cerebellum.[86] That study also found that more severe symptoms related to vmPFC hyperactivity and dACC hypoactivity during extinction recall, and suggested this vmPFC dysregulation might reflect deficits in safety signaling. However, these results were not replicated by Cano and colleagues,[88] who found no group differences during extinction or extinction recall. Sample characteristics may have contributed to lack of replication, including differences in age, symptom severity, and medication status. Few studies with inconsistent findings make it challenging to draw strong conclusions about the neural correlates of threat conditioning and extinction in OCD. However, given the shared theoretical underpinnings with behavioral treatments,[83] research should prioritize the continued study of these processes in OCD using neuroimaging.

Goal-Directed and Habitual Behavior

Compulsions have been traditionally characterized by their goal-directed nature, whereby repetitive behaviors are motivated by a desire to reduce obsessional distress.[92] A growing body of research supports the idea that impaired control of goal-directed behavior may relate to an overreliance on habits in OCD.[93,94] Although goal-directed behaviors are intentionally performed to achieve a specific outcome (reduction of obsessional distress), habits are automatic, S-R behaviors that develop with repetition.[94] Given that goal-directed action is performed to achieve a specific outcome, continued performance of a behavior when the outcome is no longer available or desired ('outcome devaluation') could be indicative of maladaptive habitual responding.[94] Neurobiological research in healthy samples indicate the caudate nucleus and OFC are involved in goal-directed control, through involvement in contingency learning and action evaluation,[95] whereas the putamen and premotor cortex are involved in the formation of stimulus-response habits.[95]

Gillan and colleagues[93] interrogated the neural correlates of habit learning in OCD using a shock avoidance task. Participants were first trained to avoid shocks, and then habitual avoidance responses were measured by removing the threat of shock. Acquisition of (goal-directed) avoidance behavior related to hyperactivity in the medial OFC/vmPFC whereas habitual avoidance responding related to increased caudate activation.[93] Further, stronger self-reported urge to habitually respond correlated with increased caudate activity. These results suggest that maladaptive habits in OCD may relate to aberrant patterns of activity in neural regions implicated in goal-directed control rather than the habit system.

Banca and colleagues[96] examined the neural correlates of avoidance responding in OCD using an individualized provocation task where participants could choose to avoid the presentation of OCD-relevant images. Hypoactivity in the vmPFC and caudate, and hyperactivity in putamen and pre-SMA was seen during symptom provocation and avoidance responding. As opposed to the shock avoidance task used by

Gillan and colleagues,[93] which required acquisition of a new habit, this paradigm leveraged existing, person-specific pathological associations. Given that avoidance responses to symptom-related stimuli would have been reinforced over a longer period of time, it's possible they had become habitual before the experiment. Thus, activation in the putamen and pre-SMA during provocation and avoidance might reflect engagement of habit systems resulting from a longer history of repetitive performance.[94,96] Although methodological differences and the low number of studies make it challenging to draw strong conclusions, OCD appears to relate to altered activity in brain regions underlying goal-directed control and habit systems. Future research using standard paradigms such as the outcome devaluation task will serve to deepen our understanding of the neurocircuitry underlying goal-directed and habitual behavior in OCD.

SUMMARY

Cognitive neuroscientific research has the ability to yield important insights into the complex psychological processes underlying OCD. This review of the current literature suggests consistent neurobiological differences in OCD during error detection and task-switching tasks. Specifically, OCD samples, compared with HCs, tend to show increased activation in response to errors and decreased activation during switching tasks in the prefrontal cortex as well as the anterior cingulate cortex, striatum, and parietal cortex. A growing body of evidence also indicates individuals with OCD show fronto-limbic dysfunction when making decisions involving ambiguity and risk. Despite the major relevance to cognitive-behavioral treatment models, neuroimaging studies examining threat conditioning, habits, and goal-directed control are limited in number and methodologically variable, thus creating difficulty in drawing conclusions. Given the multifaceted and often interrelated processes involved in the neurocognitive constructs discussed, no single paradigm is likely to fully elucidate OCD's pathophysiology. Furthermore, the well-described heterogeneity of OCD symptoms may mean that some constructs or paradigms described in this article are more relevant for certain OCD symptoms than others (ie, threat learning and extinction may be most relevant for patients with prominent harm-related obsessions). Future research on the neural mechanisms of cognitive-affective constructs in OCD would benefit from both considering the role of symptom heterogeneity and by prioritizing investigations into how aberrant processes relate to theoretically targeted treatments. Such steps would contribute to the identification of novel and personalized targets for treatment and the optimization of existing interventions.

CLINICS CARE POINTS

- Despite an increasing understanding of the pathophysiology of OCD, current treatments have remained largely unchanged over the past 30 years. Elucidation of the cognitive neuroscience underlying OCD can provide insights for enhancing treatment outcomes and identifying new targets for intervention.

- In OCD, findings demonstrating altered activation in the dorsal medial frontal cortex in response to errors has already begun to be translated into clinical trials using transcranial magnetic stimulation. Though preliminary findings have thus far been inconsistent, continuing to examine neuroscience-informed targets will help to identify effective interventions for individuals who do not respond to current treatments.

- For existing psychotherapy practice, particularly exposure and response prevention (Ex/RP), it remains pertinent to continue neuroimaging research of threat conditioning and extinction.

Too few studies have investigated the cognitive neuroscience of these domains, and given that they form the theoretical foundation for Ex/RP, future research is needed to better understand methods for fine-tuning or augmenting therapeutic strategies to optimize outcomes.

REFERENCES

1. Springer KS, Levy HC, Tolin DF. Remission in CBT for adult anxiety disorders: a meta-analysis. Clin Psychol Rev 2018;61:1–8.
2. Stern ER, Taylor SF. Cognitive neuroscience of obsessive-compulsive disorder. Psychiatric Clinics 2014;37(3):337–52.
3. Pitman RK. A cybernetic model of obsessive-compulsive psychopathology. Compr Psychiatry 1987;28(4):334–43.
4. Botvlnick MM, Braver TS, Barch DM, et al. Conflict monitoring and cognitive control. Psychol Rev 2001;108(3):624–52.
5. Garavan H, Ross TJ, Kaufman J, et al. A midline dissociation between error-processing and response-conflict monitoring. Neuroimage 2003;20(2):1132–9.
6. Taylor SF, Stern ER, Gehring WJ. Neural systems for error monitoring: recent findings and theoretical perspectives. Neuroscientist 2007;13(2):160–72.
7. Dosenbach NU, Fair DA, Miezin FM, et al. Distinct brain networks for adaptive and stable task control in humans. Proc Natl Acad Sci U S A 2007;104(26): 11073–8.
8. Sridharan D, Levitin DJ, Menon V. A critical role for the right fronto-insular cortex in switching between central-executive and default-mode networks. Proc Natl Acad Sci U S A 2008;105(34):12569–74.
9. Ullsperger M, Danielmeier C, Jocham G. Neurophysiology of performance monitoring and adaptive behavior. Physiol Rev 2014;94(1):35–79.
10. Gehring WJ, Himle J, Nisenson LG. Action-monitoring dysfunction in obsessive-compulsive disorder. Psychol Sci 2000;11(1):1–6.
11. Michael JA, Wang M, Kaur M, et al. EEG correlates of attentional control in anxiety disorders: a systematic review of error-related negativity and correct-response negativity findings. J Affect Disord 2021;291:140–53.
12. Endrass T, Ullsperger M. Specificity of performance monitoring changes in obsessive-compulsive disorder. Neurosci Biobehav Rev 2014;46(Pt 1):124–38.
13. Riesel A. The erring brain: Error-related negativity as an endophenotype for OCD-A review and meta-analysis. Psychophysiology 2019;56(4):e13348.
14. Norman LJ, Taylor SF, Liu Y, et al. Error processing and inhibitory control in obsessive-compulsive disorder: a meta-analysis using statistical parametric maps. Biol Psychiatry 2019;85(9):713–25.
15. Fitzgerald KD, Welsh RC, Gehring WJ, et al. Error-related hyperactivity of the anterior cingulate cortex in obsessive-compulsive disorder. Biol Psychiatry 2005;57(3):287–94.
16. Stern ER, Welsh RC, Fitzgerald KD, et al. Hyperactive error responses and altered connectivity in ventromedial and frontoinsular cortices in obsessive-compulsive disorder. Biol Psychiatry 2011;69(6):583–91.
17. Andrews-Hanna JR . The brain's default network and its adaptive role in internal mentation. Neuroscientist 2012;18(3):251–70.
18. Buckner RL, Andrews-Hanna JR, Schacter DL. The brain's default network: anatomy, function, and relevance to disease. Ann N Y Acad Sci 2008;1124:1–38.

19. Gusnard DA, Akbudak E, Shulman GL, et al. Medial prefrontal cortex and self-referential mental activity: relation to a default mode of brain function. Proc Natl Acad Sci U S A 2001;98(7):4259–64.
20. De Nadai AS, Fitzgerald KD, Norman LJ, et al. Defining brain-based OCD patient profiles using task-based fMRI and unsupervised machine learning. Neuropsychopharmacology 2022;1–8. https://doi.org/10.1038/s41386-022-01353-x.
21. Modirrousta M, Shams E, Katz C, et al. The efficacy of deep repetitive transcranial magnetic stimulation over the medial prefrontal cortex in obsessive compulsive disorder: results from an open-label study. Depress Anxiety 2015;32(6):445–50.
22. Carmi L, Tendler A, Bystritsky A, et al. Efficacy and Safety of Deep Transcranial Magnetic Stimulation for Obsessive-Compulsive Disorder: A Prospective Multicenter Randomized Double-Blind Placebo-Controlled Trial. Am J Psychiatry 2019;176(11):931–8.
23. Carmi L, Alyagon U, Barnea-Ygael N, et al. Clinical and electrophysiological outcomes of deep TMS over the medial prefrontal and anterior cingulate cortices in OCD patients. Brain Stimul 2018;11(1):158–65.
24. Chamberlain SR, Menzies L. Endophenotypes of obsessive-compulsive disorder: rationale, evidence and future potential. Expert Rev Neurother 2009;9(8):1133–46.
25. Schachar R, Logan GD, Robaey P, et al. Restraint and cancellation: multiple inhibition deficits in attention deficit hyperactivity disorder. J Abnorm Child Psychol 2007;35(2):229–38.
26. Aron AR, Poldrack RA. Cortical and subcortical contributions to stop signal response inhibition: role of the subthalamic nucleus. J Neurosci 2006;26(9):2424–33.
27. Buchsbaum BR, Greer S, Chang WL, et al. Meta-analysis of neuroimaging studies of the Wisconsin card-sorting task and component processes. Hum Brain Mapp 2005;25(1):35–45.
28. Aron AR, Fletcher PC, Bullmore ET, et al. Stop-signal inhibition disrupted by damage to right inferior frontal gyrus in humans. Nat Neurosci 2003;6(2):115–6.
29. Chambers CD, Bellgrove MA, Stokes MG, et al. Executive "brake failure" following deactivation of human frontal lobe. J Cogn Neurosci 2006;18(3):444–55.
30. Rubia K, Cubillo A, Smith AB, et al. Disorder-specific dysfunction in right inferior prefrontal cortex during two inhibition tasks in boys with attention-deficit hyperactivity disorder compared with boys with obsessive-compulsive disorder. Hum Brain Mapp 2010;31(2):287–99.
31. Berlin HA, Schulz KP, Zhang S, et al. Neural correlates of emotional response inhibition in obsessive-compulsive disorder: A preliminary study. Psychiatry Res Neuroimaging 2015;234(2):259–64.
32. Kang DH, Jang JH, Han JY, et al. Neural correlates of altered response inhibition and dysfunctional connectivity at rest in obsessive-compulsive disorder. Prog Neuropsychopharmacol Biol Psychiatry 2013;40:340–6.
33. Roth RM, Saykin AJ, Flashman LA, et al. Event-related functional magnetic resonance imaging of response inhibition in obsessive-compulsive disorder. Biol Psychiatry 2007;62(8):901–9.
34. de Wit SJ, de Vries FE, van der Werf YD, et al. Presupplementary motor area hyperactivity during response inhibition: A candidate endophenotype of obsessive-compulsive disorder. Am J Psychiatry 2012;169(10):1100–8.
35. Page LA, Rubia K, Deeley Q, et al. A functional magnetic resonance imaging study of inhibitory control in obsessive-compulsive disorder. Psychiatry Res 2009;174(3):202–9.

36. Shephard E, Stern ER, van den Heuvel OA, et al. Toward a neurocircuit-based taxonomy to guide treatment of obsessive-compulsive disorder. Mol Psychiatry 2021;26(9):4583–604.

37. Abramovitch A, Abramowitz JS, Mittelman A. The neuropsychology of adult obsessive-compulsive disorder: a meta-analysis. Clin Psychol Rev 2013;33(8): 1163–71.

38. Hagland P, Thorsen AL, Ousdal OT, et al. Disentangling Within- and Between-Person Effects During Response Inhibition in Obsessive-Compulsive Disorder. Front Psychiatry 2021;12:519727.

39. Kalanthroff E, Teichert T, Wheaton MG, et al. The Role of Response Inhibition in Medicated and Unmedicated Obsessive-Compulsive Disorder Patients: Evidence from the Stop-Signal Task. Depress Anxiety 2017;34(3):301–6.

40. Silveira VP, Frydman I, Fontenelle LF, et al. Exploring response inhibition and error monitoring in obsessive-compulsive disorder. J Psychiatr Res 2020;126:26–33.

41. Berlin GS, Lee H-J. Response inhibition and error-monitoring processes in individuals with obsessive-compulsive disorder. J obsessive-compulsive Relat Disord 2018;16:21–7.

42. Leopold R, Backenstrass M. Neuropsychological differences between obsessive-compulsive washers and checkers: A systematic review and meta-analysis. J Anxiety Disord 2015;30:48–58.

43. Uddin LQ. Cognitive and behavioural flexibility: neural mechanisms and clinical considerations. Nat Rev Neurosci 2021;22(3):167–79.

44. Gruner P, Pittenger C. Cognitive inflexibility in Obsessive-Compulsive Disorder. Neuroscience 2017;345:243–55.

45. Kim C, Cilles SE, Johnson NF, et al. Domain general and domain preferential brain regions associated with different types of task switching: a meta-analysis. Hum Brain Mapp 2012;33(1):130–42.

46. Uddin LQ, Yeo BTT, Spreng RN. Towards a Universal Taxonomy of Macro-scale Functional Human Brain Networks. Brain Topogr 2019;32(6):926–42.

47. Morein-Zamir S, Voon V, Dodds CM, et al. Divergent subcortical activity for distinct executive functions: stopping and shifting in obsessive compulsive disorder. Psychol Med 2016;46(4):829–40.

48. Gu BM, Park JY, Kang DH, et al. Neural correlates of cognitive inflexibility during task-switching in obsessive-compulsive disorder. Brain 2008;131:155–64.

49. Remijnse PL, van den Heuvel OA, Nielen MM, et al. Cognitive inflexibility in obsessive-compulsive disorder and major depression is associated with distinct neural correlates. PLoS One 2013;8(4):e59600.

50. Vriend C, de Wit SJ, Remijnse PL, et al. Switch the itch: a naturalistic follow-up study on the neural correlates of cognitive flexibility in obsessive-compulsive disorder. Psychiatry Res 2013;213(1):31–8.

51. Ghahremani DG, Monterosso J, Jentsch JD, et al. Neural components underlying behavioral flexibility in human reversal learning. Cereb Cortex 2010;20(8): 1843–52.

52. Remijnse PL, Nielen MM, van Balkom AJ, et al. Reduced orbitofrontal-striatal activity on a reversal learning task in obsessive-compulsive disorder. Arch Gen Psychiatry 2006;63(11):1225–36.

53. Remijnse PL, Nielen MM, van Balkom AJ, et al. Differential frontal-striatal and paralimbic activity during reversal learning in major depressive disorder and obsessive-compulsive disorder. Psychol Med 2009;39(9):1503–18.

54. Freyer T, Kloppel S, Tuscher O, et al. Frontostriatal activation in patients with obsessive-compulsive disorder before and after cognitive behavioral therapy. Psychol Med 2011;41(1):207–16.

55. Verfaillie SCJ, de Wit SJ, Vriend C, et al. The course of the neural correlates of reversal learning in obsessive–compulsive disorder and major depression: A naturalistic follow-up fMRI study. J Obsessive-Compulsive Relat Disord 2016; 9:51–8.

56. Szechtman H, Woody E. Obsessive-compulsive disorder as a disturbance of security motivation. Psychol Rev 2004;111(1):111–27.

57. Pastor-Bernier A, Stasiak A, Schultz W. Reward-specific satiety affects subjective value signals in orbitofrontal cortex during multicomponent economic choice. Proc Natl Acad Sci U S A 2021;118(30):1–11.

58. Liu X, Hairston J, Schrier M, et al. Common and distinct networks underlying reward valence and processing stages: a meta-analysis of functional neuroimaging studies. Neurosci Biobehav Rev 2011;35(5):1219–36.

59. Figee M, Vink M, de Geus F, et al. Dysfunctional reward circuitry in obsessive-compulsive disorder. Biol Psychiatry 2011;69(9):867–74.

60. Marsh R, Tau GZ, Wang Z, et al. Reward-based spatial learning in unmedicated adults with obsessive-compulsive disorder. Am J Psychiatry 2015;172(4):383–92.

61. Jung WH, Kang DH, Han JY, et al. Aberrant ventral striatal responses during incentive processing in unmedicated patients with obsessive-compulsive disorder. Acta Psychiatr Scand 2011;123(5):376–86.

62. Admon R, Bleich-Cohen M, Weizmant R, et al. Functional and structural neural indices of risk aversion in obsessive–compulsive disorder (OCD). Psychiatry Res Neuroimaging 2012;203(2):207–13.

63. Norman LJ, Carlisi CO, Christakou A, et al. Frontostriatal Dysfunction During Decision Making in Attention-Deficit/Hyperactivity Disorder and Obsessive-Compulsive Disorder. Biol Psychiatry Cogn Neurosci Neuroimaging 2018;3(8): 694–703.

64. Abramovitch A, Pizzagalli DA, Reuman L, et al. Anhedonia in obsessive-compulsive disorder: beyond comorbid depression. Psychiatry Res 2014; 216(2):223–9.

65. Kaufmann C, Beucke JC, Preusse F, et al. Medial prefrontal brain activation to anticipated reward and loss in obsessive-compulsive disorder. Neuroimage Clin 2013;2:212–20.

66. Grassi G, Pallanti S, Righi L, et al. Think twice: Impulsivity and decision making in obsessive-compulsive disorder. J Behav Addict 2015;4(4):263–72.

67. Jung WH, Kang DH, Kim E, et al. Abnormal corticostriatal-limbic functional connectivity in obsessive-compulsive disorder during reward processing and resting-state. Neuroimage Clin 2013;3:27–38.

68. Xie C, Ma L, Jiang N, et al. Imbalanced functional link between reward circuits and the cognitive control system in patients with obsessive-compulsive disorder. Brain Imaging Behav 2017;11(4):1099–109.

69. Ferreira GM, Yucel M, Dawson A, et al. Investigating the role of anticipatory reward and habit strength in obsessive-compulsive disorder. CNS Spectr 2017; 22(3):295–304.

70. Voon V, Baek K, Enander J, et al. Motivation and value influences in the relative balance of goal-directed and habitual behaviours in obsessive-compulsive disorder. Translational psychiatry 2015;5:e670.

71. Sip KE, Gonzalez R, Taylor SF, et al. Increased Loss Aversion in Unmedicated Patients with Obsessive-Compulsive Disorder. Front Psychiatry 2017;8:309.

72. Murray GK, Knolle F, Ersche KD, et al. Dopaminergic drug treatment remediates exaggerated cingulate prediction error responses in obsessive-compulsive disorder. Psychopharmacology (Berl) 2019;236(8):2325–36.

73. Norman LJ, Mannella KA, Yang H, et al. Treatment-Specific Associations Between Brain Activation and Symptom Reduction in OCD Following CBT: A Randomized fMRI Trial. Am J Psychiatry 2021;178(1):39–47.

74. Cavedini P, Gorini A, Bellodi L. Understanding obsessive-compulsive disorder: Focus on decision making. Neuropsychol Rev 2006;16(1):3–15.

75. Nisticò V, De Angelis A, Erro R, et al. Obsessive-compulsive disorder and decision making under ambiguity: A systematic review with meta-analysis. Brain Sci 2021;11(2):143.

76. Tolin DF, Abramowitz JS, Brigidi BD, et al. Intolerance of uncertainty in obsessive-compulsive disorder. J anxiety Disord 2003;17(2):233–42.

77. Wu S, Sun S, Camilleri JA, et al. Better the devil you know than the devil you don't: Neural processing of risk and ambiguity. NeuroImage 2021;236:118109.

78. Stern ER, Welsh RC, Gonzalez R, et al. Subjective uncertainty and limbic hyperactivation in obsessive-compulsive disorder. Hum Brain Mapp 2013;34(8):1956–70.

79. Moreira PS, Macoveanu J, Marques P, et al. Altered response to risky decisions and reward in patients with obsessive–compulsive disorder. J Psychiatry Neurosci 2020;45(2):98–107.

80. Luigjes J, Figee M, Tobler PN, et al. Doubt in the insula: risk processing in obsessive-compulsive disorder. Front Hum Neurosci 2016;10:283.

81. Rotge JY, Langbour N, Dilharreguy B, et al. Contextual and behavioral influences on uncertainty in obsessive-compulsive disorder. Cortex 2015;62:1–10.

82. Naaz F, Chen L, Gold AI, et al. Neural correlates of doubt in decision-making. Psychiatry Res Neuroimaging 2021;317:111370.

83. Foa EB, Yadin E, Lichner TK. Exposure and response (ritual) prevention for obsessive-compulsive disorder: Therapist guide. New York, NY: Oxford University Press; 2012.

84. Cooper SE, Dunsmoor JE. Fear conditioning and extinction in obsessive-compulsive disorder: a systematic review. Neurosci Biobehav Rev 2021;129:75–94.

85. Greco JA, Liberzon I. Neuroimaging of Fear-Associated Learning. Neuropsychopharmacology 2016;41(1):320–34.

86. Milad MR, Furtak SC, Greenberg JL, et al. Deficits in conditioned fear extinction in obsessive-compulsive disorder and neurobiological changes in the fear circuit. JAMA Psychiatry 2013;70(6):608–18 [quiz: 554].

87. Apergis-Schoute AM, Gillan CM, Fineberg NA, et al. Neural basis of impaired safety signaling in obsessive compulsive disorder. Proc Natl Acad Sci 2017;114(12):3216–21.

88. Cano M, Martínez-Zalacaín I, Gimenez M, et al. Neural correlates of fear conditioning and fear extinction and its association with cognitive-behavioral therapy outcome in adults with obsessive-compulsive disorder. Behav Res Ther 2021;144:103927.

89. Craig AD. How do you feel–now? The anterior insula and human awareness. Nat Rev Neurosci 2009;10(1):59–70.

90. Kalisch R, Gerlicher AM. Making a mountain out of a molehill: on the role of the rostral dorsal anterior cingulate and dorsomedial prefrontal cortex in conscious threat appraisal, catastrophizing, and worrying. Neurosci Biobehav Rev 2014;42:1–8.

91. Bragdon LB, Eng GK, Belanger A, et al. Interoception and obsessive-compulsive disorder: a review of current evidence and future directions. Front Psychiatry 2021;12:686482.
92. Rachman S, Rachman SJ, Hodgson RJ. Obsessions and compulsions. Englewood Cliffs, NJ: Prentice Hall; 1980.
93. Gillan CM, Apergis-Schoute AM, Morein-Zamir S, et al. Functional neuroimaging of avoidance habits in obsessive-compulsive disorder. Am J Psychiatry 2015; 172(3):284–93.
94. Gillan CM. Recent developments in the habit hypothesis of OCD and compulsive disorders. In: Fineberg NA, Robbins TW, editors. The neurobiology and treatment of OCD: accelerating progress. Cham Switzerland: Springer; 2021. p. 147–67.
95. de Wit S, Watson P, Harsay HA, et al. Corticostriatal connectivity underlies individual differences in the balance between habitual and goal-directed action control. J Neurosci 2012;32(35):12066–75.
96. Banca P, Voon V, Vestergaard MD, et al. Imbalance in habitual versus goal directed neural systems during symptom provocation in obsessive-compulsive disorder. Brain 2015;138(Pt 3):798–811.

Neuroinflammation in Obsessive-Compulsive Disorder

Sydenham Chorea, Pediatric Autoimmune Neuropsychiatric Disorders Associated with Streptococcal Infections, and Pediatric Acute Onset Neuropsychiatric Syndrome

Allison Vreeland, PhD[a,b,1,*], Margo Thienemann, MD[a,b,1],
Madeleine Cunningham, PhD[c,2], Eyal Muscal, MD, MS[d,3],
Christopher Pittenger, MD, PhD[e,4], Jennifer Frankovich, MD, MS[b,f,1]

KEYWORDS

- Pediatric acute-onset neuropsychiatric syndrome
- Pediatric autoimmune neuropsychiatric
disorder associated with streptococcal infections • Obsessive compulsive disorder

KEY POINTS

- Sydenham chorea (SC), pediatric autoimmune neuropsychiatric disorders associated with streptococcal infections (PANDAS), and pediatric acute-onset neuropsychiatric syndrome (PANS) are believed to be postinfectious, immune-mediated syndromes that manifest with obsessive-compulsive disorder (OCD) symptoms and likely have overlapping pathogenic mechanisms.

Continued

[a] Division of Child and Adolescent Psychiatry and Child Development, Department of Psychiatry, Stanford University School of Medicine, Stanford, CA, USA; [b] Stanford Children's Health, PANS Clinic and Research Program, Stanford University School of Medicine, Stanford, CA, USA; [c] Department of Microbiology and Immunology, University of Oklahoma Health Sciences Center, Oklahoma City, OK, USA; [d] Department of Rheumatology, Texas Children's Hospital, Houston, TX, USA; [e] Department of Psychiatry, Yale University School of Medicine, New Haven, CT, USA; [f] Division of Pediatrics, Department of Allergy, Immunology, Rheumatology, Stanford University School of Medicine, Stanford, CA, USA

[1] Present address: Stanford Univeristy, School of Medicine, 700 Welch Road, Suite 301, Palo Alto, CA 94304.
[2] Present address: University of Oklahoma Helath Sciences Center, Biomedical Research Center Room 217, 975 NE 10th Street, Oklahoma City, OK 73104.
[3] Present address: Texas Medical Center, 6701 Fannin Street, 11th Floor, Houston, TX, 77030.
[4] Present address: Connecticut Mental Health Center, 34 Park Street, W333b, New Haven, CT 06519.
* Corresponding author. 700 Welch Road, Suite 301, Palo Alto, CA 94304.
E-mail address: vreeland@stanford.edu

Psychiatr Clin N Am 46 (2023) 69–88
https://doi.org/10.1016/j.psc.2022.11.004
0193-953X/23/© 2022 Elsevier Inc. All rights reserved.

Continued

- Features that distinguish PANDAS and PANS from idiopathic OCD and other psychiatric syndromes include: an abrupt and severe symptom onset, a relapsing and remitting course, and specified comorbid symptoms.
- PANDAS and PANS continue to be a provisional diagnosis with provisional treatments, which include use of immunomodulatory therapies and antibiotics. These treatments are also considered provisional until randomized placebo, control trials establish safety and efficacy.
- Psychiatric and behavioral interventions have been shown to significantly reduce OCD symptoms in children with PANDAS and PANS.
- Future research should consider the relapsing-remitting course, the disease state (flare vs remission vs flare on chronic), and the trajectory of the patients enrolled in studies (ie, new-onset flare vs resolving flare, flare on chronic vs chronic static, etc.).

INTRODUCTION

Postinfectious neuroinflammation has been implicated in models of acute onset obsessive-compulsive disorder (OCD) in children since the description of pediatric autoimmune neuropsychiatric disorders associated with streptococcal infections (PANDAS).[1] Centuries before then, Sydenham chorea (SC) was recognized and eventually confirmed to be caused by a post-streptococcal autoimmune process.[2] Pediatric acute-onset neuropsychiatric syndrome (PANS) (defined in 2015) has a broader definition than PANDAS and is agnostic to the triggering event. Triggers of most autoimmune/inflammatory diseases are often not knowable in individual cases. With SC, PANDAS and PANS, cortico-basal ganglia-thalamo-cortical (CBGTC) circuities are thought to become disrupted by immune dysfunction. Antibody studies[3–16] imaging studies,[17–20] and response to immunomodulation[21] support this proposed pathogenic model, but much work remains to be done to discover and validate specific diagnostic and predictive biomarkers and treatment pathways.

This article aimed to outline current research that provides evidence of an association of PANDAS and PANS with inflammation, immune dysregulation, and/or autoimmunity. We begin by discussing SC as an accepted model of a post-infection autoimmune response leading to neuropsychiatric symptoms. Data supporting neuroinflammation in SC strongly overlap with data in PANDAS and PANS, including a similar autoantibody profile, imaging data showing alterations in the basal ganglia, and observable data regarding the efficacy of immunomodulation. We then review the current clinical diagnostic criteria for PANDAS and PANS, as well as currently recommended evaluation pathways to rule out other diagnoses with established interventions. Next, we outline the accumulating evidence that neuroinflammation plays a role in these disorders, including work in animal models with patient-derived anti-neuronal autoantibodies and imaging studies showing changes in the basal ganglia. We conclude by providing current treatment recommendations for PANDAS and PANS and an agenda for future research targeting phase-specific mechanisms involved in the development and perpetuation of inflammation.

Background

Sydenham chorea
Sydenham chorea (SC) is a post-streptococcal neurologic manifestation of acute rheumatic fever and is characterized by involuntary choreic movements and

prominent behavior changes.[22] Sydenham chorea occurs in 25% of acute rheumatic fever cases.[23] The average age of onset is between 9.2 years and 11.7 years; there are very few reports of SC cases in adults.[10,24,25] SC is seen most frequently in areas of the world where household crowding is common and where access to health care is limited as these are factors are associated with the undertreatment of streptococcal infections.[26]

Obsessive-compulsive symptoms affect roughly 80% of SC patients[27–29] along with sudden personality changes and additional neuropsychiatric symptoms (restlessness, irritability, emotional lability, distractibility, anxiety, night terrors, and outbursts of inappropriate and/or violent behavior).[30–33]

SC is thought to result from a Group A beta-hemolytic streptococcal (Group A Strep)-induced autoimmune process in which the CBGTC circuits are disrupted by cross-reactive antibodies through the process of molecular mimicry.[10] It is believed that Group A Strep-induced antibodies cross-react with dopamine 1 and 2 receptors (D1R and D2R),[3,6,8,34,35] tubulin (the fundamental protein of microtubules), and lyso-ganglioside (ganglioside-monosialic acid [GM1]) and are elevated in patients with SC compared with controls.[10] Furthermore, sera and cerebrospinal fluid from patients with SC induce activation of CaM Kinase II (CaMKII; a key protein kinase downstream from dopamine and another neuronal receptor signaling).[10]

Several SC studies implicate abnormalities in the basal ganglia structures. Volumetric MRI analyses have shown increased volume in the caudate, putamen, and globus pallidus in 24 children with early-stage SC when compared with controls.[36] In addition, multiple MRI analyses have revealed both abnormal T_1 and T_2 signals in the basal ganglia of SC subjects.[37–43] Importantly, as is the case with all inflammatory diseases, grouping patients according to illness stage/phase is critical to identifying structural abnormalities. Not surprisingly, studies with pooled MRIs of subjects in different stages (active/early-stage SC, chronic phase, and remitted SC) show a high variance in volume across subjects; however, when volumes are averaged across stages, the finding of swelling (seen in the acute phase) is washed out.[44] Generally speaking, initial inflammatory events have been more closely associated with acute swelling of tissues, whereas atrophy develops at later stages.

The standard of care for the treatment of SC consists of eliminating Group A Strep in the patient and close contacts (people living in the home), immunomodulatory therapy (corticosteroids and intravenous immune globulin [IVIG]), and psychiatric care.[28,45,46] Autoantibodies associated with SC, imaging studies pointing toward basal ganglia pathology, and mounting evidence supporting successful treatment with immunomodulation indicate that SC (and the SC-associated psychiatric symptoms including OCD) is the result of an inflammatory brain disorder.

Pediatric Autoimmune Neuropsychiatric Disorders Associated with Streptococcal Infections and Pediatric Acute-Onset Neuropsychiatric Syndrome

Much like SC, PANDAS and PANS are believed to be postinfectious, immune-mediated syndromes that manifest with OCD symptoms and likely have overlapping pathogenic mechanisms. An abrupt and severe symptom onset, a relapsing and remitting course, and specified comorbid symptoms define and distinguish PANDAS and PANS from idiopathic OCD and other psychiatric syndromes. The dramatic sudden onset logically suggests a triggering event (like an infection), similar to the way streptococcal infection is thought to trigger SC in rheumatic fever. However, in clinical practice, establishing the diagnosis of a preceding or associated Group A Strep infection to diagnose PANDAS at presentation and/or relapse is difficult since patients often come to clinical attention after the "window of opportunity to detect Group A

Strep infection" has passed and since diagnostic approaches to detect current or recent Group A Strep are imperfect. Although establishing a causal link between infections and neuropsychiatric symptoms in human diseases is a key part of untangling pathogenic mechanisms, it is only possible through epidemiologic studies and depends on animal model studies for proof of principle. Nevertheless, frequent temporal correlations between coincident infections and clinical deterioration as well as responses to antibiotic therapy can strengthen a clinician's suspicion that symptoms are a result of a postinfectious inflammatory process. However, clinicians should be aware that in most cases of postinfectious inflammatory disorders, relapses are on average 3 months in duration and can self-resolve[47]; thus, "response" to any treatment (antibiotic, SSRI, behavioral, etc.) should be interpreted with caution. In addition, clinical deterioration in the absence of detectable/remembered infection (ie, subclinical or subtle infections) does not exclude the possibility of postinfectious inflammatory causes as many viruses and even certain "rheumatic strains" of Group A Strep can present with mild symptoms.

Researchers and clinicians have hypothesized multiple pathogenic factors leading to PANDAS and PANS, with Group A Strep and resultant neuroinflammation being the most well studied.[48] As most children who are infected with Group A Strep do not develop PANDAS or PANS, other factors, such as timing of infection, trauma, or underlying hereditary and genetic factors (eg, the presence of specific HLA haplotypes, microbiome differences, prior infections, smoldering inflammation, underlying immune dysregulation and/or immune deficiency, and exposure to rheumatogenic strains of Group A Strep) may predispose an individual child to PANDAS or PANS. Indeed, families with a history of autoimmune diseases and rheumatic fever have a higher incidence of PANDAS, PANS, and OCD.[49–51]

As has been seen in medicine generally, recognizing and treating these syndromes early is likely to yield better long-term outcomes. PANDAS and PANS are diagnosed clinically by ascertaining the course of illness and identifying symptoms (**Table 1**). Interpretation of the clinical presentation may present challenges because flaring children are highly dysregulated, may be anguished and raging, and are often unable to articulate thoughts and feelings necessary for accurate diagnosis. Thus, clinicians rely heavily on parents' reports; parents are good reporters of their children's external behaviors though may be less accurate about their children's internal experiences and thoughts.[52] To date, no specific laboratory biomarker has been identified to reliably diagnose PANDAS and PANS, which is similar to most pediatric rheumatological diseases (including the many subtypes of juvenile arthritis and periodic fever syndromes) that are not characterized by specific blood inflammatory markers despite clear physical exam markers. Lack of specific inflammation-related biomarkers in rheumatic disorders does not preclude a need for early clinical diagnosis and therapy. Nonetheless, without any clear blood and imaging diagnostic markers, proof of diagnosis and study of immune-mediated psychiatric disorders remain nuanced and controversial.

History

The first description of 50 children with PANDAS was published in 1998 in which children were, by definition, reported to experience neuropsychiatric symptom exacerbations in temporal association with Group A Strep infection.[1] However, clinicians observed that many relapses of PANDAS did not coincide with Group A Strep infections. As a result, a new diagnostic criterion was developed by expert consensus to describe patients who closely resembled the PANDAS symptom presentation but did not have evidence of Group A Strep infection. The resulting new PANS criteria modified the symptom requirements, including being agnostic to the specific

Table 1	
PANDAS and PANS clinical classification criteria	
PANDAS Criteria 1998	**PANS Criteria 2012**
1. Presence of diagnosis of OCD and/or tic disorder	1. Abrupt, dramatic onset of OCD or severely restricted food intake

2. Pediatric onset
3. Episodic course
4. Association with group A beta-hemolytic streptococcus infection
5. Association with neurologic abnormalities
	2. Concurrent presence of additional neuropsychiatric symptoms, (with similarly severe and acute onset), from at least two of the following seven categories
	  A. Anxiety
	  B. Emotional lability and/or depression
	  C. Irritability, aggression, and/or severely oppositional behaviors
	  D. Behavioral (developmental) regression
	  E. Deterioration in school performance
	  F. Sensory or motor difficulties
	  G. Somatic signs or symptoms, including sleep disturbances, enuresis, or urinary frequency
	3. Symptoms are not better explained by a known neurologic or medical disorder, such as Sydenham chorea, systemic lupus erythematosus, Tourette syndrome, or others

infectious trigger. The PANS criteria recognized the possibility of triggers beyond Group A Strep, including other infections, stress, metabolic disturbances, and other neuroinflammatory triggering events.[53] Current PANDAS and PANS criteria are listed in **Table 1**.

Demographic information from the first and subsequent cohorts of PANDAS cases revealed the mean age of symptom onset as 6-year-old for cases with primary tics and 7-year-old for those with primary OCD,[1] with a 3 to 1 prevalence of boys.[54] Epidemiologic studies of PANDAS/PANS are sparse; one published study and the experience of the authors suggest that these disorders are rare. Children with PANDAS or PANS comprised 5% of patients in a Canadian outpatient pediatric OCD clinic, making the estimated prevalence of PANDAS and PANS 5% of one to 4% (the prevalence of pediatric OCD) of the pediatric population.[55]

First-degree relatives of children with PANDAS have been noted to have up to a 10-fold increase in rates of OCD, tic disorders, and acute rheumatic fever; this suggests that children with PANDAS may inherit a specific vulnerability to non-pyogenic post-streptococcal sequelae.[50] Family histories of patients with PANS reveal a remarkably high incidence of both psychiatric disorders (51%–78%) and autoimmune disorders (67%–80%) [49,51]; however, rates of familial psychiatric disorders are reported to be much lower when parents self-report through an online survey.[56]

Patients with PANS often also have coexisting autoimmune and/or inflammatory diseases, most commonly inflammatory back pain (21%) and reactive or persistent arthritis (28%).[57] PANDAS has also been associated with changes in the gut microbiome, including higher percentage of Bacteroidetes, Rikenellaceae, and

Odoribacteriaceae and a deficit of Saccharibacteria, Turicibacteraceae, and Tissierel-laceae.[58] Animal models indicate that these alterations in the gut microbiome influence and regulate microglia; it is, therefore, posited that these alterations influence brain functions and behavior[59] and predispose patients to arthritis.[60]

Evaluation

Although clear clinical diagnostic criteria and treatment recommendations exist for both PANDAS and PANS,[61-67] diagnosis of these disorders remains challenging. This is largely due to the heterogeneous presentation of symptoms and the potential subjectivity and difficulty in accurate history gathering, including details about the disease course.[68] In addition, signs, symptoms, and co-morbidities in this patient group overlap with many other psychiatric conditions (OCD, anorexia nervosa, avoidant/restrictive food intake disorder, transient tic disorder, bipolar disorder, Sydenham chorea, Tourette syndrome, autoimmune encephalitis, systemic autoimmune disease, Wilson's disease), thus complicating the differential diagnosis. As PANDAS and PANS diagnoses are ones of exclusion, it is important to complete a comprehensive diagnostic workup to rule out the wide range of other psychiatric and pediatric conditions.[61] The diagnostic evaluation serves to:

1. Identify treatable components of symptoms.
2. Explore triggers and drivers of the symptoms.
3. Differentiate from other disorders that have a more defined immunomodulatory treatment path (eg, Sydenham chorea, autoimmune encephalitis, systemic autoimmune disease) and psychiatric disorders (eg, non-PANS OCD, tics, and Tourette syndrome).

Although animal models of PANDAS strongly point to postinfectious immune-mediated etiology,[12,69-72] the diagnosis of PANDAS and PANS is not based on physical or laboratory indicators of infection or autoimmunity, but on those of clinical course (ie, the unique characteristics of the clinical presentation). History and physical examination can help to exclude other medical conditions and co-morbid conditions, which can inform treatment including chorea and hung-up knee jerk for Sydenham chorea, constitutional systems for thyroid disease, skin rashes, and arthritis for systemic autoimmune diseases like lupus, cerebral spinal fluid and imaging characteristics that go along with autoimmune encephalitis and lupus, and abdominal tenderness, anemia, and stool findings which go along with inflammatory bowel conditions, etc. Furthermore, collecting a family history including a review of neurologic diseases, psychiatric disorders, autoimmune and autoinflammatory diseases, immunodeficiency syndromes, and frequent infections may provide important clues to genetic susceptibilities.[61]

It is encouraged that all patients meeting PANS criteria have the following: complete blood cell count with manual differential, erythrocyte sedimentation rate and C-reactive protein, comprehensive metabolic panel, urinalysis (to assess hydration status, infection, and signs of glomerulonephritis) and other infection evaluations (throat culture, anti-streptolysin O, anti-DNAse B, mycoplasma titers, and assessment of sinusitis and otitis media).[61] Given findings linking PANDAS, PANS, SC, and idiopathic OCD, and the fact that autoimmunity and Group A Strep have been associated with OCD in epidemiologic studies,[73] PANDAS and PANS specialists encourage that diagnostic testing for PANDAS and PANS to include checking for inflammatory markers, particularly those suggested by results of history, physical exam, family history, and other laboratory findings.[49,57,61,73-79]

Brain MRI (eg, structural, diffusion-weighted imaging [DWI], and fluid-attenuated inversion recovery [FLAIR] sequences) and cerebral spinal fluid evaluation are indicated when abnormal neurologic signs are present (eg, focal neurologic symptoms, chorea, encephalopathy or epilepsy), when other conditions are suspected (eg, central nervous system [CNS] small vessel vasculitis, lupus, and autoimmune encephalitis), or when the patient has severe headaches, gait disturbances, cognitive deterioration, memory impairment, or psychosis.[61] For particularly severe cases, MRI including contrast enhancements may be useful in demonstrating inflammatory changes in the basal ganglia.[18,80] Identification of clinically available specific and reliable biomarkers will provide better diagnostic accuracy.

Current Evidence

The prevailing model of PANDAS and PANS posits that symptoms result from an immune response to an infectious trigger. As part of the immune response, it is thought that cross-reactive antibodies and other immune-mediators breaches a compromised blood-brain barrier and target brain cells and/or brain receptors and possibly other tissues in the body (blood vessels, joints, etc.) akin to SC and acute rheumatic fever. In a variety of PANDAS animal models, antibodies are associated with neurovascular inflammation and injury, with the basal ganglia being the most consistently reported structure affected.[12,69–72]

Autoantibodies in patients with PANDAS have been found to bind to cholinergic interneurons (CINs) (in mouse brain) and reduce their function both metabolically and electrically.[72,81] These CIN autoantibody findings have been reproduced in four separate cohorts. Specifically, CIN autoantibodies in PANDAS patients have been shown to have higher binding levels than age- and gender-matched healthy control subjects.[72] This elevated CIN autoantibody binding in patients with PANDAS has been shown to reduce in parallel with symptom improvement (pre-vs post-IVIG treatment),[81,82] which provides indirect evidence that binding of IgG to CINs in the basal ganglia may contribute to the symptoms of PANDAS.[72]

Clinical studies also demonstrate higher levels of autoantibodies in patients with PANDAS and SC compared with controls.[5,10–12] As is the case in autoantibody studies in most rheumatologic disorders, binding patterns have exhibited heterogenicity across cohorts and have been detected in separate but related patient populations. Serum samples from patients with PANDAS exhibit higher titers of dopamine D1 and D2 receptor autoantibodies (D1R and D2R),[7] lysoganglioside,[7,83] and tubulin.[12] In addition, Chain and colleagues[5] demonstrated the same antineuronal autoantibody titers and CaMKII activation in both sera and CSF of PANDAS patients in the early-acute phase of PANDAS. This human data, coupled with post-streptococcal animal model data, suggests that the movement and behavior abnormalities seen in PANDAS and PANS involve dopaminergic pathways.[4,14,16,84,85]

Autoantibody research provides further evidence for the contribution of autoimmunity in the pathogenesis of PANDAS and PANS. Nonetheless, additional studies are needed to elucidate more specific pathogenic pathways and to determine how individuals are immunogenetically predisposed to react to specific infectious triggers (Group A Strep vs other microbial triggers). In addition, further work must be done both to determine how the various and heterogeneous antibody profiles can be used to aid in diagnosis and to refine research subject classification (as has been done for other complex heterogeneous rheumatic diseases like lupus and Sjorgren's syndrome). Finally, more work must be done to streamline the laborious and expensive cell-based assays into clinically useful, reliable high throughput assays.

Imaging

Changes in the basal ganglia are the most prominent finding in neuroimaging studies concerning PANDAS and PANS (**Table 2**). One volumetric brain MRI study showed higher volumes of the caudate, putamen, and globus pallidus in patients with early-stage PANDAS ($n = 34$) compared with age- and sex-matched controls ($n = 82$),[18] which is a similar finding as to what was reported by the same author (using the same control group) in Sydenham chorea. However, no correlation was found between basal ganglia size and symptom severity or duration of symptoms. In another study, basal ganglia structure volumes were not significantly different from controls, though the range of volumes was greater.[20] This null finding may reflect that the patients in the Zheng and colleagues study were in different phases of their illness (new-acute $n = 12$ [35%], chronic $n = 7$ [21%], flare on chronic $n = 15$ [44%]), which is a notable distinction from the Giedd and colleagues[18] study where all 34 subjects were in the early-stage of their illness.

Heterogenous findings in neuroimaging studies of PANDAS and PANS are expected as the variability likely relates to the stage of the disease at the time of the MRI scan, a phenomenon commonly appreciated in rheumatological diseases (eg, lupus nephritis and juvenile arthritis) where the initial presentation of inflammation (acute/early phase) involves more fluid/swelling (ie, enlarged structures on imaging) and is followed by atrophy in the more chronic stage. This phenomenon has also been demonstrated in animal models and in multiple sclerosis.[86,87] Thus, although increased basal ganglia volume is reported in early-stage (new-onset) PANDAS patients, diminished volume of the basal ganglia is reported in adults and children with chronic OCD.[88–90] In addition, in rheumatologic disorders, the degree of swelling does not necessarily correlate with symptom severity or disease course severity; for example, children with psoriatic arthritis can have a severe/aggressive disease course despite having minimal swelling.[91] Thus, it is unsurprising that the Giedd and colleagues[18] study found no correlation between basal ganglia size and symptom severity. Evidence of basal ganglia involvement in PANDAS is further supported by:

1. A study measuring diffusivity in patients with PANS. Increased diffusivity suggests a less intact cell membrane that allows for increased water molecule diffusion within the tissues. Researchers found increased median diffusivity in the patients with PANS compared with controls with deep gray matter (eg, the basal ganglia) demonstrating the most profound increases in diffusivity.[20]
2. A study using multivariate pattern analysis (MVPA) of MRI data. Greater gray matter volume and reduced white matter volume was found in the basal ganglia of patients with PANDAS compared with controls.[17] Additional group differences, including volume differences in the frontal lobe, parietal lobe, temporal lobes, subcortical areas, and cerebellum, were also found.

PET imaging is another imaging methodology that can provide direct evidence of neuroinflammation by quantifying brain receptors, such as microglia. Microglia are resident immune cells in the brain; their activation in neurologic disease has classically been associated with inflammation, neuronal damage, and neurodegeneration. A small but important PET imaging study points toward microglial activation in the basal ganglia in children with PANDAS.[19] In this study, ligand-translocator protein (TSPO) receptor binding potential was calculated both for the basal ganglia and for the thalamus; TSPO is known to be highly expressed by activated microglia, but it is expressed at a lower level in quiescent microglia.[92] Binding potential values were found to be increased in the bilateral caudate and bilateral lentiform nucleus in patients

Table 2
Neuroimaging findings in PANDAS and PANS

Citation	Neuroimaging Technique (Disease Stage and Cohort)	Study Groups	Results
Giedd et al,[18] 2000	MRI (early-stage PANDAS)	PANDAS ($n = 34$) Age and sex matched healthy controls ($n = 82$)	Larger caudate, putamen and globus pallidus volume (PANDAS vs controls)
Zheng et al,[20] 2020	MRI (mixed-stage PANS).	PANS ($n = 34$) Age and sex matched patient controls ($n = 64$)	Increased diffusivity throughout the brain, most prominently in the thalamus, basal ganglia and amygdala (PANS vs controls)
Kumar et al,[19] 2015	PET (mixed-stage PANDAS)	PANDAS ($n = 17$) Tourette ($n = 12$) Adult controls[a] ($n = 15$)	Activated microglia in bilateral caudate (PANDAS & Tourette) and bilateral lentiform nucleus (PANDAS only)
Cabrera et al,[17] 2019	MRI (mixed-stage PANDAS)	PANS ($n = 14$) Matched healthy controls ($n = 14$)	Greater gray matter volume and reduced white matter volume in the basal ganglia (PANDAS vs controls)

[a] Owing to ethical considerations, a pediatric control group was not available. However, pediatric brain C-[R]-PK11195 (PK) values have been reported to be less than or at most equal to normal adult values; thus, pediatric brain PK values that exceed adult values can be safely and reasonably considered to be abnormal.

with PANDAS and to be increased in the bilateral caudate in patients with Tourette compared with adult controls. This is a particularly impressive finding as microglial activation increases as humans age.[93]

Although measures of brain volume, microstructural differences, and microglial activation can distinguish between patient groups and controls, these technologies are not currently available to clinicians to aid in the diagnosis of individual patients. In fact, in this population, routine non-research grade MRIs typically are normal or "incidental" findings.[20,68,94] Although signs of central nervous system inflammation are more often seen in conventional imaging of children with active neuropsychiatric systemic lupus erythematosus or autoimmune encephalitis, these findings may not be seen during active PANDAS or PANS disease. We hope that besides their utility in identifying structural abnormalities and informing pathophysiological mechanisms, neuroimaging studies will be useful as a clinical tool, for not only improving diagnosis but also for disease staging (early vs late disease), subtyping OCD (Tourette vs PANDAS/PANS vs chronic OCD vs other) and for measuring treatment response based on illness stage and subtype.

Therapeutic Options

Based on the proposed pathophysiology of PANDAS and PANS, logical treatment strategies have been proposed but randomized clinical trials with rigorous methodology are lacking. Current clinical management of SC, PANDAS, and PANS focuses on three important target areas:

1. Treatment of active and clinically apparent infection (eg, streptococcal pharyngitis, impetigo, peri-anal strep, sinusitis, otitis media, paronychia, abscess, mycoplasma, etc.) and clearance of Group A Strep from the home in cases of SC, PANDAS, and post-strep PANS.
2. Treatment of postinfectious inflammation (eg, corticosteroids, NSAIDS, IVIG).
3. Treatment of psychiatric symptoms (eg, behavior management, cognitive behavior therapy [CBT], psychotropic medication).[28,62,64,66,67,95,96]

When possible, clinicians should be guided by standard evidence-based interventions for the treatment of the identified infection and of the presenting clinical disorders (eg, gold-standard treatments for OCD, anxiety, rage, ADHD, sleep dysregulation, pain dysregulation, immunodeficiency, etc.). Specifically, studies examining the effects of CBT on symptoms of OCD in patients with PANDAS and PANS have shown a significant decrease in OCD symptom severity, including in patients who were incomplete responders to antibiotic treatment.[95,96] Importantly, clinicians should also thoughtfully tailor interventions for the PANDAS and PANS populations. For example, some children with PANS may be in extreme distress (due to agitation, anxiety, exhaustion due to lack of sleep, hyperactivation, rage, etc.) and may not be able to begin CBT; in these situations, the parents can meet with a therapist to obtain coaching on how to use CBT in the home. In regard to psychiatric treatment, one retrospective review study suggests that children with PANS may tolerate lower than typical doses of psychotropic medications.[97]

Observational studies have reported that interventions that treat the active infection and that include IVIG infusions have led to rapid and clinically significant improvement of symptoms.[21,64,65,98–103] Importantly, immunomodulation in PANS requires a comprehensive approach in a center with experience assessing different types of neuroinflammation.[63–65] Furthermore, although an early study reported the benefit of IVIG treatment,[21] these findings were not replicated.[82] This may reflect the heterogeneity in the disease of the enrolled subjects (immunogenetic predisposition, disease stage, pre-treatment path, etc.) and varied methodologies used. Additional randomized studies are needed in pediatric neuroinflammatory disease.

A recent systematic review of PANS treatments (anti-inflammatory, antibacterial and immunomodulatory) concluded that "available evidence neither supports nor excludes potential beneficial effects but supports that such treatment can result in adverse effects".[104] The review identified seven studies from 1998 to 2020 that met criteria for methodological directness, risk of bias, and precision. Known biases exist for all observational studies and many clinical trials (especially when the drug has clear physiologic symptoms during administration); this review highlights these known biases – for example, one of several concerns regarding IVIG trials includes the fact that blinding subjects for treatment conditions is difficult due to the prominent and common side effects of IVIG treatment (nausea, vomiting, and headache). Despite the fact that these biases exist for all observational studies and clinical trials that employ similar treatments and methodologies as those used in PANS, tremendous progress has been made in effectively treating other pediatric inflammatory conditions (eg, juvenile dermatomyositis, juvenile arthritis, and rare neuroinflammatory conditions such as childhood autoimmune encephalitis, central nervous system vasculitis, febrile infection-related epilepsy syndrome and other catastrophic epilepsy syndromes, and pediatric neuropsychiatric systemic lupus erythematosus). Even though these other conditions faced the exact same challenges that we are currently facing with PANS, these previously disabling conditions are now generally considered curable if early aggressive treatment is employed. However, this same progress and optimism has not been applied to PANDAS and PANS. Although the medical field unbiasedly identifies and treats other neuroinflammatory conditions including Sydenham chorea and autoimmune encephalitis, there is a large clinical prejudice (and bias in the literature) to not identify or treat PANDAS and PANS.[105–108] The field needs to reflect on whether this prejudice exists due to the purely psychiatric nature of PANDAS and PANS or due to previous controversies in the field.

Nonetheless, in practice, the severity and urgency of symptoms, the concern of brain injury and atrophy due to brain inflammation, and the possibility of chronic disabling psychiatric symptoms has led some clinicians to consider treatments despite minimal supporting evidence (in individual cases) for an inflammatory syndrome. This is especially true for patients who have repeatedly failed standard psychiatric approaches and are crippled by their psychiatric condition (ie, cannot participate in school, enjoy hobbies or sports, or spend time with family, friends, and live in a chronic state of mental anguish). For these patients and their families, the risks of IVIG, plasmapheresis, steroids, and antibiotics may pale in comparison to the severity of the child's illness; many of these families are willing to engage in a risk/benefit discussion with their clinician. The possibility of improvement in these scenarios often mirrors the presumed risk/benefit/lack of evidence scenario that encompasses the same set of treatments for Sydenham chorea and various forms of pediatric autoimmune encephalitis.

When children with PANDAS and PANS present with agitation, time-consuming and interfering compulsions, and violent or life-threatening behavior/mood outbursts/changes, both they and their families suffer.[109] Most have significant school absenteeism and many parents miss work. Some patients even threaten to jump out of cars and windows or threaten to run away. In these extreme conditions when hospitalization is necessary, medical-psychiatric hospital units are the best equipped to deliver both medical and psychiatric care of the agitated child; unfortunately, these units are rare in most countries.

Although there is insufficient evidence to plainly propose any specific treatment for PANDAS and PANS, expert consensus treatment recommendations have been proposed using psychiatric and behavioral interventions,[67] immunomodulatory therapies,[64] and antibiotics.[62,65] A key to successful treatment is a multidisciplinary approach, which poses a great challenge in our current medical care systems. International work in pediatric autoimmune encephalitis, pediatric neuropsychiatric systemic lupus erythematosus, and immune-mediated epilepsy syndromes gives us both a roadmap and hope for the future of enhanced care for children with PANDAS and PANS.

SUMMARY

SC, PANDAS, and PANS are postinfectious neuroinflammatory diseases that involve the basal ganglia and have OCD as a major manifestation. These conditions are associated with a range of autoantibodies, which are thought to be triggered by infections (most notably Group A Strep), to cross-react with neural antigens within the basal ganglia, and to modulate neuronal activity and behavior based on animal models using human sera.[70,72] MRI and PET imaging studies of patients with SC/PANDAS/PANS support the organic nature of these disorders and also point toward involvement of the basal ganglia and beyond.[17–20,110] Classically defined autoimmune disease and arthritis in patients with PANDAS/PANS and family members are common,[49,51] lending support to the syndromes' link to inflammation/immune-dysregulation and/ or autoimmunity. As is true for many childhood rheumatological diseases and neuroinflammatory diseases, SC, PANDAS and PANS lack clinically available, rigorous diagnostic biomarkers and randomized clinical trials.

The course of SC, PANDAS, and PANS is most commonly characterized as relapsing and remitting; single episodes and chronic courses are rare. The tendency for these disorders to be relapsing-remitting should be considered carefully when reporting cross-sectional data (ie, imaging results) and response to treatment in observational studies, and when planning clinical trials. Not only do we need to consider the disease state (flare vs remission vs flare on chronic), but we also need to understand the trajectory of the patients enrolled in studies (ie, new-onset flare vs resolving flare, flare on chronic vs chronic static, etc.).

Despite the lack of biomarker and treatment research, there is still the pressing need to provide care for children with severe psychiatric symptoms who also require workups for inflammatory brain disease and other possible "medical" interventions. These cases require the expertise of academic centers with wards capable of managing severe behavior challenges (such wards are rare) and that allow for cross-disciplinary coordination (eg, pediatrics, rheumatology, neurology, and psychiatry).[57,65] Because of the urgent need to treat these acutely ill patients, we have published diagnostic and treatment recommendations[62,64,67] based on the strategies used for other inflammatory brain conditions.

It is essential to investigate all contributing factors of an abruptly deteriorated child, beyond just streptococcal infections. Frankovich and colleagues[57] reported five cases of PANS likely reflecting multiple immune-activation pathways (eg, underlying immunodeficiency, autoimmunity, systemic inflammation [arthritis and gut inflammation], and various infections). The varied presentation of PANS highlights the importance of organic disease evaluations for managing and treating all abruptly deteriorating patients. In addition to biological contributors, trauma and psychosocial stressors should be evaluated and addressed.

Future studies that integrate neuroimaging, inflammation, immunogenetic, and clinical data (noting the stage in the clinical course) remain critical to better understanding and treating SC, PANDAS, PANS, and all other postinfectious/immune-mediated behavioral disorders.

CLINICS CARE POINTS

- It is imperative to not only treat the psychiatric symptoms but to also treat active and clinically apparent infections. In some cases, postinfectious inflammation may need to be addressed with immunomodulation. In the case of Sydenham chorea (SC), pediatric autoimmune neuropsychiatric disorders associated with streptococcal infections (PANDAS), and post-strep pediatric acute-onset neuropsychiatric syndrome (PANS), eliminating Group A Strep from both the patient and close contacts (eg, housemates) is essential.

- There are few trials that have evaluated the efficacy of antibiotics and immunomodulatory therapies. Thus, it is important to weigh the risks/benefits of antibiotics and immunomodulatory therapy when a patient is presenting with disabling neuropsychiatric symptoms.

- Cognitive behavioral therapy (CBT) should be used to address obsessive-compulsive disorder symptoms in PANDAS and PANS; furthermore, it is appropriate to use CBT in conjunction with other interventions (eg, immunomodulation and antibiotic treatments).

- Patients with SC, PANDAS, and PANS may tolerate lower doses of antidepressants and antipsychotics at initial presentation and early in a flare, but doses can be escalated over time.

- When children with PANDAS and PANS present with severe symptoms, hospitalization may be necessary; medical-psychiatric hospital units are best equipped.

DISCLOSURE

The authors have no financial conflicts of interests to disclose.

REFERENCES

1. Swedo SE, Leonard HL, Garvey M, et al. Pediatric autoimmune neuropsychiatric disorders associated with streptococcal infections: Clinical description of the first 50 cases. Am J Psychiatry 1998;155(2):264–71.
2. Taranta A, Stollerman GH. The relationship of Sydenham's chorea to infection with group A streptococci. Am J Med 1956;20(2):170–5.
3. Ben-Pazi H, Stoner J, Cunningham M. Dopamine receptor autoantibodies correlate with symptoms in Sydenham's chorea. PLoS One 2013;8(9):e73516.
4. Brimberg L, Benhar I, Mascaro-Blanco A, et al. Behavioral, pharmacological, and immunological abnormalities after streptococcal exposure: a novel rat model of sydenham chorea and related neuropsychiatric disorders. Neuropsychopharmacology 2012;37(9):2076–87.
5. Chain J, Alvarez K, Mascaro-Blanco A, et al. Autoantibody biomarkers for basal ganglia encephalitis in sydenham chorea and pediatric autoimmune neuropsychiatric disorder associated with streptococcal infections. Front Psychiatry 2020;11:564.
6. Cox CJ, Sharma M, Leckman JF, et al. Brain human monoclonal autoantibody from Sydenham chorea targets dopaminergic neurons in transgenic mice and

signals dopamine d2 receptor: Implications in human disease. J Immunol 2013; 191(11):5524–41.

7. Cox CJ, Zuccolo AJ, Edwards EV, et al. Antineuronal Antibodies in a Heterogeneous Group of Youth and Young Adults with Tics and Obsessive-Compulsive Disorder. J Child Adolesc Psychopharmacol 2015;25(1):76–85.

8. Dale RC, Merheb V, Pillai S, et al. Antibodies to surface dopamine-2 receptor in autoimmune movement and psychiatric disorders. Brain 2012;135(Pt 11): 3453–68.

9. Hoffman KL, Hornig M, Yaddanapudi K, et al. A murine model for neuropsychiatric disorders associated with group A beta-hemolytic streptococcal infection. J Neurosci 2004;24(7):1780–91.

10. Kirvan CA, Swedo SE, Heuser JS, et al. Mimicry and autoantibody-mediated neuronal cell signaling in Sydenham chorea. Nat Med 2003;9(7):914–20.

11. Kirvan CA, Swedo SE, Snider LA, et al. Antibody-mediated neuronal cell signaling in behavior and movement disorders. J Neuroimmunology 2006; 179(1):173–9.

12. Kirvan CA, Swedo SE, Kurahara D, et al. Streptococcal mimicry and antibody-mediated cell signaling in the pathogensis of Sydenham's chorea. Autoimmunity 2006;39(1):21–9.

13. Kirvan CA, Cox CJ, Swedo SE, et al. Tubulin is a neuronal target of autoantibodies in Sydenham's chorea. J Immunol 2007;178:7412–21.

14. Lotan D, Benhar I, Alvarez K, et al. Behavioral and neural effects of intra-striatal infusion of anti-streptococcal antibodies in rats. Brain Behav Immun 2014;38: 249–62.

15. Singer HS, Mascaro-Blanco A, Alvarez K, et al. Neuronal antibody biomarkers for Sydenham's chorea identify a new group of children with chronic recurrent episodic acute exacerbations of tic and obsessive compulsive symptoms following a streptococcal infection. PLoS One 2015;10(3):e0120499.

16. Yaddanapudi K, Hornig M, Serge R, et al. Passive transfer of streptococcus-induced antibodies reproduces behavioral disturbances in a mouse model of pediatric autoimmune neuropsychiatric disorders associated with streptococcal infection. Mol Psychiatry 2010;15(7):712–26.

17. Cabrera B, Romero-Rebollar C, Jiménez-Ángeles L, et al. Neuroanatomical features and its usefulness in classification of patients with PANDAS. CNS Spectrums 2019;24(5):533–43.

18. Giedd Jay N, Rapoport JL, Garvey MA, et al. MRI assessment of children with obsessive-compulsive disorder or tics associated with streptococcal infection. Am J Psychiatry 2000;157(2):281–3.

19. Kumar A, Williams MT, Chugani HT. Evaluation of Basal Ganglia and Thalamic Inflammation in Children With Pediatric Autoimmune Neuropsychiatric Disorders Associated With Streptococcal Infection and Tourette Syndrome: A Positron Emission Tomographic (PET) Study Using 11C-[R]-PK11195. J Child Neurol 2015;30(6):749–56.

20. Zheng J, Frankovich J, McKenna ES, et al. Association of Pediatric Acute-Onset Neuropsychiatric Syndrome With Microstructural Differences in Brain Regions Detected via Diffusion-Weighted Magnetic Resonance Imaging. JAMA Netw Open 2020;3(5):e204063.

21. Perlmutter SJ, Leitman SF, Garvey MA, et al. Therapeutic plasma exchange and intravenous immunoglobulin for obsessive-compulsive disorder and tic disorders in childhood. Lancet 1999;354(9185):1153–8.

22. Stollerman GH, Lewis AJ, Schultz I, et al. Relationship of immune response to group A streptococci to the course of acute, chronic and recurrent rheumatic fever. Am J Med 1956;20(2):163–9.
23. Loiselle CR, Singer HS. Genetics of Childhood Disorders: XXXI. Autoimmune Disorders, Part 4: Is Sydenham Chorea an Autoimmune Disorder? J Am Acad Child Adolesc Psychiatry 2001;40(10):1234–6.
24. Cardoso F, Eduardo C, Silva AP, et al. Chorea in Fifty Consecutive Patients with Rheumatic Fever. Movement Disord 1997;12(5):701–3.
25. Faustino PC, Terreri MTRA, da Rocha A, et al. Clinical, laboratory, psychiatric and magnetic resonance findings in patients with Sydenham chorea. Neuroradiology 2003;45(7):456–62.
26. Jaine R, Baker M, Venugopal K. Acute rheumatic fever associated with household crowding in a developed country. The Pediatr Infect Dis J 2011;30(4):315–9. https://doi.org/10.1097/INF.0b13e3181fbd85b.
27. Asbahr FR, Negrão AB, Gentil V, et al. Obsessive-Compulsive and Related Symptoms in Children and Adolescents With Rheumatic Fever With and Without Chorea: A Prospective 6-Month Study. Am J Psychiatry 1998;155(8):1122–4.
28. Garvey MA, Swedo SE. Sydenham's Chorea Clinical and Therapeutic Update. Adv Exp Med Biol 1997;418:115–20.
29. Maia DP, Teixeira AL, Cunningham MCQ, et al. Obsessive compulsive behavior, hyperactivity, and attention deficit disorder in Sydenham chorea. Neurology 2005;64(10):1799–801.
30. Bruetsch WL. The histopathology of psychoses with subacute bacterial and chronic verrucose rheumatic endocarditis. Am J Psychiatry 2006;95(2):346–7.
31. Ebaugh FG. Neuropsychiatric aspects of chorea in children. J Am Med Assoc 1926;87:1083–8.
32. Greenfield JG, Wolfsohn JM. The pathology of Syndenham's chorea. The Lancet 1922;200(5168):603–6.
33. Swedo SE. Sydenham's Chorea: A Model for Childhood Autoimmune Neuropsychiatric Disorders. JAMA: The J Am Med Assoc 1994;272(22):1788–91.
34. Chain JL, Cox CJ, Alvarez KM, et al. Anti-neuronal and anti-microbial immunity link CaMKII and autism spectrum disorder with pediatric acute-onset neuropsychiatric syndrome. The J Immunol 2018;200(1):166–263.
35. Dale RC, Brilot FB. Autoimmune basal ganglia disorders. J Child Neurol 2012;27(11):1470–81.
36. Giedd JN, Rapoport JL, Kruesi MJP, et al. Sydenham chorea: Magnetic resonance imaging of the basal ganglia. Neurology 1995;45(12):2199–202. https://doi.org/10.1212/WNL.45.12.2199.
37. Castillo M, Kwock L, Arbelaez A. Sydenham's chorea: MRI and proton spectroscopy. Neuroradiology 1999;41(12):943–5.
38. Emery ES, Vieco PT. Sydenham chorea: Magnetic resonance imaging reveals permanent basal ganglia injury. Neurology 1997;48(2):531–3.
39. Kienzle GD, Breger RK, Chun RWM, et al. Sydenham chorea: MR manifestations in two cases. Am J Neuroradiology 1991;12:73–6.
40. Konagaya M, Konagaya Y. MRI in hemiballism due to Sydenham's chorea. J Neurol Neurosurg Psychiatry 1992;55(3):238–9.
41. Ikuta N, Hirata M, Sasabe F, et al. High-signal basal ganglia on T1-weighted images in a patient with Sydenham's chorea. Diagn Neuroradiology 1998;40:659–61, s.
42. Robertson WC Jr, Smith CD. Sydenham's chorea in the age of MRI: A case report and review. Pediatr Neurol 2002;27(1):65–7.

43. Moreau C, Devos D, Delmaire C, et al. Progressive MRI abnormalities in late recurrence of Sydenham's chorea. J Neurol 2005;252:1341–4.

44. Williams KA, Swedo SE. Postinfectious autoimmune disorders: Sydenham's chorea, PANDAS and beyond. Brain Res 2015;1617:144–54.

45. Dean SL, Singer HS. Treatment of Sydenham's Chorea: A Review of the Current Evidence. Tremor and Other Hyperkinetic Movements 2017;7:1–13. https://doi.org/10.7916/D8W95GJ2.

46. Walker KG, Wilmshurst JM. An update on the treatment of Sydenham's chorea: The evidence for established and evolving intervention. Ther Adv Neurol Disord 2010;3(5):301–9. https://doi.org/10.1177/1756285610382063.

47. Brown K, Farmer C, Farhadian B, et al. Pediatric acute-onset neuropsychiatric syndrome response to oral corticosteroid bursts: An observational study of patients in an academic community-based PANS clinic. J Child Adolesc Psychopharmacol 2017;27(7):629–39.

48. Orefici G, Cardona F, Cox CJ, et al. Pediatric autoimmune neuropsychiatric disorders associated with streptococcal infections (PANDAS). In: Ferrettl JJ, Stevens DL, Fischetti VA, editors. Streptococcus Pyogenes: Basic Biology to clinical manifestations [Internet]. Oklahoma City (OK): University of Oklahoma Health Sciences Cdenter; 2016.

49. Chan A, Phu T, Farhadian B, et al. Familial clustering of immune-mediated diseases in children with abrupt-onset obsessive compulsive disorder. J Child Adolesc Psychopharmacol 2020;30(5):345–6.

50. Lougee L, Perlmutter SJ, Nicolson R, et al. Psychiatric Disorders in First-Degree Relatives of Children With Pediatric Autoimmune Neuropsychiatric Disorders Associated With Streptococcal Infections (PANDAS). J Am Acad Child Adolesc Psychiatry 2000;39(9):1120–6.

51. Murphy TK, Storch EA, Turner A, et al. Maternal history of autoimmune disease in children presenting with tics and/or obsessive–compulsive disorder. J Neuroimmunology 2010;229(1–2):243–7.

52. Achenbach TM, McConaughy SH, Howell CT. Child/Adolescent Behavioral and Emotional Problems: Implications of Cross-Informant Correlations for Situational Specificity. Psychol Bull 1987;101(2):213–32.

53. Swedo SE, Leckman JF, Rose NR. From research subgroup to clinical syndrome: modifying the PANDAS criteria to describe PANS (pediatric acute-onset neuropsychiatric syndrome). Pediatr Ther 2012;2(2).

54. Kalra SK, Swedo SE. Children with obsessive-compulsive disorder: are they just "little adults". The J Clin Invest 2009;119(4):737–46.

55. Jaspers-Fayer F, Han SHJ, Chan E, et al. Prevalence of acute-onset subtypes in pediatric obsessive-compulsive disorder. J Child Adolesc Psychopharmacol 2017;27(4):332–41.

56. Calaprice D, Tona J, Parker-Athill EC, et al. A Survey of Pediatric Acute-Onset Neuropsychiatric Syndrome Characteristics and Course. J Child Adolesc Psychopharmacol 2017;27(7):607–18.

57. Frankovich J, Thienemann M, Pearlstein J, et al. Multidisciplinary clinic dedicated to treating youth with pediatric acute-onset neuropsychiatric syndrome: Presenting characteristics of the first 47 consecutive patients. J Child Adolesc Psychopharmacol 2015;25(1):38–47.

58. Baj J, Sitarz E, Forma A, et al. Alterations in the Nervous System and Gut Microbiota after β-Hemolytic Streptococcus Group A Infection-Characteristics and Diagnostic Criteria of PANDAS Recognition. Int J Mol Sci 2020;21(4):1476. https://doi.org/10.3390/ijms21041476.

59. Wang Y, Wang Z, Wang Y, et al. The Gut-Microglia Connection: Implications for Central Nervous System Diseases. Front Immunol 2018;9:2325.
60. El Menofy NG, Ramadan M, Abdelbary ER, et al. Bacgterial compositional shifts of gut microbiomes in patients with rheumatoid arthritis in association with disease activity. Microorganisms 2022;10:1820.
61. Chang K, Frankovich J, Cooperstock M, et al. Clinical Evaluation of Youth with Pediatric Acute-Onset Neuropsychiatric Syndrome (PANS): Recommendations from the 2013 PANS Consensus Conference. J Child Adolesc Psychopharmacol 2015;25(1):3–13. Available at: https://Home.Liebertpub.Com/Cap.
62. Cooperstock MS, Swedo SE, Pasternack MS, et al. Clinical Management of Pediatric Acute-Onset Neuropsychiatric Syndrome: Part III—Treatment and Prevention of Infections. J Child Adolesc Psychopharmacol 2017;27(7):594–606.
63. de Bruijn MAAM, Bruijstens AL, Bastiaansen AEM, et al. Pediatric autoimmune encephalitis: Recognition and diagnosis. Neurol Neuroimmunology, Neuroinflammation 2020;7:e682.
64. Frankovich J, Swedo S, Murphy T, et al. Clinical Management of Pediatric Acute-Onset Neuropsychiatric Syndrome: Part II—Use of Immunomodulatory Therapies. J Child Adolesc Psychopharmacol 2017;27(7):574–93. https://doi.org/10.1089/CAP.2016.0148.
65. Pfeiffer HCV, Wickstrom R, Skov L, et al. Clinical guidance for diagnosis and management of suspected pediatric acute-onset neuropsychiatric syndrome in the Nordic countries. Acta Paediatr 2021;110:3389.
66. Swedo SE, Frankovich J, Murphy TK. Overview of treatment of pediatric acute-onset neuropsychiatric syndrome. J Child Adolesc Psychopharmacol 2017;27(7):562–5.
67. Thienemann M, Murphy T, Leckman J, et al. Clinical Management of Pediatric Acute-Onset Neuropsychiatric Syndrome: Part I—Psychiatric and Behavioral Interventions. J Child Adolesc Psychopharmacol 2017;27(7):566–73.
68. Gagliano A, Galati C, Ingrassia M, et al. Pediatric Acute-Onset Neuropsychiatric Syndrome: A Data Mining Approach to a Very Specific Constellation of Clinical Variables. J Child Adolesc Psychopharmacol 2020;30(8):495–511.
69. Aron AM, Freeman JM, Carter S. The natural history of Sydenham's chorea: Review of the literature and long term evaluation on cardiac sequelae. Am J Med 1965;38:89–93.
70. Cutforth T, DeMille M, Agalliu I, et al. CNS autoimmune disease after Streptococcus pyogenes infections: Animal models, cellular mechanisms and genetic factors. Future Neurol 2016;11(1):63–76.
71. Husby G, Van De Rijn I, Zabriskie B, et al. Antibodies reacting with cytoplasm of subthalamic and caudate nuclei neurons in chorea and acute rheumatic fever. The J Exp Med 1976;144(4):1094–110.
72. Xu J, Liu RJ, Fahey S, et al. Antibodies from children with PANDAS bind specifically to striatal cholinergic interneurons and alter their activity. Am J Psychiatry 2021;178(1):48–64.
73. Mataix-Cols D, Frans E, Pérez-Vigil A, et al. (2017). A total-population multigenerational family clustering study of autoimmune diseases in obsessive–compulsive disorder and Tourette's/chronic tic disorders. Mol Psychiatry 2018;23(7):1652–8.
74. Dale RC. Autoimmunity and the basal ganglia: New insights into old diseases. QJM: An Int J Med 2003;96(3):183–91.
75. Gerentes M, Pelissolo A, Rajagopal K, et al. Obsessive-Compulsive Disorder: Autoimmunity and Neuroinflammation. Curr Psychiatry Rep 2019;21(8):1–10.

76. Pérez-Vigil A, Fernández de la Cruz L, Brander G, et al. The link between auto-immune diseases and obsessive-compulsive and tic disorders: A systematic review. Neurosci Biobehavioral Rev 2016;71:542–62.

77. Rodríguez N, Morer A, González-Navarro EA, et al. Altered frequencies of Th17 and Treg cells in children and adolescents with obsessive-compulsive disorder. Brain Behav Immun 2019;81:608–16.

78. Westwell-Roper C, Williams KA, Samuels J, et al. Immune-Related Comorbidities in Childhood-Onset Obsessive Compulsive Disorder: Lifetime Prevalence in the Obsessive Compulsive Disorder Collaborative Genetics Association Study. J Child Adolesc Psychopharmacol 2019;29(8):615–24.

79. Williams K, Shorser-Gentile L, Sarvode Mothi S, et al. Immunoglobulin A Dysgammaglobulinemia Is Associated with Pediatric-Onset Obsessive-Compulsive Disorder. J Child Adolesc Psychopharmacol 2019;29(4):268–75.

80. Giedd Jay N, Rapoport JL, Leonard HL, et al. Case Study: Acute Basal Ganglia Enlargement and Obsessive-Compulsive Symptoms in an Adolescent Boy. J Am Acad Child Adolesc Psychiatry 1996;35(7):913–5.

81. Frick LR, Rapanelli M, Jindachomthong K, et al. Differential binding of antibodies in PANDAS patients to cholinergic interneurons in the striatum. Brain Behav Immun 2018;69:304–11.

82. Williams KA, Swedo SE, Farmer CA, et al. Randomized, Controlled Trial of Intravenous Immunoglobulin for Pediatric Autoimmune Neuropsychiatric Disorders Associated With Streptococcal Infections. J Am Acad Child Adolesc Psychiatry 2016;55(10):860–7, e2.

83. Fallon B, Strobino B, Reim S, et al. Anti-lysoganglioside and other anti-neuronal autoantibodies in post-treatment Lyme disease and erythema migrans after repeat infection. Brain Behav Immun – Health 2020;2:100015.

84. Macrì S, Proietti Onori M, Laviola G. Theoretical and practical considerations behind the use of laboratory animals for the study of Tourette syndrome. Neurosci Biobehavioral Rev 2013;37(6):1085–100.

85. Spinello C, Laviola G, Macrì S. Pediatric autoimmune disorders associated with streptococcal infections and Tourette's syndrome in preclinical studies. Front Neurosci 2016;10.

86. Rodriguez-Paez AC, Brunschwig JP, Bramlett HM. Light and electron microscopic assessment of progressive atrophy following moderate traumatic brain injury in the rat. Acta Neuropathologica 2005;109(6):603–16.

87. Simon JH. From enhancing lesions to brain atrophy in relapsing MS. J Neuroimmunology 1999;98(1):7–15.

88. Arnold P, Kronenberg S. Biological Models and Treatments for Obsessive-Compulsive and Related Disorders for Children and Adolescents. In: Abramowitz JS, McKay D, Storch EA, editors. The Wiley Handbook Obsessive Compulsive Disordll. John Wiley & Sons, Ltd; 2017. p. 1061–96.

89. Peterson B, Riddle MA, Cohen DJ, et al. Reduced basal ganglia volumes in Tourette's syndrome using three-dimensional reconstruction techniques from magnetic resonance images. Neurology 1993;43:941–9.

90. Szeszko PR, MacMillan S, McMeniman M, et al. Brain structural abnormalities in psychotropic drug-naive pediatric patients with obsessive-compulsive disorder. Am J Psychiatry 2004;161(6):1049–56. JPEG.

91. De Somer L, Lambot K, Wouters C, et al. Juvenile idiopathic arthritis with dry synovitis: Clinical and imaging aspects in a cohort of 6 patients. Pediatr Rheumatol 2011;9:P173.

92. Ching AS, Kuhnast B, Damont A, et al. Current paradigm of the 18-kDa translocator protein (TSPO) as a molecular target for PET imaging in neuroinflammation and neurodegernative diseases. Insights into Imaging 2012;3:111–9.

93. Harry GJ. Microglia during development and aging. Pharmacol Ther 2013; 139(3):313–26.

94. Gamucci A, Uccella S, Sciarretta L, et al. PANDAS and PANS: Clinical, Neuropsychological, and Biological Characterization of a Monocentric Series of Patients and Proposal for a Diagnostic Protocol. J Child Adolesc Psychopharmacol 2019;29(4):305–12.

95. Nadeau JM, Jordan C, Selles RR, et al. A pilot train of cognitive-behavioral therapy augmentation of antibiotic treatment in youth with Pediatric Acute-Onset Neuropsychiatric Syndrome-related obsessive-compulsive disorder. J Child Adolesc Psychopharmacol 2015;25(4):XX.

96. Storch EA, Murphy TK, Geffken GR, et al. Cognitive-behavioral therapy for PANDAS-related obsessive-compulsive disorder: Findings from a preliminary waitlist controlled open trail. Child Adolesc Psychiatry 2006;45(10):1171–8.

97. Thienemann M, Park M, Chan A, et al. Patients with abrupt early-onset OCD due to PANS tolerate lower doses of antidepressants and antipsychotics. J Psychiatr Res 2021;135:270–8.

98. Hajjari P, Huldt Oldmark M, Fernell E, et al. Paediatric acute-onset neuropsychiatric syndrome (PANS) and intravenous immunoglobulin (IVIG): Comprehensive open-label trial in ten children. BMC Psychiatry 2022;22:535.

99. Mahony T, Sidell D, Gans H, et al. Improvement of psychiatric symptoms in youth following resolution of sinusitis. Int Jouranl Pediatr Otorhinolaryngol 2017;92:38–44.

100. Melamed I, Kobayashi RH, O'Connor M, et al. Evaluation of Intravenous Immunoglobulin in Pediatric Acute-Onset Neuropsychiatric Syndrome. J Child Adolesc Psychopharmacol 2021;31(2):118–28.

101. Murphy TK, Snider LA, Mutch PJ, et al. Relationship of movements and behaviors to Group A Streptococcus infections in elementary school children. Biol Psychiatry 2007;61(3):279–84. https://doi.org/10.1016/j.biopsych.2006.08.031.

102. Murphy TK, Parker-Athill EC, Lewin AB, et al. Cefdinir for recent-onset pediatric neuropsychiatric disorders: A pilot randomized trial. J Child Adolesc Psychopharmacol 2015;25(1):57–64. https://doi.org/10.1089/cap.2014.0010.

103. Murphy TK, Brennan EM, Johnco C, et al. A double-blind randomized placebo-controlled pilot study of azithromycin in youth with acute-onset obsessive-compulsive disorder. J Child Adolesc Psychopharmacol 2017;27(7):640–51. https://doi.org/10.1089/cap.2016/0190.

104. Johnson M, Ehlers S, Fernell E, et al. Anti-inflammatory, antibacterial and immunomodulatory treatment in children with symptoms corresponding to the research condition PANS (Pediatric Acute-onset Neuropsychiatric Syndrome): A systematic review. PloS one 2021;16(7):e0253844.

105. Bertsias GK, Ioannidis JPA, Aringer M, et al. EULAR recommendations for the management of systemic lupus erythematosus with neuropsychiatric manifestations: Report of a task force of the EULAR standing committee for clinical affairs. Ann Rheum Dis 2010;69(12):2074–82.

106. Koh S, Wirrell E, Vezzani A, et al. Proposal to optimize evaluation and treatment of Febrile infection-related epilepsy syndrome (FIRES): A report from FIRES workshop. Epilepsia Open 2021;6(1):62–72.

107. Nosadini M, Thomas T, Eyre M, et al. International consensus recommendations for the treatment of pediatric NMDAR antibody encephalitis. Nuerology Neuro-immunology & Neuroinflammation 2021;8(5):e1052.
108. Titulaer MJ, McCracken L, Gabilondo I, et al. Treatment and prognostic factors for long-term outcome in patients with anti-NMDA receptor encephalitis: An observational cohort study. Lancet Neurol 2013;12(2):157–65.
109. Frankovich J, Leibold CM, Farmer C, et al. The burden of caring for a child or adolescent with pediatric acute-onset neuropsychiatric syndrome (PANS): An observational longitudinal study. J Clin Psychiatry 2018;80(1):17m12091.
110. Ehrlich DJ, Walker RH. Functional neuroimaging and chorea: a systematic review. J Clin Movement Disord 2017;4:8.

Childhood Obsessive–Compulsive Disorder

McKenzie Schuyler, BS[a], Daniel A. Geller, MD[a,b],*

KEYWORDS

- Obsessive–compulsive disorder • Child and adolescent • Pediatric • Development
- Psychopathology

KEY POINTS

- Most cases of obsessive compulsive disorder (OCD) begin in childhood or adolescence.
- OCD affecting children and adolescents is associated with distinct clinical correlates, familial loading, and outcomes compared with adult-onset cases.
- Scales to address childhood OCD and related conditions are available and useful in clinical care.
- Outcomes for childhood OCD are generally better than adult-onset with substantial proportions becoming subclinical or achieving remission.

INTRODUCTION

Obsessive–compulsive disorder (OCD) is a potentially debilitating psychiatric condition characterized by intrusive thoughts (obsessions) and stereotyped behaviors (compulsions) that cause pronounced distress and impairment or are overly time-consuming.[1] Decades of research have shown that OCD affecting children and adolescents is associated with distinct clinical correlates, familial loading, and outcomes compared with adult-onset cases, such that it has been suggested to be a developmental subtype of the disorder.[2] Currently, the diagnostic and statistical manual of mental Disorders, 5th edition (DSM-5) diagnostic criteria for childhood OCD are the same as those for adult OCD.[1] However, there are two "specifiers" that are particularly relevant for childhood-onset cases. One specifier refers to "tic-associated" OCD which is more frequently seen in youth and in males, where comorbid tic disorders including Tourette syndrome are common. The second specifier alludes to "poor insight" which may be noted in very young patients whose ability to recognize and articulate the ego dystonic nature of their obsessions may be limited.

a Department of Psychiatry, Massachusetts General Hospital, 185 Cambridge Street, Suite 2000, Boston, MA 02114, USA; b Harvard Medical School, 25 Shattuck Street, Boston, MA 02115, USA
* Corresponding author.
E-mail address: dan.geller@mgh.harvard.edu

Psychiatr Clin N Am 46 (2023) 89–106
https://doi.org/10.1016/j.psc.2022.10.002
0193-953X/23/© 2022 Elsevier Inc. All rights reserved.

Because childhood OCD may impact progress of normal developmental milestones and impair long-term achievement, early recognition of the condition and adequate treatment by specialized clinicians is particularly important.[3,4] It is generally held that early recognition and intervention can limit and mitigate impairment and negative outcomes associated with childhood OCD.[3] In the past, the lag between onset and diagnosis was substantial, often several years,[5] and some cases in epidemiologic surveys had not been previously identified.[6,7] One aim of dissemination of the unique presentation of childhood OCD is therefore to reduce the time between onset, diagnosis, and intervention. Specific symptoms are highly variable and are often hidden from adult observers, especially teachers and peers, when partial insight of irrational behavior leads to inhibition of overt compulsions in public. As well, cases of early-onset OCD are associated with later development of other psychiatric disorders, including anxiety, mood, eating, and other "OCD-related" disorders, pointing to a critical need for early intervention.[8]

As OCD affecting youth differs in several important ways from OCD in adults, this article highlights those distinctions and their clinical and research relevance.

Prevalence/Incidence

Early epidemiologic studies identified a prevalence of childhood OCD between 0.25% and 3%,[6,7,9] with a more recent Danish population-based study of nearly 2 million individuals finding a prevalence of 0.84%[10] (**Fig. 1**). These rates are similar to prevalence estimates in adults ranging from 1% to 3%.[11] Despite the frequent occurrence of OCD in children, it may exist undetected by caretakers for some time if children struggle to communicate their experiences or lack the insight necessary to recognize their obsessions and compulsions as irrational.[12] Conversely, children may intentionally hide their symptoms, delaying discovery of the problem.[13] This may result in underestimates of true prevalence.

Age at Onset Versus Age at Ascertainment

The incidence of OCD, which refers to new cases per annum, seems to occur in a bimodal distribution, with the first onset peak occurring at 9 to 10 years of age (with an SD of ± 2.5 years) and the second occurring in the early 20s[14,15] (**Fig. 2**). OCD is more likely to manifest before adulthood, with over 50% of cases beginning in childhood or adolescence according to a recent international multisite report.[16] Thus, most adults with OCD have had their illness for many years, underscoring the chronic nature of the disorder. One puzzling aspect of the steady prevalence across the life span is that it does not increase as new cases are added to the clinically affected population with time and advancing age. From this, we may surmise that cases "leaving" the affected population (ie, those whose OCD becomes subclinical or remits), more or less equal those "entering" from new incidence. This is a notable feature of childhood OCD which generally has a better outcome than adult-onset cases (see *Clinical Outcomes*).

Gender

Although several studies have observed a male preponderance of 60% to 70% in childhood OCD,[17–19] the more recent Danish population-based study identified a slight female preponderance of 56%.[20] This pattern is in line with studies indicating that most adult OCD patients are female.[21] However, many of the most common comorbid conditions associated with childhood OCD (**Fig. 3**) show a distinct male preponderance.[22,23] Age of ascertainment may account for these gender prevalence differences based on improvement and remission in younger or comorbid cases.[5]

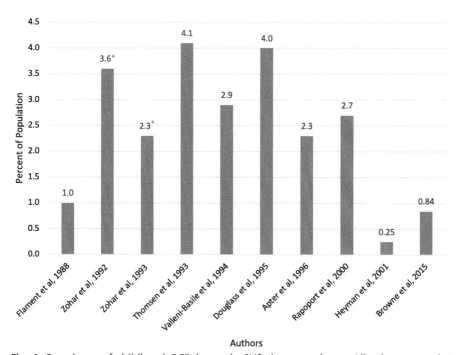

Fig. 1. Prevalence of childhood OCD by study. [a]Lifetime prevalence. All others are point prevalence. (*Data from* Refs.[6,7,9,10,114–119])

THE ROLE OF FAMILY AND HEREDITY

Both genetic and environmental factors are important for the manifestation of some psychiatric disorders, including OCD. Heritability estimates for OCD in adults and children are at most 47% and 65%, respectively, suggesting that environmental and epigenetic factors are equally important for clinical manifestation of OCD.[24] Childhood OCD specifically is associated with greater familial and genetic risk such that it represents a more familial subgroup than cases of adult OCD.[25,26] Although the first-degree relatives of childhood-onset probands have a risk as high as 26%, risk for OCD drops to 12% for relatives of adult-onset probands.[25,27,28]

Beyond family and twin studies, genome-wide association studies have more recently been used in an attempt to identify specific genes associated with OCD,[29,30] with the first statistically significant genome-wide single-nucleotide polymorphism reported in the last year.[31] Like most psychiatric disorders, OCD is polygenic, with small additive effects from variation in multiple loci.[32] Genes involved in serotonergic (eg, HTR2C[33]) and glutamatergic (eg, SLC1A1[34]) signaling have been associated with OCD. See also chapter 3, Genetics of OCD, in this volume.

Family Involvement

Pediatric OCD often affects a child's entire family and familial responses to the disorder can play a significant role in its course.[35] Up to 97% of families report participating in OCD-related symptoms and behaviors, which has been termed family accommodation (FA).[35–37] FA can include giving reassurance, facilitating rituals, assisting with avoidance, and modifying schedules or routines around symptoms.[38] Family members who engage in accommodation often intend to help children in some way,

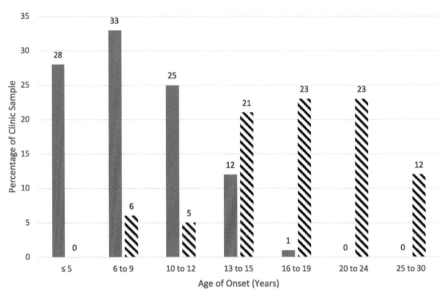

Fig. 2. Bimodal distribution of age at onset of OCD. [a]*Data from* Geller D, Biederman J, Faraone SV, et al. Clinical correlates of obsessive compulsive disorder in children and adolescents referred to specialized and non-specialized clinical settings. *Depress Anxiety.* 2000;11(4):163-168. doi:10.1002/1520-6394(2000)11:4<163::AIDDA3> 3.0.CO;2-3). [b]*Data from* Rasmussen SA, Eisen J. The epidemiology and clinical features of obsessive compulsive disorder. *Psychiatr Clin.* 1992;15(4):743-758. doi:10.1016/S0193-953X(18)30205-3.

such as by assuaging anxiety or reducing the time involved in symptoms.[39] However, FA is counterproductive to long-term symptom relief, as it ultimately maintains symptoms by reinforcing reliance on the obsessive-compulsive behaviors and family help.[40] Likewise, FA interferes with successful exposures that can lead to fear extinction learning.[41] Scales to assess FA are available and useful in clinical care (see *Assessment*).

CLINICAL FINDINGS
Childhood Obsessive–Compulsive Disorder Symptoms

Efforts to organize similar OCD symptoms into groups using factor or cluster analysis have led to identification of "symptom dimensions." Those observed in childhood OCD are congruent with the four main symptom dimensions identified in adults: (1) symmetry/ordering, (2) contamination/cleaning, (3) hoarding symptoms, and (4) aggressive/sexual/religious obsessions.[42,43] Although the factor structure of OCD is stable across the lifespan, studies comparing OCD symptomatology in children, adolescents, and adults have found that obsessions and compulsions tend to relate to the developmental stage of the patient.[19]

In accordance with this, children and adolescents tend to have higher rates of fears about disastrous or harmful events befalling themselves or loved ones, reflecting developmental concerns around separation from attachment figures such as parents or guardians.[4,19] Similarly, it is more common for youth to involve primary caregivers in compulsions and rituals (eg, through seeking reassurance or participation in a

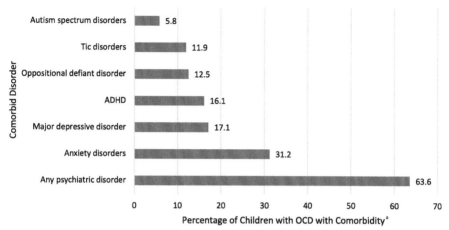

Fig. 3. Comorbid disorders in childhood OCD. [a]*Data from* Sharma E, Sharma LP, Balachander S, et al. Comorbidities in obsessive-compulsive disorder across the lifespan: A systematic review and meta-analysis. *Front Psychiatry.* 2021;12:703701. doi:10.3389/fpsyt.2021.703701.

behavior). In adolescence, normal developmental anxiety around sexuality, morality, and religion become prevalent, and these themes are often reflected in the obsessional content of adolescent patients.[19,44,45] Indeed, religious and sexual obsessions are overrepresented in adolescents compared with their younger counterparts.[19,45]

Over a quarter of youth with OCD also display hoarding symptoms.[46–48] There is some evidence that pediatric hoarding symptoms are more likely in females and are associated with specific clinical correlates such as magical thinking and ordering/arranging compulsions.[43,47] Concerns about contamination and cleanliness are also common among children and adolescents.[45] Finally, symptoms from the symmetry and ordering dimension may occur more frequently in very young children, perhaps related to greater comorbidity with tic disorders.[49,50]

Insight

The concept of insight in OCD refers to the extent to which an individual recognizes the excessive, irrational nature of their obsessions and compulsions.[1] Although the diagnosis of OCD in adults requires an assessment of level of insight, this is not the case for pediatric populations.[1] Insight may be difficult to measure in pediatric OCD patients, especially in young children, due to a limited ability to convey intrusive thoughts which drive their compulsions. Some studies have found that when youth are capable of demonstrating insight, it is limited,[19,51] whereas others have reported comparable insight to adults.[45] Overall, younger children also show less resistance and less control over OCD symptoms compared with their older counterparts[52] which may be reflected in higher scalar severity scores.

Comorbid Conditions

Comorbidity is extremely common with 64% of children with OCD meeting criteria for another psychiatric condition according to a recent meta-analysis (see **Fig. 3**).[22] As in adults with OCD, major depressive disorder and anxiety disorders are frequent comorbid conditions.[22] However, of particular note for children with OCD are neurodevelopmental and tic disorders, including attention-deficit hyperactivity disorder (ADHD), conduct disorders, autism spectrum disorder, and Tourette syndrome. Compared with the general population, these conditions are found more frequently in children with OCD, especially in male individuals.[22,23]

The presence of comorbid diagnoses can elevate impairment above and beyond that due to OCD. Youth who exhibit other psychiatric disorders in addition to OCD may experience more severe obsessive–compulsive symptoms,[53] educational impairment,[54] and emotional adjustment difficulties.[55] Likewise, comorbidity can have an adverse impact on OCD treatment response and remission. One study found that children with comorbid conduct disorder, major depression, and ADHD had lower response rates to cognitive behavioral therapy (CBT),[56] whereas another study found that children with oppositional defiant disorder, tics, and ADHD showed worse response to Selective serotonin reuptake inhibitor (SSRI) treatment.[23]

Pediatric Autoimmune Neuropsychiatric Disorders Associated with Streptococcal Infections and Pediatric Acute-Onset Neuropsychiatric Syndrome

Pediatric Autoimmune Neuropsychiatric Disorders Associated with Streptococcal Infections (PANDAS) refers to an acute onset of OCD or tics in children thought to be caused by an autoimmune reaction and inflammatory pathophysiology following infection with group A streptococcus.[57] The first cases of this putative condition were described in 1998 by Swedo and colleagues who drew comparisons to patients with Sydenham's chorea experiencing obsessive–compulsive symptoms.[57] PANDAS is a subcategory of Pediatric Acute-Onset Neuropsychiatric Syndrome (PANS), a diagnosis later proposed by Swedo and colleagues to encompass children with fulminant onset of OCD or food restriction not necessarily associated with a strep infection.[58] PANS is also accompanied by a variety of neuropsychiatric symptoms, such as emotional lability, behavioral regression, and urinary frequency.[58] OCD that is associated with PANDAS/PANS may involve distinct treatment approaches in addition to conventional treatments, including the use of antibiotics and anti-inflammatory agents to modulate immune responses.

Many studies have explored the underlying pathophysiology of PANDAS/PANS, searching for autoantibodies against neuronal targets, but without consistency. However, recent work has implicated elevated immunoglobulin G (IgG) antibody binding to cholinergic interneurons from the striatum in PANDAS.[59,60] Further, intravenous immunoglobulin (IVIG) treatment reduced IgG binding to these interneurons, and this correlated with improvements in patients' symptoms.[59] See chapter 5 for more information.

Functional Impairment

Pediatric OCD is associated with significant functional impairment in the school, home, and social environments. Close to 90% of children and adolescents endorse impairment in at least one of these functional domains and nearly 50% exhibit impairment in all three areas.[61] Impairment in this group is associated with the presence of depressive symptoms, higher levels of FA, and poorer insight.[62]

In the school environment, impairment presents idiosyncratically; for instance, affected youth may struggle to get to school on time, be prepared for class, or concentrate on assignments depending on the nature of their obsessive–compulsive symptoms. Indeed, a recent study found that children reported being most significantly affected by their OCD within the school domain.[63] Beyond this, youth with OCD may exhibit some relative neurocognitive deficits (eg, in processing speed, visuospatial abilities, and working memory) compared with non-OCD controls, yet performance on neurocognitive tasks remains in the normative range.[64]

Likewise, the majority of parents of youth with OCD endorse home and family problems related to their child's condition.[61,65] This may involve disruptions to family routines and relationships, with negative effects even extending into parents' occupational lives.[66] Families of children with OCD report more strain and stress, parental guilt and fear, and parental anxiety.[67,68] In the interpersonal domain, youth with OCD may have trouble making and keeping friends, or participating in typical activities with peers.[61]

ASSESSMENT

Detecting and assessing OCD in children and adolescents are important to ensure timely intervention. Several measures have been developed for this purpose. Two recent reviews discuss these measures and their psychometric properties in detail.[69,70] See also chapter 2, Assessment of OCD.

Children's Yale–Brown Obsessive–Compulsive Scale

The Children's Yale–Brown Obsessive–Compulsive Scale (CY-BOCS) is a semi-structured interview of OCD symptom severity over the past week administered by clinicians.[71] The CY-BOCS is the gold-standard measure for assessing OCD symptoms in children and quantifying change in symptoms over time.[70] It includes a checklist of past and current obsessions and compulsions and a 10-item severity scale capturing time occupied, degree of functional interference, subjective distress, resistance, and degree of control. A recent study examining Y-BOCS severity benchmarks for OCD across the lifespan identified subclinical OCD as corresponding to a total score of 0 to 13, mild OCD to 14 to 21, moderate OCD to 22 to 29, and severe OCD to 30 to 40.[72] Positive treatment response is defined as a $\geq 35\%$ score reduction, whereas symptom remission is defined as a raw score of ≤ 12 posttreatment.[73] The CY-BOCS II was recently created to address criticisms of the psychometric properties of the original CY-BOCS.[74] The initial examination of CY-BOCS II found strong reliability and validity.[74]

Obsessive–Compulsive Inventory–Child Version

The child version of the Obsessive–Compulsive Inventory (OCI-CV) is a 21-item self-report measure to assess childhood OCD symptoms occurring over the past month.[75] Cut-off scores of 10 and 11 are suggested in primary care settings and psychiatric clinics, respectively.[76] The OCI-CV includes six subscales: doubting/checking, hoarding, neutralizing, obsessing, washing, and ordering. However, with the release of the DSM-5, hoarding was excluded from obsessive–compulsive diagnostic criteria, prompting an update to the OCI-CV called the OCI-CV-Revised.[77] A study of the OCI-CV-Revised suggested cut-off scores of 6 and 8 to distinguish between children with OCD and children with no diagnoses and those with other psychiatric diagnoses, respectively.[77] For the original OCI-CV, treatment response is considered a 20% to 25% score reduction, and remission is considered a 55% to 65% reduction.[78]

Child Behavior Checklist—Obsessive–Compulsive Subscale

The Obsessive–Compulsive Scale of the Child Behavior Checklist (CBCL-OCS) is a short 8-item measure derived from factor analysis of the CBCL used to screen for OCD.[79] Parents rate items on a three-point scale (0 = not true to 2 = very or often true). A cut-off score of 4.5 is recommended to best distinguish between OCD and other internalizing disorders, while a cut-off score of 3.5 is recommended to discriminate between OCD and externalizing disorders.[80] However, a cut-off score of 4.5-5 is recommended to best identify OCD in the general population.[81,82] The CBCL-OCS has been found to have good sensitivity and specificity for obsessive–compulsive symptoms.[83] The CBCL-OCS provides an effective and quick way to screen for OCD in variety of clinical settings, including pediatrician and family practitioner offices.

Child Obsessive–Compulsive Impact Scale–Revised

The Child Obsessive–Compulsive Impact Scale–Revised is used to assess functional impairment related to childhood OCD.[84] There are parallel parent- and child-report versions where respondents rate 33 items on a four-point scale (0 = not at all to 3 = very much). The parent-report version examines the domains of daily living skills, school, social, and family/activities, whereas the youth-report version examines school, social, and activities. Both versions have demonstrated sensitivity to treatment response.[85]

Family Accommodation Scale–Parent Report

The Family Accommodation Scale–Parent Report (FAS-PR) is a 13-item self-report scale used to assess the extent to which family members have accommodated a child's obsessive-compulsive symptoms over the past month.[36] The FAS-PR is identical in scoring and content to the original FAS, which is clinician interview-based.[86] Parents/guardians rate items on a five-point Likert-type scale (0 = never to 4 = daily) and there are four subscales: modification of routines, participation in rituals, parent distress associated with accommodating, and the child's reaction to family attempts to refrain from accommodation.[36] Several studies examining accommodation in childhood OCD has used the FAS-PR.[36,41,87]

Children's Depression Rating Scale–Revised

The Children's Depression Rating Scale–Revised (CDRS-R) is a 17-item semi-structured interview used to assess depression in children ages 6 to 12 years.[88] Clinicians rate items on a scale of 1 to 7 or 1 to 5, with a higher score indicating more significant difficulties. A score of 40 or above is generally considered indicative of depression, whereas a score of 28 or less is often used as indicative of remission in clinical trials.[89] The CDRS-R has been found to have good reliability and validity and to be sensitive to treatment response.[89]

Screen for Child Anxiety-Related Emotional Disorders

The Screen for Child Anxiety-Related Emotional Disorders (SCARED) is a 41-item measure to screen for childhood anxiety disorders, with parallel parent- and child-report versions.[90,91] The items are rated on a three-point Likert-type scale (0 = not true to 2 = true or often true) and the measure consists of five factors: somatic/pain, general anxiety, separation anxiety, social phobia, and school phobia.[91] A cut-off score of 25 has been suggested to identify children with clinically significant anxiety.[91] The SCARED shows good discriminant validity and diagnostic utility and is freely available.[92]

Yale Global Tic Severity Scale

The Yale Global Tic Severity Scale (YGTSS) is the gold-standard scale for the assessment of number, frequency, intensity, complexity, and interference of motor and phonic tics during the past week in children, adolescents, and adults.[93,94] The YGTSS consists of five index scores: total motor tic score, total phonic tic score, total tic score, overall impairment rating, and global severity score. Treatment response is defined as a 35% reduction in the total tic score or a raw decrease of 6 to 7 points.[95]

TREATMENT

The first-line treatment for children with OCD is CBT, supported by a robust body of evidence including randomized controlled trials (RCTs) and meta-analyses.[96] The Pediatric OCD Treatment Study (POTS) is a well-known three-site RCT involving children and adolescents with OCD. The POTS I examined the efficacy of CBT, sertraline, and combination therapy in affected children aged 7 to 17 years, finding that patients treated with either CBT alone or in combination with medication exhibited a significantly greater probability of improvement.[97] The rates of remission for patients treated with either combination therapy, CBT alone, or sertraline alone were 53.6%, 39%, and 21.4%, respectively.[97] The study found large to moderate effect sizes (expressed as Hedge g) of 1.4, 0.97, and 0.67 for combined treatment, CBT alone, and sertraline alone, respectively.[97] Significant site differences in degree of response emerged for CBT and sertraline, but not for combined treatment, "suggesting that combined treatment is less susceptible to setting-specific variations in treatment outcome".[97] Similarly, the POTS II examined the effects of augmenting medication treatment with traditional CBT versus a brief control form of CBT delivered in the context of medication management for children with OCD aged 7 to 17 years.[98] The POTS II identified combined CBT and medication management as the superior form of treatment compared with medication management alone and medication management plus brief CBT.[98] In the combined treatment group, 68.6% of youth were considered responders, which was significantly greater than 34% in the plus brief CBT group and 30% in the medication alone group.[98] Finally, POTS Jr examined the efficacy of family-based CBT versus a family-based control relaxation treatment (RT) for very young children aged 5 to 8 years with OCD.[99] The POTS Jr found CBT to be superior to the control RT in reducing OCD symptoms and functional impairment, with 72% and 41% of children in the respective groups being rated as "much improved" or "very much improved" on the Clinical Global Impressions–Improvement scale posttreatment.[99] Effect sizes for the CBT and control RT were 0.84 and 0.42, respectively, indicating large and medium effects.[99] The POTS Jr also provides evidence for the usefulness and tolerability of exposure and response prevention (ERP) for very young affected children, given that the CBT condition was ERP-based.[99] In a recent systematic review and meta-analysis of CBT for children and adolescents with OCD, Uhre and colleagues found that, compared with no intervention, CBT significantly decreased OCD severity and improved functioning, although approximately half of the patients treated did not fully remit.[96]

As can be gleamed from the data presented above, CBT for childhood OCD is generally more efficacious than medication treatment. However, some children may benefit from psychopharmacotherapy, such as those who do not respond to or cannot reliably access CBT. Monotherapy with serotonin reuptake inhibitors (SRIs) has shown efficacy compared with placebo according to numerous RCTs, though with moderate effect sizes.[100–102] For instance, though the POTS I found sertraline to be inferior to CBT, it was significantly better than placebo.[97] There is evidence for the efficacy of the antidepressant selective SRIs (SSRIs) sertraline,[103] paroxetine,[104] fluoxetine,[105] fluvoxamine,[106] and citalopram[107] as well as the SRI clomipramine.[108] A recent meta-analysis identified clomipramine as providing the greatest benefit compared with placebo over the SSRIs.[108] It should be noted that SSRI use in youth with depression has been associated with suicidal ideation, resulting in a United States Food and Drug Administration (FDA) black box warning on antidepressants.[109] However, all the noted increase in suicidal ideation occurred in youth in the depression treatment trials rather than the OCD treatment trials. Further, SSRI use in children comes with an increased risk of behavioral activation (eg, insomnia, irritability, hyperactivity), making psychopharmacological management increasingly complex for young patients.[110]

In comparing CBT and medication treatment, Sanchez-Meca and colleagues found the following effect sizes: $d = 1.704$ for CBT plus medication, $d = 1.203$ for CBT alone, and $d = 0.745$ for medication alone.[111] These findings are in line with the effect sizes identified by the POTS I. Overall, this work suggests that combination treatment may be most effective for children with OCD, followed by CBT alone, which has been supported by other studies.[101] In general, parents and family members should be involved in treatment whenever possible, as successful treatment depends especially on the reduction of family members' accommodation of symptoms. To this end, family psychoeducation and parent training sessions can be incorporated into the overall treatment plan.

Given that childhood OCD is frequently accompanied by comorbid conditions, obsessive–compulsive symptoms often cannot be treated in isolation. The most effective treatment will integrate management of all co-occurring conditions, taking into account unique behavioral and pharmacotherapy approaches for each comorbidity.

CLINICAL OUTCOMES

Outlook for childhood OCD is generally optimistic, especially when few or no comorbid conditions are present and when families can reduce accommodation. Compared with their adult counterparts, children with OCD show higher rates of partial and full remission.[112] A recent 3-year prospective follow-up study of children and adolescents treated for OCD found that the probability of achieving partial remission was 53%, whereas the probably of achieving full remission was 27%.[112] For adult patients, those probabilities were 34% and 13%, respectively.[112] Further, for the children who responded to initial CBT treatment, 79% maintained remission on year later.[112] The Nordic Long-term OCD Treatment Study evaluated a stepped treatment approach (ie, CBT followed by either continued CBT or sertraline for non-responders) in a large sample of affected children and adolescents.[113] At 3-year follow-up, 90% of participants were responders and 73% were in clinical remission.[113] The extended treatment option (either CBT or sertraline) did not affect treatment outcomes, suggesting that these evidence-based treatments have long-term beneficial effects.[113]

SUMMARY

There are several facets of childhood OCD that differentiate it from the condition in adults. In children experiencing this disorder, obsessional content often reflects developmental stage and neurodevelopmental comorbidities are frequently present. Likewise, children may show less insight and more FA which should be targets of treatment. Given these complexities, the management of OCD in youth generally calls for specialist knowledge and care. Symptoms can affect all aspects of a child's life, including school performance, relationships with friends and family, and ability to engage in age-appropriate activities. CBT and SSRIs have been shown to be effective by a robust body of clinical research and can lead to sustained symptom relief.

CLINICS CARE POINTS

- Most cases of obsessive–compulsive disorder (OCD) begin during childhood or adolescence, though there is often a substantial lag between onset of symptoms and detection by adults and clinicians. Early recognition and intervention are needed to alleviate distress and impairment with as little delay as possible.

- There are validated measures available that can be used by providers to screen for obsessive–compulsive symptoms in children. There are also validated measures to track obsessive–compulsive symptoms over the course of treatment and to assess related symptoms such as tics, depression, anxiety, and family accommodation.

- Children often involve parents and family members in their obsessive–compulsive symptomatology. Such family accommodation counters the principles of treatment and works to maintain symptoms. Effective treatment will involve family psychoeducation and reduction of accommodation.

- Cognitive behavioral therapy involving exposure and response prevention is the first-line treatment for obsessive-compulsive symptoms in children. There are several indications for medication use in children with OCD and in these cases selective serotonin reuptake inhibitors are the first-line choice.

DISCLOSURE

The authors have no disclosures.

REFERENCES

1. American Psychiatric Association. Obsessive-compulsive and related disorders. *Diagnostic and statistical manual of mental disorders*. 5th edition 2013.
2. Geller D, Biederman J, Jones J, et al. Is juvenile obsessive-compulsive disorder a developmental subtype of the disorder? A review of the pediatric literature. J Am Acad Child Adolesc Psychiatry 1998;37(4):420–7.
3. Fineberg NA, Dell'Osso B, Albert U, et al. Early intervention for obsessive compulsive disorder: An expert consensus statement. *Eur Neuropsychopharmacol* 2019;29(4):549–65.
4. Geller DA, Homayoun S, Johnson G. Developmental considerations in obsessive compulsive disorder: Comparing pediatric and adult-onset cases. Front Psychiatry 2021;12:1–15.
5. Geller D, Biederman J, Faraone SV, Bellorde CA, Kim GS, Hagermoser LM. Disentangling chronological age from age of onset in children and adolescents with obsessive compulsive disorder. Int J Neuropsychopharmacol 2001;4:169–78.
6. Flament MF, Whitaker A, Rapoport J, et al. Obsessive-compulsive disorder in adolescence: An epidemiological study. J Am Acad Child Adolesc Psychiatry 1988;27(6):764–71.
7. Heyman I, Fombonne E, Simmons H, Ford T, Meltzer H, Goodman R. Prevalence of obsessive-compulsive disorder in the British nationwide survey of child mental health. Br J Psychiatry 2001;179(4):324–9.
8. Pinto A, Mancebo MC, Eisen JL, Pagano ME, Rasmussen SA. The Brown Longitudinal Obsessive-Compulsive Study: Clinical features and symptoms of the sample at intake. J Clin Psychiatry 2006;67(5):703–11.
9. Rapoport J, Inoff-Germain G, Weissman MM, et al. Childhood obsessive-compulsive disorder in the NIMH MECA study: Parent versus child identification of cases. J Anxiety Disord 2000;14(6):535–48.
10. Browne HA, Hansen SN, Buxbaum JD, et al. Familial clustering of tic disorders and obsessive-compulsive disorder. JAMA Psychiatry 2015;72(4):359–66.

11. Fontenelle LF, Mendlowicz MV, Versiani M. The descriptive epidemiology of obsessive–compulsive disorder. Prog Neuropsychopharmacol Biol Psychiatry 2006;30(3):327–37.

12. Storch E, De Nadai A, Jacob M, et al. Phenomenology and correlates of insight in pediatric obsessive-compulsive disorder. Compr Psychiatry 2014;55(3): 613–20.

13. Swedo SE, Rapoport JL, Leonard H, Lenane M, Cheslow D. Obsessive-compulsive disorder in children and adolescents: Clinical phenomenology of 70 consecutive cases. Arch Gen Psychiatry 1989;46(4):335–41.

14. Geller D, Biederman J, Faraone SV, et al. Clinical correlates of obsessive compulsive disorder in children and adolescents referred to specialized and non-specialized clinical settings. Depress Anxiety 2000;11(4):163–8.

15. Rasmussen SA, Eisen J. The epidemiology and clinical features of obsessive compulsive disorder. Psychiatr Clin 1992;15(4):743–58.

16. Dell'Osso B, Benatti B, Hollander E, et al. Childhood, adolescent and adult age at onset and related clinical correlates in obsessive-compulsive disorder: a report from the International College of Obsessive-Compulsive Spectrum Disorders (ICOCS). Int J Psychiatry Clin Pract 2016;20(4):210–7.

17. Mancebo MC, Garcia AM, Pinto A, et al. Juvenile-onset OCD: clinical features in children, adolescents and adults. Acta Psychiatr Scand 2008;118(2):149–59.

18. Masi G, Millepiedi S, Mucci M, et al. A naturalistic study of referred children and adolescents with obsessive-compulsive disorder. J Am Acad Child Adolesc Psychiatry 2005;44(7):673–81.

19. Geller D, Biederman J, Agranat A, et al. Developmental aspects of obsessive compulsive disorder: Findings in children, adolescents and adults. J Nerv Ment Dis 2001;189(7):471–7.

20. Dalsgaard S, Thorsteinsson E, Trabjerg BB, et al. Incidence Rates and Cumulative Incidences of the Full Spectrum of Diagnosed Mental Disorders in Childhood and Adolescence. JAMA Psychiatry 2019. https://doi.org/10.1001/jamapsychiatry.2019.3523.

21. Mathis M, Alvarenga P, Funaro G, et al. Gender differences in obsessive-compulsive disorder: A literature review. Rev Bras Psiquiatr 2011;33(4):390–9.

22. Sharma E, Sharma LP, Balachander S, et al. Comorbidities in obsessive-compulsive disorder across the lifespan: A systematic review and meta-analysis. Front Psychiatry 2021;12:703701.

23. Geller DA, Biederman J, Stewart ES, et al. Impact of comorbidity on treatment response to paroxetine in pediatric obsessive-compulsive disorder: Is the use of exclusion criteria empirically supported in randomized clinical trials? J Child Adolesc Psychopharmacol 2003;13(1):S19–29.

24. van Grootheest DS, Cath DC, Beekman AT, et al. Twin studies on obsessive-compulsive disorder: A review. Twin Res Hum Genet 2005;8(5):450–8.

25. Nestadt G, Samuels J, Riddle M, et al. A family study of obsessive compulsive disorder. Arch Gen Psychiatry 2000;57(4):358–63.

26. Taylor S. Early versus late onset obsessive-compulsive disorder: evidence for distinct subtypes. Clin Psychol Rev 2011;31(7):1083–100.

27. Hanna G, Himle JA, Curtis GC, et al. A family study of obsessive-compulsive disorder with pediatric probands. Am J Med Genet 2005;134B(1):13–9.

28. Pauls D, Alsobrook J II, Goodman W, et al. A family study of obsessive-compulsive disorder. Am J Psychiatry 1995;152(1):76–84.

29. Mattheisen M, Samuesl JF, Wang Y, et al. Genome-wide assocation study in obsessive-compulsive disorder: Results from the OCGAS. Mol Psychiatry 2015;20:337–44.
30. Stewart S, Yu D, Scharf J, et al. Genome-wide association study of obsessive-compulsive disorder. Mol Psychiatry 2013;18:788–98.
31. Strom NI, Yu D, Gerring ZF, et al. Genome-wide association study identifies new locus associated with OCD. bioRxiv 2021. https://doi.org/10.1101/2021.10.13.21261078.
32. Cross-Disorder Group of the Psychiatric Genomic Consortium. Genomic relationships, novel loci, pleiotropic mechanisms across eight psychiatric disorders. Cell 2019;179(7):1469–82, e11.
33. Sinopoli VM, Erdman L, Burton CL, et al. Serotonin system gene variants and regional brain volume differences in pediatric OCD. Brain Imaging Behav 2020;14(5):1612–25.
34. Arnold P, Sicard T, Burroughs E, et al. Glutamate transporter gene SLC1A1 associated with obsessive-oompulsive disorder. Arch Gen Psychiatry 2006;63(7):717–20.
35. Lebowitz ER, Panza KE, Su J, et al. Family accommodation in obsessive-compulsive disorder. Expert Rev Neurother 2012;12(2):229–38.
36. Peris TS, Bergman RL, Langley A, et al. Correlates of accommodation of pediatric obsessive-compulsive disorder: parent, child, and family characteristics. J Am Acad Child Adolesc Psychiatry 2008;47(10):1173–81.
37. Stewart E, Beresin C, Haddad S, et al. Predictors of family accommodation in obsessive-compulsive disorder. Ann Clin Psychiatry 2008;20(2):65–70.
38. Wu MS, Lewin AB, Murphy TK, et al. Phenomenological considerations of family accommodation: Related clinical characteristics and family factors in pediatric obsessive–compulsive disorder. J Obsessive Compuls Relat Disord 2014;3(3):228–35.
39. Wu MS, Geller DA, Schneider SC, et al. Comorbid psychopathology and the clinical profile of family accommodation in pediatric OCD. Child Psychiatry Hum Dev 21 2019;50(5):717–26.
40. Jacoby RJ, Smilansky H, Shin J, et al. Longitudinal trajectory and predictors of change in family accommodation during exposure therapy for pediatric OCD. J Anxiety Disord 2021;83:102463.
41. Storch EA, Geffken GR, Merlo LJ, et al. Family accommodation in pediatric obsessive-compulsive disorder. J Clin Child Adolesc Psychol 2007;36(2):207–16.
42. Stewart SE, Rosario MC, Brown TA, et al. Principal components analysis of obsessive-compulsive disorder symptoms in children and adolescents. Biol Psychiatry 2007;61(3):285–91.
43. Mataix-Cols D, Nakatani E, Micali N, et al. Structure of obsessive-compulsive symptoms in pediatric OCD. J Am Acad Child Adolesc Psychiatry 2008;47(7):773–8.
44. Fernández de la Cruz L, Barrow F, Bolhuis K, et al. Sexual obsessions in pediatric obsessive-compulsive disorder: Clinical characteristics and treatment outcomes. Depress Anxiety 2013;30(8):732–40.
45. Farrell L, Barrett P, Piacentini J. Obsessive-compulsive disorder across the developmental trajectory: Clinical correlates in children, adolescents and adults. Behav Change 2006;23(2):103–20.
46. Hojgaard D, Skarphedinsson G, Ivarsson T, et al. Hoarding in children and adolescents with obsessive-compulsive disorder: prevalence, clinical correlates,

and cognitive behavioral therapy outcome. Eur Child Adolesc Psychiatry 2019; 28(8):1097–106.

47. Storch EA, Lack CW, Merlo LJ, et al. Clinical features of children and adolescents with obsessive-compulsive disorder and hoarding symptoms. Compr Psychiatry 2007;48(4):313–8.

48. Rozenman M, McGuire J, Wu M, et al. Hoarding symptoms in children and adolescents with obsessive-compulsive disorder: Clinical features and response to cognitive behavioral therapy. J Am Acad Child Adolesc Psychiatry 2019;58(8): 799–805.

49. Labad J, Menchon JM, Alonso P, et al. Gender differences in obsessive-compulsive symptom dimensions. Depress Anxiety 2008;25(10):832–8.

50. Nakatani E, Krebs G, Micali N, et al. Children with very early onset obsessive-compulsive disorder: Clinical features and treatment outcome. J Child Psychol Psychiatry 2011;52(12):1261–8.

51. Storch EA, Milsom VA, Merlo LJ, et al. Insight in pediatric obsessive-compulsive disorder: associations with clinical presentation. Psychiatry Res 2008;160(2): 212–20.

52. Selles RR, Storch E, Lewin A. Variations in symptom prevalence and clinical correlates in younger versus older youth with obsessive-compulsive disorder. Child Psychiatry Hum Dev 2014;45(6):666–74.

53. Storch EA, Larson MJ, Merlo LJ, et al. Comorbidity of pediatric obsessive-compulsive disorder and anxiety disorders: Impact on symptom severity and impairment. J Psychopathol Behav Assess 2008;30(2):111–20.

54. Geller DA, Coffey BJ, Faraone S, et al. Does comorbid attention-deficit/ hyperactivity disorder impact the clinical expression of pediatric obsessive compulsive disorder? CNS Spectr 2003;8(4):259–64.

55. Sukhodolsky DG, do Rosario-Campos MC, Scahill L, et al. Adaptive, emotional, and family functioning of children with obsessive-compulsive disorder and comorbid attention deficit hyperactivity disorder. Am J Psychiatry 2005;162(2): 1125–32.

56. Storch EA, Merlo LJ, Larson MJ, et al. Impact of comorbidity on cognitive-behavioral therapy response in pediatric obsessive-compulsive disorder. J Am Acad Child Adolesc Psychiatry 2008;47(5):583–92.

57. Swedo SE, Leonard HL, Garvey M, et al. Pediatric autoimmune neuropsychiatric disorders associated with streptococcal infections: Clinical description of the first 50 cases. Am J Psychiatry 1998;155(2):264–71.

58. Swedo SE, Leckman JF, Rose NR. From research subgroup to clinical syndrome: Modifying the PANDAS criteria to describe PANS (pediatric acute-onset neuropsychiatric syndrome). Pediatr Therapeut 2012;2(2):1–8.

59. Xu J, Liu R-J, Fahey S, et al. Antibodies from children with PANDAS bind specifically to striatal cholinergic interneurons and alter their activity. Am J Psychiatry 2021;178(1):48–64.

60. Frick L, Rapanelli M, Jindachomthong K, et al. Differential binding of anitbodies in PANDAS patients to cholinergic interneurons in the striatum. Brain Behav Immun 2018;69:304–11.

61. Piacentini J, Bergman L, Keller M, et al. Functional impairment in children and adolescents with obsessive-compulsive disorder. J Child Adolesc Psychopharmacol 2003;13(1):S61–9.

62. Storch EA, Larson MJ, Muroff J, et al. Predictors of functional impairment in pediatric obsessive-compulsive disorder. J Anxiety Disord 2010;24(2):275–83.

63. du Plessis LJ, Lochner C, Louw D, et al. A comprehensive view of functional impairment in children and adolescents with obsessive-compulsive disorder adds value. Early Interv Psychiatry 2021;1–8.

64. Geller DA, Abramovitch A, Mittelman A, et al. Neurocognitive function in paediatric obsessive-compulsive disorder. World J Biol Psychiatry 2018;1–10.

65. Valderhaug R, Ivarsson T. Functional impairment in clinical samples of Norwegian and Swedish children and adolescents with obsessive-compulsive disorder. Eur Child Adolesc Psychiatry 2005;14(3):164–73.

66. Stewart SE, Hu YP, Leung A, et al. A multisite study of family functioning impairment in pediatric obsessive-compulsive disorder. J Am Acad Child Adolesc Psychiatry 2017;56(3):241–9.

67. Murphy YE, Flessner CA. Family functioning in paediatric obsessive compulsive and related disorders. Br J Clin Psychol 2015;54(4):414–34.

68. Storch EA, Lehmkuhl H, Pence SL, et al. Parental experiences of having a child with obsessive-compulsive disorder: Associations with clinical characteristics and caregiver adjustment. J child Fam Stud 2009;18(3):249–58.

69. Bennett SD, Coughtrey AE, Shafran R, et al. Measurement issues: The measurement of obsessive-compulsive disorder in children and young people in clinical practice. Child Adolesc Ment Health 2017;22(2):100–12.

70. Rapp AM, Bergman RL, Piacentini J, et al. Evidence-based assessment of obsessive-compulsive disorder. J Cent Nerv Syst Dis 2016;2016(8):13–29.

71. Scahill L, Riddle M, McSwiggin-Hardin M, et al. Children's Yale-Brown Obsessive Compulsive Scale: Reliability and validity. J Am Acad Child Adolesc Psychiatry 1997;36(6):844–52.

72. Cervin M, Mataix-Cols D. Empirical severity benchmarks for obsessive-compulsive disorder across the lifespan. World Psychiatry 2022;21(2):315–6.

73. Farhat L, Vattimo E, Ramakrishnan D, et al. Systematic review and meta-analysis: An empirical approach to defining treatment response and remission in pediatric obsessive-compulsive disorder. J Am Acad Child Adolesc Psychiatry 2022;61(4):495–507.

74. Storch EA, McGuire JF, Wu MS, et al. Development and psychometric evaluation of the Children's Yale-Brown Obsessive-Compulsive Scale Second Edition. J Am Acad Child Adolesc Psychiatry 2019;58(1):92–8.

75. Foa E, Coles M, Huppert J, et al. Development and validation of a child version of the Obsessive Compulsive Inventory. Behav Ther 2010;41(1):121–32.

76. Rough H, Hanna B, Gillett C, et al. Screening for pediatric obsessive-compulsive disorder using the Obsessive-Compulsive Inventory - Child Version. Child Psychiatry Hum Dev 2020;51(6):888–99.

77. Abramovitch A, Abramowitz JS, McKay D, et al. The OCI-CV-R: A revision of the Obsessive-Compulsive Inventory - Child Version. J Anxiety Disord 2022;86:102532.

78. McGuire JF, Geller DA, Murphy TK, et al. Defining treatment outcomes in pediatric obsessive-compulsive disorder using a self-report scale. Behav Ther 2019;50(2):314–24.

79. Nelson EC, Hanna GL, Hudziak JJ, et al. Obsessive-compulsive scale of the Child Behavior Checklist: Specificity, sensitivity, and predictive power. Pediatrics 2001;108(1):e14.

80. Storch E, Murphy T, Bagner D, et al. Reliability and validity of the Child Behavior Checklist Obsessive-Compulsive Scale. J Anxiety Disord 2006;20(4):473–85.

81. Hudziak J, Althoff R, Stanger C, et al. The Obsessive Compulsive Scale of the Child Behavior Checklist predicts obsessive-compulsive disorder: A receiver

operating characteristic curve analysis. J Child Adolesc Psychiatry 2006;47(2): 160–6.

82. Ivarsson T, Larsson B. The Obsessive-Compulsive Symptom (OCS) scale of the Child Behavior Checklist: A comparison between Swedish children with Obsessive-Compulsive Disorder from a specialized unit, regular outpatients and a school sample. J Anxiety Disord 2007;22(7):1172–9.

83. Geller DA, Doyle R, Shaw D, et al. A quick and reliable screening measure for OCD in youth: reliability and validity of the obsessive compulsive scale of the Child Behavior Checklist. Compr Psychiatry 2006;47(3):234–40.

84. Piacentini J, Peris T, Bergman L, et al. Functional impairment in childhood OCD: development and psychometrics properties of the Child Obsessive-Compulsive Impact Scale-Revised (COIS-R). J Clin Child Adolesc Psychol 2007;36(4): 645–53.

85. Piacentini J, Bergman R, Chang S, et al. Controlled comparison of family cognitive behavioral therapy and psychoeducation/relaxation training for child obsessive-compulsive disorder. J Am Acad Child Adolesc Psychiatry 2011; 50(11):1149–61.

86. Calvocoressi L, Mazure C, Kasl S, et al. Family accommodation in obsessive-compulsive disorder symptoms: Instrument development and assessment of family behavior. J Nerv Ment Dis 1999;187(10):636–42.

87. Merlo LJ, Lehmkuhl HD, Geffken GR, et al. Decreased family accommodation associated with improved therapy outcome in pediatric obsessive-compulsive disorder. J Consult Clin Psychol 2009;77(2):355–60.

88. Poznanski E, Grossman J, Buchsbaum Y, et al. Preliminary studies of the reliability and validity of the Children's Depression Rating Scale. J Am Acad Child Psychiatry 1984;23(2):191–7.

89. Mayes T, Bernstein I, Haley C, et al. Psychometric properties of the Children's Depression Rating Scale–Revised in adolescents. J Child Adolesc Psychopharmacol 2010;20(6):513–6.

90. Birmaher B, Khetarpal S, Brent D, et al. The Screen for Child Anxiety Related Emotional Disorders (SCARED): Scale construction and psychometric characteristics. J Am Acad Child Adolesc Psychiatry 1997;36(4):545–53.

91. Birmaher B, Brent D, Chiappetta L, et al. Psychometric properties of the Screen for Child Anxiety Related Emotional Disorders (SCARED): A replication study. J Am Acad Child Adolesc Psychiatry 1999;38(10):1230–6.

92. Rappaport B, Pagliaccio D, Pine D, et al. Discriminant validity, diagnostic utility, and parent-child agreement on the Screen for Child Anxiety Related Emotional Disorders (SCARED) in treatment- and non-treatment-seeking youth. J Anxiety Disord 2017;51:22–31. https://doi.org/10.1016/j.janxdis.2017.08.006.

93. Leckman J, Riddle M, Hardin M, et al. The Yale Global Tic Severity Scale: Initial testing of a clinician-rated scale of tic severity. J Am Acad Child Adolesc Psychiatry 1989;28(4):566–73.

94. Haas M, Jakubovski E, Fremer C, et al. Yale Global Tic Severity Scale (YGTSS): Psychometric quality of the gold standard for tic assessment based on the large-scale EMTICS study. Front Psychiatry 2021;12:626459.

95. Storch E, De Nadai A, Lewin A, et al. Defining treatment response in pediatric tic disorders: A signal detection analysis of the Yale Global Tic Severity Scale. J Child Adolesc Psychopharmacol 2011;21(6):621–7.

96. Uhre CF, Uhre VF, Lonfeldt NN, et al. Systematic review and meta-analysis: Cognitive-behavioral therapy for obsessive-compulsive disorder in children and adolescents. J Am Acad Child Adolesc Psychiatry 2020;59(1):64–77.

97. The Pediatric OCD Treatment Study (POTS) Team. Cognitive-behavior therapy, sertraline, and their combination for children and adolescents with obsessive-compulsive disorder: The pediatric OCD treatment study (POTS) randomized controlled trial. JAMA 2004;292(16):1969–76.

98. Franklin M, Sapyta J, Freeman J, et al. Cognitive behavior therapy augmentation of pharmacotherapy in pediatric obsessive-compulsive disorder: The pediatric OCD treatment study II (POTS II) randomized controlled trial. JAMA 2011; 306(11):1224–32.

99. Freeman J, Sapyta J, Garcia A, et al. Family-based treatment of early childhood obsessive-compulsive disorder:The pediatric obsessive-compulsive disorder treatment study for young children (POTS Jr)—A randomized clinical trial. JAMA Psychiatry 2014;71(6):689–98.

100. Geller DA, Biederman J, Stewart SE, et al. Which SSRI? A meta-analysis of pharmacotherapy trials in pediatric obsessive compulsive disorder. Am J Psychiatry 2003;160(11):1919–28.

101. Ivarsson T, Skarphedinsson G, Kornor H, et al. The place of and evidence for serotonin reuptake inhibitors (SRIs) for obsessive compulsive disorder (OCD) in children and adolescents: Views based on a systematic review and meta-analysis. Psychiatry Res 2015;227(1):93–103.

102. Kotapati VP, Khan AM, Dar S, et al. The effectiveness of selective serotonin reuptake inhibitors for treatment of obsessive-compulsive disorder in adolescents and children: A systematic review and meta-analysis. Front Psychiatry 2019; 10:523.

103. March JS, Biederman J, Wolkow R, et al. Sertraline in children and adolescents with obsessive-compulsive disorder: A multicenter randomized control trial. JAMA 1998;280(20):1752–6.

104. Geller DA, Wagner KD, Emslie G, et al. Paroxetine treatment in children and adolescents with obsessive-compulsive disorder: A randomized, multicenter, double-blind, placebo-controlled trial. J Am Acad Child Adolesc Psychiatry 2004;43(11):1387–96.

105. Geller DA, Hoog SL, Heiligenstein JH, et al. Fluoxetine treatment for obsessive-compulsive disorder in children and adolescents: A placebo-controlled clinical trial. J Am Acad Child Adolesc Psychiatry 2001;40(7):773–9.

106. Riddle MA, Reeve EA, Yaryura-Tobias JA, et al. Fluvoxamine for children and adolescents with obsessive-compulsive disorder: A randomized, controlled, multicenter trial. J Am Acad Child Adolesc Psychiatry 2001;40(2):222–9.

107. Alaghband-Rad J, Hakimshooshtary M. A randomized controlled clinical trial of citalopram versus fluoxetine in children and adolescents with obsessive-compulsive disorder. Eur Child Adolesc Psychiatry 2009;18(3):131–5.

108. Varigonda A, Jakubovski E, Bloch M. Systematic review and meta-analysis: early treatment responses of selective serotonin reuptake inhibitors and clomipramine in pediatric obsessive-compulsive disorder. J Am Acad Child Adolesc Psychiatry 2016;55(10):851–9.

109. Fornaro M, Anastasia A, Valchera A, et al. The FDA "black box" warning on antidepressant suicide risk in young adults: More harm than benefits? Front Psychiatry 2019;10:294.

110. Luft M, Lamy M, DelBello M, et al. Antidepressant-induced activation in children and adolescents: Risk, recognition, and management. Curr Probl Pediatr Adolesc Health Care 2018;48(2):50–62.

111. Sanchez-Meca J, Rosa-Alcazar AI, Iniesta-Sepulveda M, et al. Differential efficacy of cognitive-behavioral therapy and pharmacological treatments for

pediatric obsessive-compulsive disorder: a meta-analysis. J Anxiety Disord 2014;28(1):31–44.

112. Mancebo MC, Boisseau CL, Garnaat SL, et al. Long-term course of pediatric obsessive-compulsive disorder: 3 years of prospective follow-up. Compr Psychiatry 2014;55(7):1498–504.

113. Melin K, Skarphedinsson G, Thomsen P, et al. Treatment gains are sustainable in pediatric obsessive-compulsive disorder: Three-year follow-up from the NordLOTS. J Am Acad Child Adolesc Psychiatry 2020;59(2):244–53.

114. Zohar A, Ratzoni G, Binder M, et al. An epidemiological study of obsessive-compulsive disorder and related disorders in Israeli adolescents. J Am Acad Child Adolesc Psychiatry 1992;31(6):1057–61.

115. Zohar A, Ratzoni G, Binder M, et al. An epidemiological study of obsessive-compulsive disorder. and anxiety disorders in Israeli adolescents. Psychiatr Genet 1993;3:184.

116. Thomsen P. Obsessive-compulsive disorder in children and adolescents: self-reported obsessive-compulsive behaviour in pupils in Denmark. Acta Psychiatr Scand 1993;88:212–7.

117. Valleni-Basile L, Garrison CZ, Jackson KL, et al. Frequency of obsessive-compulsive disorder in a community sample of young adolescents. J Am Acad Child Adolesc Psychiatry 1994;33(6):782–91.

118. Douglass HM, Moffitt TE, Dar R, et al. Obsessive-compulsive disorder in a birth cohort of 18-year-olds: prevalence and predictors. J Am Acad Child Adolesc Psychiatry 1995;34:1424–31.

119. Apter A, Fallon TJ, King RA, et al. Obsessive-compulsive characteristics: from symptoms to syndrome. J Am Acad Child Adolesc Psychiatry 1996;35(7):907–12.

The Pharmacological Treatment of Obsessive-Compulsive Disorder

Christopher Pittenger, MD, PhD*

KEYWORDS

- Obsessive-compulsive disorder (OCD) • Pharmacotherapy
- Selective serotonin reuptake inhibitor (SSRI) • Clomipramine • Neuroleptic
- Glutamate

KEY POINTS

- Pharmacotherapy with selective serotonin reuptake inhibitors (SSRIs) and appropriate cognitive-behavioral therapy with exposure and response prevention (CBT/ERP) are both first-line treatments for obsessive-compulsive disorder (OCD); they can be administered alone or in combination.
- The SSRIs and the older tricyclic drug clomipramine have been robustly shown to be of benefit in OCD. Other antidepressants are less effective or have not been adequately studied.
- Optimal SSRI response requires high doses and a long duration of treatment.
- The best-supported augmentation strategy is the addition of low doses of neuroleptic, especially risperidone and aripiprazole.
- Several other augmentation strategies have been investigated and are sometimes used in refractory disease, but none have a solid evidentiary basis.

INTRODUCTION

Obsessive-compulsive disorder (OCD) is an enormous source of morbidity and public health impact, in the United States and worldwide.[1,2] It affects approximately 1.3% of the population—one person in 80—in any given year, and 2.7%—more than one person in 40—over the course of a lifetime.[3,4] Half of patients with OCD describe their symptoms as causing severe distress or impairment.[5]

OCD is defined by the presence of obsessions and/or compulsions.[6] Obsessions are defined as recurrent and persistent thoughts, images, or urges that are typically experienced as intrusive and unwanted and as irrational or excessive, that lead to

Departments of Psychiatry, Psychology, and Child Study Center, and Center for Brain and Mind Health, Yale University
* Corresponding author. 34 Park Street, Room 335, New Haven, CT 06519.
E-mail address: christopher.pittenger@yale.edu

Psychiatr Clin N Am 46 (2023) 107–119
https://doi.org/10.1016/j.psc.2022.11.005
0193-953X/23/© 2022 Elsevier Inc. All rights reserved.

marked distress or significant impairment. In many cases, they can be understood as common intrusive thoughts that are maladaptively interpreted as powerful and important.[7] Compulsions are repetitive or stereotyped actions, manifest or mental, that are performed to mitigate the anxiety or distress associated with obsessions but are clearly irrational or excessive. Most individuals with OCD have both obsessions and compulsions, and there is usually a functional relationship between the two.[7] Most individuals with OCD have good insight into the excessive and maladaptive nature of their obsessions and compulsions; unfortunately, this insight does little to reduce the insistent nature of the symptoms.[8]

A robust evidence base defines first- and second-line pharmacological and psychotherapeutic treatment strategies for individuals with OCD, and a majority of patients can achieve a reasonable therapeutic response when appropriately treated.[9] Several practice guidelines have been published, and they agree, for the most part, on early steps of treatment.[10–14] First-line treatment consists of pharmacotherapy with selective serotonin reuptake inhibitors (SSRIs) or cognitive behavioral therapy using the technique of exposure with response prevention (CBT/ERP), alone or in combination. Unfortunately, a substantial minority of patients, around 30%, do not adequately respond to standard treatments. Evidence to guide further treatment when first- and second-line treatment prove inadequate is limited.

This article summarizes standard strategies for the pharmacotherapy of adult OCD, and some of the less well-established options when first- and second-line treatments provide insufficient relief, or are not tolerated. Although the focus here is on pharmacotherapy, comprehensive treatment planning should always consider the role of appropriate psychotherapy. Optimal treatment of moderate or severe illness, or of OCD symptoms complicated by comorbidity, typically requires that both modalities be used. This review does not seek to be comprehensive; the reader is referred to other recent reviews for more exhaustive summaries of the recent literature and to current treatment guidelines for more details.[10,11,14–16] The goal here is to summarize the issues that are most relevant to the practicing psychiatrist, focusing on questions about pharmacotherapy that arise when formulating a treatment plan, both for first-line treatment and for refractory symptoms.

FIRST-LINE PHARMACOLOGICAL TREATMENT OF OCD: SSRI MONOTHERAPY

All clinical guidelines and expert opinion agree that monotherapy with the SSRIs is the first-line pharmacotherapy of choice.[9–15,17] The efficacy of SSRI treatment in OCD, compared with placebo, has been shown in multiple studies and summarized by definitive meta-analyses.[9,18] In contrast, other monotherapies have been disappointing (with the exception of clomipramine, to which we return below). Trials of combined serotonin-norepinephrine reuptake inhibitors (SNRIs) have been small and have yielded decidedly mixed results.[19] There have been no controlled trials of bupropion, but clinical experience suggests a lack of efficacy—indeed, that it can even worsen anxiety. There have been no trials of the newer agents agomelatine, brexanolone, vortioxetine, and vilazadone.

Which SSRI is best?

When contemplating initiation of an SSRI in clinical practice, a first question is which agent to choose. There are six SSRIs available in the United States: fluoxetine, fluvoxamine, sertraline, paroxetine, citalopram, and escitalopram. Only the first four of these are approved by the US Food and Drug Administration for use in OCD, but the latter two are also well supported by controlled data and are frequently used off-label.[9,14]

Escitalopram is also approved for the treatment of OCD in Europe. Fluvoxamine was the first SSRI shown to be effective for OCD,[20] and for many years it was marketed as the preferred medication for this indication. However, comparison of controlled studies does not support this practice and suggests that all six SSRIs are of similar efficacy.[9,21] Indeed, fluvoxamine tends to have more side effects and more interactions with other medications than some of the other SSRIs.

Given that they are of similar efficacy, other factors influence the choice of agent. Patient preference, due to past success, use by a family member, or other factors, can be determinative. Pharmacokinetics can be an important factor; fluoxetine has the longest half-life of the available SSRIs and so can be a good choice for individuals who have difficulty taking their medication regularly, whereas paroxetine has the shortest half-life.

Side effects can be a consideration; some are class effects and are shared across all of the agents, whereas others are off-target effects that are specific to one or another agent. Common side effects across the class include nausea, changes in bowel habits, increased anxiety/agitation with dose change, sleep changes, and sexual side effects. An increase in suicidal thinking has been seen in children and adolescents; it is less clear that this is a problem when treating adults. Agent-specific side effects include anticholinergic effects (more pronounced with fluvoxamine and paroxetine), weight gain (same), and prolongation of the QT interval (most pronounced with citalopram). This last effect led to a black-box warning and restricted dosing range for citalopram, especially in older patients; although expert opinions vary as to the necessity of this warning,[22] it has steered many practitioners away from the use of citalopram, especially at high doses. Periodic EKG monitoring is advisable. Similar concerns have been raised for escitalopram.

Pharmacogenetic testing is available, at a cost, and purports to inform the choice of medication for individual patients. However, the utility of these analyses has not been clearly shown, and they cannot generally be recommended.[23] It is to be hoped that with advancing knowledge the predictive value of genetic testing will improve.

SSRI Dosing

Although SSRI doses in the standard antidepressant range (eg, fluoxetine 10 to 40, sertraline 50 to 200) can be of benefit in OCD, multiple-dose studies and meta-analysis have shown that higher doses produce, on average, greater benefit, with only a small increase in dropout due to side effects (**Figs. 1 and 2**).[24] Therefore, a common practice is to push the dose to higher levels than one would in the treatment of depression, if problematic side effects do not emerge. When SSRI treatment at moderate dose produces a measurable but incomplete response and there are not problematic side effects, increasing the dose may be a better next step than switching SSRIs or adding an augmentation agent. A caveat must again be made in the case of citalopram, for which increasing the dose is contraindicated by the black-box warning and the concern about QTc prolongation at higher doses.

Commonly used high doses of the SSRIs, as listed in recent treatment guidelines, are 60 to 80 mg/dy of fluoxetine, 30 to 40 mg/dy of escitalpram, 300 mg/dy of fluvoxamine, and 60 mg/dy of paroxetine.[10] Higher doses may be used in select cases.

Duration of Treatment

Response to SSRI treatment is slower in OCD than in depression. Indeed, clinical lore has been that there is no response to SSRI treatment until after many weeks. Such a pattern would have implications for plausible drug mechanisms. Recent meta-analysis suggests, however, that this is not the case; rather, benefit seems to begin shortly after the initiation of treatment but to accrue slowly, such that clinically measurable change,

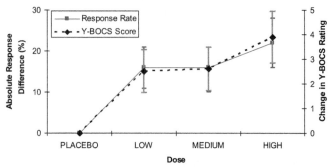

Fig. 1. SSRI dose–response relationship. *, different from placebo at *P* <.05; #, different from low dose at *P* <.05; ^, different from medium dose at *P* <.05. (*From* Bloch MH, McGuire J, Landeros-Weisenberger A, Leckman JF, Pittenger C. Meta-analysis of the dose-response relationship of SSRI in obsessive-compulsive disorder. Mol Psychiatry. 2010 Aug;15(8):850-5. https://doi.org/10.1038/mp.2009.50. Epub 2009 May 26. PMID: 19468281; PMCID: PMC2888928.)

at both the individual and the group level, is not identifiable with confidence until after several weeks.[25] A typical SSRI trial lasts 8 to 12 weeks; a common error in clinical practice is to declare a trial a failure and a patient refractory to SSRI treatment without reaching adequate medication dosage and duration. Although most research studies end at 12 weeks, improvement can continue beyond this point, and response rates in longer trials are higher.[26–28] Because other pharmacological options, to which we turn below, often have more side effects than the SSRIs, it is important to optimize an SSRI trial before moving on.

What happens when SSRIs fail? A first SSRI trial, of adequate dose and duration, is of benefit to perhaps 40% of patients treated, though the exact percentage varies from study to study. There are several options to pursue when initial response is inadequate:

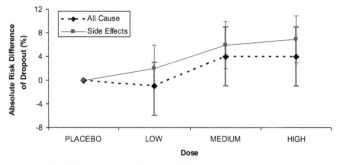

Fig. 2. SSRI dose–tolerability relationship. *, different from placebo at *P* <.05; #, different from low dose at *P* <.05. (*From* Bloch MH, McGuire J, Landeros-Weisenberger A, Leckman JF, Pittenger C. Meta-analysis of the dose-response relationship of SSRI in obsessive-compulsive disorder. Mol Psychiatry. 2010 Aug;15(8):850-5. https://doi.org/10.1038/mp. 2009.50. Epub 2009 May 26. PMID: 19468281; PMCID: PMC2888928.)

- Ensure that dose and duration of the trial are adequate (see above).
- Ensure that the patient is in fact taking the medication on a daily basis as prescribed. Although there are not careful studies examining the impact of irregular medication compliance on efficacy, the reduction in benefit may be substantial. This may be minimized by using an agent with a longer half-life, such as fluoxetine, though again there is little rigorous data to back up this expert guidance.
- Initiate, optimize, or increase the intensity of CBT/ERP.
- Consider a trial of a second SSRI. Clinical experience, and studies in major depressive disorder, suggest that the likelihood of response to a second SSRI after failing to respond to a first is reduced, perhaps 10% to 20%[29]; nevertheless, because of their favorable side effect profile, a second SSRI trial is often chosen as the next step.
- Consider switching to clomipramine monotherapy (see below).
- Consider augmentation with a second agent (see below).

Duration of treatment. When SSRI treatment does work well, a new question arises: how long should one treat? Moderate to severe OCD is often a chronic condition,[30] and long-term treatment is generally advised.[6,14] Relapse following the discontinuation of effective treatment is common.[31] Cognitive-behavioral therapy may mitigate the risk of relapse following SSRI discontinuation.[32,33]

CLOMIPRAMINE

The older tricyclic drug clomipramine was the first antidepressant shown to be of benefit in the treatment of OCD[34-37]; its efficacy is supported by a large literature and is borne out by recent meta-analyses.[9] Interestingly, other tricyclics do not appear to be of benefit; for example, in an early randomized comparison trial, benefit was seen in OCD patients treated with clomipramine but not those treated with amitriptyline.[38] Clomipramine is the most serotonergic of the tricyclics, which may explain its particular efficacy in the treatment of OCD.

Clomipramine vs SSRIs. Clomipramine is widely believed to be slightly superior to the SSRIs in the treatment of OCD, and it is often recommended as an option for the treatment of SSRI-refractory symptoms.[10] Superiority to the SSRIs was suggested by early meta-analyses,[21,39,40] though it was never been proven in head-to-head trials. More recently it has been suggested that the appearance of greater response to clomipramine in controlled trials may be an artifact of the fact that these trials were older and on a largely treatment-naïve population; the most recent meta-analyses do not show superiority of clomipramine over SSRIs.[9] Nevertheless, clomipramine monotherapy is often used as a second- or third-line treatment, when response to initial SSRI monotherapy is inadequate.[6,14]

Management of clomipramine. Clomipramine is not typically used as a first-line treatment because it has more side effects and is more difficult to manage than the SSRIs. Common problematic side effects relate to anticholinergic and histaminergic effects and include weight gain, dry mouth, and sedation.[41] Potential toxic effects at higher doses include arrhythmia and a lowering of the seizure threshold.[42] Because of these potential adverse effects, regular monitoring of serum levels is advised; levels outside of this range are associated with poor outcomes and more side effects.[43]

Clomipramine as an augmentation agent. Some investigators have examined the addition of clomipramine to SSRI treatment, or of an SSRI to clomipramine.[29] The logic is that the benefits of the agents might be combined while minimizing the risk of the side effects associated with higher clomipramine doses. However, the literature on this pharmacological strategy is sparse.

Modulating the metabolism of clomipramine. Clomipramine has an active metabolite, desmethylclomipramine (DCMI), that contributes to toxicity.[44] Conversion of clomipramine to DCMI is mediated by several cytochrome P450 enzymes in the liver and can be reduced by medications that inhibit the relevant enzymes (CYP1A2, CYP2C19, and CYP3A4), including fluvoxamine.[45] This has led to the suggestion that coadministration of a low dose of fluvoxamine with a therapeutic dose of clomipramine can bias metabolism to give higher serum levels of clomipramine relative to DCMI.[45,46] This pharmacological strategy has not been tested in controlled studies.

AUGMENTATION: NEUROLEPTICS

Unfortunately, many individuals with OCD do not achieve substantial improvement of their symptoms with SSRI or clomipramine treatment alone. No other agents have been shown to be of benefit when used as monotherapy. Therefore, third-line pharmacological treatment entails augmentation—the addition of a second agent. Although again emphasizing the importance of optimizing psychotherapy in individuals who are refractory to initial attempts at treatment,[47] we now turn to a summary of available pharmacological augmentation strategies.

The best-proven pharmacological augmentation strategy is the addition of a low dose of a D2 antagonist—a first- or second-generation neuroleptic or antipsychotic. This was first shown with the potent first-generation/typical neuroleptic haloperidol.[48] Subsequent work has examined augmentation with several second-generation/atypical neuroleptics, including risperidone, olanzapine, quetiapine, and aripiprazole. Most studies have been small, and outcomes have varied; but meta-analysis convincingly shows the benefit of augmentation,[9,49–51] which is included as a principal second-line pharmacological strategy in major guidelines.[10,14] Neuroleptic augmentation has not been approved for this purpose by the US FDA, and so the use of these agents in OCD is off-label.

Interestingly, neuroleptic monotherapy does *not* appear to be of benefit, though few studies have examined it rigorously.[52] In fact, atypical neuroleptics, especially clozapine, can worsen or precipitate obsessive-compulsive symptoms.[9,53] A few case reports suggest that aripiprazole, uniquely, may be of benefit in some cases of OCD, and that it may be less likely to produce treatment-emergent OCD symptoms.[54] More work is needed here.

Which neuroleptic? As noted, studies of neuroleptic augmentation in OCD have been small, and the literature is not sufficiently robust to systematically compare the efficacy of the different agents. With this caveat, the best results have been reported for risperidone (three positive studies, one negative) and aripiprazole (two positive studies).[55] Only a single study of haloperidol augmentation has been reported; it was positive.[48] Results have been less promising, and not statistically significant in meta-analysis, for olanzapine, quetiapine, and paliperidone.[55] There have been no studies with the newer agents brexpiprazole, asenapine, iloperidone, or lurasidone. Therefore, although more work is needed to formulate definitive guidance, the current literature favors the use of risperidone or aripiprazole.

The earliest studies of neuroleptic augmentation in OCD were motivated in part by the efficacy of the high-potency D2 antagonists haloperidol, pimozide, and risperidone in the treatment of tic disorders, which are commonly comorbid with OCD. In these early studies, especially the first controlled study with haloperidol, greater benefit was seen in individuals with a history of tics.[48,49] This does not appear to be the case in more recent studies with the atypical neuroleptics, although analysis is limited by the fact that most studies did not stratify patients by presence or history of comorbid tics.[51] Although the data remain inconclusive, it is reasonable to select a higher-potency agent such as haloperidol or risperidone when treating a patient with current or historical comorbid tics.

Aripiprazole has a well-established role in the treatment of mood dysregulation, either depression or bipolar disorder.[56,57] It is therefore reasonable to select aripiprazole augmentation when treating a patient with refractory OCD and mood instability. However, there is not strong evidence to support this recommendation, which is best considered expert opinion.

Neuroleptic dosing. Early studies of haloperidol and risperidone used lower doses than are typically employed in the treatment of psychosis: typically ~6 mg for haloperidol and 0.5 to 2 mg for risperidone.[55] Aripiprazole doses have similarly been on the low end of the usual range at 10 to 15 mg. Meta-regression across published studies finds no association between augmentation dose and clinical response.[55] Thus, given the side effect profile of these agents, it is sensible to start with low doses, and to increase only slowly. This is in contrast to the higher doses of SSRIs that are generally recommended.

Neuroleptic discontinuation. When patients improve following neuroleptic augmentation, discontinuation may lead to relapse,[58] although the literature on this point is sparse. Therefore, if symptoms improve following initiation of neuroleptic augmentation, discussions of discontinuation should be approached with caution. On the other hand, a majority of OCD patients treated with neuroleptic augmentation will not respond—this strategy is effective in only 30% of patients, compared with 12.5% of those treated with placebo augmentation.[55] Given the often problematic side effects of neuroleptics, it is important not to leave patients on ineffective treatment. Available data suggest that the response to neuroleptic augmentation in OCD, when it occurs, is more rapid than the response to SSRI or clomipramine monotherapy; the mean duration of treatment in published trials is ~8 weeks.[55] Therefore, if there is no clear clinical benefit following 6 to 8 weeks of treatment, discontinuation should be considered.

AUGMENTATION: GLUTAMATE MODULATORS

There has been substantial interest over the past 20 years in the potential utility of modulators of the neurotransmitter glutamate as an augmentation strategy in refractory OCD.[17,59] The literature remains mixed, with no large definitive studies published to date. Nevertheless, several agents have been studied and merit consideration when better-established pharmacological strategies have proven inadequate.

Memantine. Memantine, a noncompetitive antagonist of the NMDA-class glutamate receptor, is used in the treatment of moderate-severity Alzheimer's disease.[60] Motivated by the hypothesis that elevated glutamate contributes to pathophysiology in some individuals with OCD,[59] several studies have examined the addition of memantine to standard pharmacotherapy in the treatment of refractory symptoms. A few studies have also examined memantine as monotherapy.[61] Doses have typically followed those used in Alzheimer's disease, most commonly 20 mg (10 mg twice daily). The literature on memantine in OCD is muddied by a cluster of four studies from a single geographic area, in Iran, that reported robust response rates far in excess of what others have observed, even in open-label studies.[62] The generalizability of these findings has been questioned[63]; robust controlled studies from a range of clinical and geographical contexts are needed to clarify the role of memantine in the treatment of refractory OCD.

Riluzole. Riluzole is approved for the treatment of amyotrophic lateral sclerosis and has been studied in several psychiatric conditions.[64] It has multiple effects on glutamate neurotransmission but may work primarily by enhancing glutamate reuptake by glial cells, buffering dysregulated or excessive levels of the neurotransmitter.[65] Early open-label reports[66,67] and two small controlled studies in adults[68,69] suggest benefit, though another controlled study in children was negative.[70] Riluzole is typically used at the standard dose of 100 mg (50 mg twice daily), though doses up to 200 mg daily have been reported. Side effects include nausea, sedation, and reversible effects on the liver that require monitoring. Riluzole has a strong negative food effect and must be taken on an empty stomach; this complicates compliance. More studies of this agent are needed.

Ketamine. The dissociative anesthetic ketamine was found to work as a rapidly acting antidepressant over twenty years ago and is now widely used clinically for this purpose.[28] A few studies have examined its use in OCD, with mixed results. A first open-label trial in refractory patients, many with comorbidities and many on other medications, found benefit to depressive symptoms but not to OCD.[71] A subsequent controlled trial in less sick patients, with limited comorbidities and on no medication, did find a rapid and robust benefit.[72] Ongoing clinical experience suggests that the benefit in refractory OCD is limited, though a minority of patients may experience significant improvement.[73] Current data support the use of ketamine to treat severe comorbid depression in individuals with OCD; its role in the treatment of OCD symptoms themselves is less clear, and more controlled studies are needed. Ketamine is typically administered intravenously in a specialized center. Experience in OCD with intranasal delivery of ketamine is limited[74]; there have been no studies with oral ketamine or with intranasal esketamine (Spravato), which is FDA-approved for the treatment of depression.

CONCLUSION

Pharmacotherapy remains a mainstay of the treatment of OCD. When deployed in conjunction with appropriate psychotherapy (CBT/ERP), evidence-based pharmacotherapy can support substantial symptom improvement in 60% to 70% of individuals suffering from OCD. Unfortunately, definitive evidence-based guidance is only available for first- and second-line treatment decisions. For a substantial minority of patients, the prescriber must turn to treatment strategies for which the evidentiary base is decidedly thin. Careful weighing of the probability of response, the strength of the evidence, and possible side effects is essential. More research is needed to extend current guidance and to develop novel interventions for the many patients whose symptoms do not respond to current tools.

DISCLOSURE

Dr C. Pittenger consults for Biohaven Pharmaceuticals, Ceruvia Lifesciences, Transcend Therapeutics, Freedom Biosciences, and Nobilis Therapeutics and receives research funding from Biohaven, Transcend, and Freedom. He has filed patents for neurofeedback and psychedelics in the treatment of obsessive-compulsive disorder, unrelated to the current work.

CLINICS CARE POINTS

- CBT with exposure and pharmacotherapy with the SSRIs are both first-line treatments for obsessive-compulsive disorder.

- All SSRIs are of equivalent efficacy as monotherapy in the treatment of OCD, though pharmacokinetics and side effects differ.
- High doses and long duration of treatment are typically required for optimal SSRI response.
- The tricyclic antidepressant clomipramine is effective as monotherapy and may be superior to SSRIs in some cases, but it has a higher side effect burden.
- CBT with extinction should always be considered when SSRI response is inadequate.
- Augmentation of SSRIs with low-dose neuroleptics can be of benefit in some patients.
- Augmentation of SSRIs with any of several glutamate modulating agents shows promise in research studies, but more investigation is needed.

REFERENCES

1. Hollander E, Doernberg E, Shavitt R, et al. The cost and impact of compulsivity: a research perspective. Eur Neuropsychopharmacol 2016;26(5):800–9.
2. Boisseau CL, Schhwartzman CM, Rasmussen SA. Quality of life and psychosocial functioning in OCD. In: Pittenger C, editor. Obsessive-compulsive disorder: phenomenology, pathophysiology, and treatment. New York: Oxford University Press; 2017. p. 57–64.
3. Kessler RC, Petukhova M, Sampson NA, et al. Twelve-month and lifetime prevalence and lifetime morbid risk of anxiety and mood disorders in the United States. Int J Methods Psychiatr Res 2012;21(3):169–84.
4. Torres AR, Fontenelle LH, Shhavitt RG, et al. Epidemiology, comorbidity, and burden of OCD. In: Pittenger C, editor. Obsessive-compulsive disorder: phenomenology, pathophysiology, and treatment. New York: Oxford University Press; 2017. p. 35–46.
5. Ruscio AM, Stein DJ, Chiu WT, et al. The epidemiology of obsessive-compulsive disorder in the National Comorbidity Survey Replication. Mol Psychiatry 2010; 15(1):53–63.
6. American Psychiatric Association. American Psychiatric Association. DSM-5 Task Force. *Diagnostic and statistical manual of mental disorders : DSM-5*. 5th ed. Washington, D.C.: American Psychiatric Association; 2013.
7. Pittenger C, Gruner P, Adams TA, et al. The dynamics of obsessive-compulsive disorder: A heuristic framework. In: Pittenger C, editor. Obsessive-compulsive disorder: phenomenology, pathophysiology, and treatment. New York: Oxford University Press; 2017. p. 669–82.
8. Hamblin RJ, Park JM, Wu MS, et al. Variable insight in OCD. In: Pittenger C, editor. Obsessive-compulsive disorder: phenomenology, pathophysiology, and treatment. New York: Oxford University Press; 2017. p. 129–36.
9. Skapinakis P, Caldwell DM, Hollingworth W, et al. Pharmacological and psychotherapeutic interventions for management of obsessive-compulsive disorder in adults: a systematic review and network meta-analysis. Lancet Psychiatry 2016;3(8):730–9.
10. Koran LM, Hanna GL, Hollander E, et al. Practice guideline for the treatment of patients with obsessive-compulsive disorder. Am J Psychiatry 2007;164(7 Suppl):5–53.
11. (NICE) NIoCE. Obsessive-compulsive disorder: core interventions in the treatment of obsessive-compulsive disorder and body dysmorphic disorder31. London: British Psychiatric Society & Royal College of Psychiatrists; 2006.

12. Bandelow B, Zohar J, Hollander E, et al. World Federation of Societies of Biological Psychiatry (WFSBP) guidelines for the pharmacological treatment of anxiety, obsessive-compulsive and post-traumatic stress disorders - first revision. World J Biol Psychiatry 2008;9(4):248–312.

13. Janardhan Reddy YC, Sundar AS, Narayanaswamy JC, et al. Clinical practice guidelines for Obsessive-Compulsive Disorder. Indian J Psychiatry 2017; 59(Suppl 1):S74–90.

14. Bandelow B, Allgulander C, Baldwin DS, et al. World Federation of Societies of Biological Psychiatry (WFSBP) guidelines for treatment of anxiety, obsessive-compulsive and posttraumatic stress disorders - Version 3. Part II: OCD and PTSD. World J Biol Psychiatry 2022;1–17. https://doi.org/10.1080/15622975. 2022.2086296.

15. Pittenger C, Brennan BP, Koran L, et al. Specialty knowledge and competency standards for pharmacotherapy for adult obsessive-compulsive disorder. Psychiatry Res 2021;300.

16. Skapinakis P, Caldwell DM, Hollingworth W, et al. Pharmacological and psychotherapeutic interventions for management of obsessive-compulsive disorder in adults: a systematic review and network meta-analysis. Focus (Am Psychiatr Publ). 2021;19(4):457–67.

17. Pittenger C. Pharmacotherapeutic strategies and new targets in OCD. Curr Top Behav Neurosci 2021;49:331–84.

18. Soomro GM, Altman D, Rajagopal S, et al. Selective serotonin re-uptake inhibitors (SSRIs) versus placebo for obsessive compulsive disorder (OCD). Cochrane database Syst Rev 2008;(1):CD001765.

19. Dell'Osso B, Nestadt G, Allen A, et al. Serotonin-norepinephrine reuptake inhibitors in the treatment of obsessive-compulsive disorder: a critical review. J Clin Psychiatry 2006;67(4):600–10.

20. Goodman WK, Price LH, Rasmussen SA, et al. Efficacy of fluvoxamine in obsessive-compulsive disorder. A double-blind comparison with placebo. Arch Gen Psychiatry 1989;46(1):36–44.

21. Geller DA, Biederman J, Stewart SE, et al. Which SSRI? A meta-analysis of pharmacotherapy trials in pediatric obsessive-compulsive disorder. Am J Psychiatry 2003;160(11):1919–28.

22. Hutton LMJ, Cave AJ, St-Jean R, et al. Should we be worried about QTc prolongation using citalopram? A review. J Pharm Pract 2017;30(3):353–8.

23. Zai G. Pharmacogenetics of obsessive-compulsive disorder: an evidence-update. Curr Top Behav Neurosci 2021;49:385–98.

24. Bloch MH, McGuire J, Landeros-Weisenberger A, et al. Meta-analysis of the dose–response relationship of SSRI in obsessive-compulsive disorder. Mol Psychiatry 2010;15(8):850–5.

25. Issari Y, Jakubovski E, Bartley CA, et al. Early onset of response with selective serotonin reuptake inhibitors in obsessive-compulsive disorder: a meta-analysis. J Clin Psychiatry 2016;77(5):e605–11.

26. Fineberg NA, Tonnoir B, Lemming O, et al. Escitalopram prevents relapse of obsessive-compulsive disorder. Eur Neuropsychopharmacol 2007;17(6–7): 430–9.

27. Rasmussen S, Hackett E, DuBoff E, et al. A 2-year study of sertraline in the treatment of obsessive-compulsive disorder. Int Clin Psychopharmacol 1997;12(6): 309–16.

28. Stein DJ, Andersen EW, Tonnoir B, et al. Escitalopram in obsessive-compulsive disorder: a randomized, placebo-controlled, paroxetine-referenced, fixed-dose, 24-week study. Curr Med Res Opin 2007;23(4):701–11.

29. Reid JE, Reghunandanan S, Roberts A, et al. Standard evidence-based pharmacological treatment for OCD. In: Pittenger C, editor. Obsessive-compulsive disorder: phenomenology, pathophysiology, and treatment. New York: Oxford University Press; 2017. p. 443–62.

30. Rufer M, Hand I, Alsleben H, et al. Long-term course and outcome of obsessive-compulsive patients after cognitive-behavioral therapy in combination with either fluvoxamine or placebo: a 7-year follow-up of a randomized double-blind trial. Eur Arch Psychiatry Clin Neurosci 2005;255(2):121–8.

31. Ravizza L, Barzega G, Bellino S, et al. Drug treatment of obsessive-compulsive disorder (OCD): long-term trial with clomipramine and selective serotonin reuptake inhibitors (SSRIs). Psychopharmacol Bull 1996;32(1):167–73.

32. Foa EB, Simpson HB, Gallagher T, et al. Maintenance of wellness in patients with obsessive-compulsive disorder who discontinue medication after exposure/response prevention augmentation: a randomized clinical trial. JAMA Psychiatry 2022;79(3):193–200.

33. Simpson HB, Liebowitz MR, Foa EB, et al. Post-treatment effects of exposure therapy and clomipramine in obsessive-compulsive disorder. Depress Anxiety 2004;19(4):225–33.

34. DeVeaugh-Geiss J, Landau P, Katz R. Preliminary results from a multicenter trial of clomipramine in obsessive-compulsive disorder. Psychopharmacol Bull 1989; 25(1):36–40.

35. Marks IM, Stern RS, Mawson D, et al. Clomipramine and exposure for obsessive-compulsive rituals: i. Br J Psychiatry 1980;136:1–25.

36. Insel TR, Murphy DL, Cohen RM, et al. Obsessive-compulsive disorder. A double-blind trial of clomipramine and clorgyline. Arch Gen Psychiatry 1983;40(6): 605–12.

37. Fineberg NA, Gale TM. Evidence-based pharmacotherapy of obsessive-compulsive disorder. Int J Neuropsychopharmacol 2005;8(1):107–29.

38. Ananth J, Pecknold JC, van den Steen N, et al. Double-blind comparative study of clomipramine and amitriptyline in obsessive neurosis. Prog Neuropsychopharmacol 1981;5(3):257–62.

39. Eddy KT, Dutra L, Bradley R, et al. A multidimensional meta-analysis of psychotherapy and pharmacotherapy for obsessive-compulsive disorder. Clin Psychol Rev 2004;24(8):1011–30.

40. Greist JH, Jefferson JW, Kobak KA, et al. Efficacy and tolerability of serotonin transport inhibitors in obsessive-compulsive disorder. A meta-analysis. Arch Gen Psychiatry 1995;52(1):53–60.

41. Hollander E, Kaplan A, Allen A, et al. Pharmacotherapy for obsessive-compulsive disorder. Psychiatr Clin North Am 2000;23(3):643–56.

42. Wilson M. Tripp J. Clomipramine. Island, FL: StatPearls Publishing; 2022. StatPearls. Treasure.

43. Pfuhlmann B, Gerlach M, Burger R, et al. Therapeutic drug monitoring of tricyclic antidepressants in everyday clinical practice. J Neural Transm Suppl 2007;(72): 287–96.

44. Balant-Gorgia AE, Gex-Fabry M, Balant LP. Clinical pharmacokinetics of clomipramine. Clin Pharmacokinet 1991;20(6):447–62.

45. Szegedi A, Wetzel H, Leal M, et al. Combination treatment with clomipramine and fluvoxamine: drug monitoring, safety, and tolerability data. J Clin Psychiatry 1996; 57(6):257–64.
46. Fung R, Elbe D, Stewart SE. Retrospective Review of fluvoxamine-clomipramine combination therapy in obsessive-compulsive disorder in children and adolescents. J Can Acad Child Adolesc Psychiatry 2021;30(3):150–5.
47. Simpson HB, Foa EB, Liebowitz MR, et al. Cognitive-behavioral therapy vs risperidone for augmenting serotonin reuptake inhibitors in obsessive-compulsive disorder: a randomized clinical trial. JAMA Psychiatry 2013;70(11):1190–9.
48. McDougle CJ, Goodman WK, Leckman JF, et al. Haloperidol addition in fluvoxamine-refractory obsessive-compulsive disorder. A double-blind, placebo-controlled study in patients with and without tics. Arch Gen Psychiatry 1994;51(4):302–8.
49. Bloch MH, Landeros-Weisenberger A, Kelmendi B, et al. A systematic review: antipsychotic augmentation with treatment refractory obsessive-compulsive disorder. Mol Psychiatry 2006;11(7):622–32.
50. Skapinakis P, Papatheodorou T, Mavreas V. Antipsychotic augmentation of serotonergic antidepressants in treatment-resistant obsessive-compulsive disorder: a meta-analysis of the randomized controlled trials. Eur Neuropsychopharmacol 2007;17(2):79–93.
51. Veale D, Miles S, Smallcombe N, et al. Atypical antipsychotic augmentation in SSRI treatment refractory obsessive-compulsive disorder: a systematic review and meta-analysis. BMC Psychiatry 2014;14:317.
52. McDougle CJ, Barr LC, Goodman WK, et al. Lack of efficacy of clozapine monotherapy in refractory obsessive-compulsive disorder. Am J Psychiatry 1995; 152(12):1812–4.
53. Lykouras L, Alevizos B, Michalopoulou P, et al. Obsessive-compulsive symptoms induced by atypical antipsychotics. A review of the reported cases. Prog Neuropsychopharmacol Biol Psychiatry 2003;27(3):333–46.
54. Crapanzano C, Francesco Laurenzi P, Casolaro I, et al. Antipsychotic Monotherapy in Obsessive-Compulsive Disorder. Psychiatr Danub 2022;34(1):106.
55. Dold M, Aigner M, Lanzenberger R, et al. Antipsychotic augmentation of serotonin reuptake inhibitors in treatment-resistant obsessive-compulsive disorder: an update meta-analysis of double-blind, randomized, placebo-controlled trials. Int J Neuropsychopharmacol 2015;18(9):pyv047. https://doi.org/10.1093/ijnp/pyv047.
56. Kishi T, Ikuta T, Matsuda Y, et al. Pharmacological treatment for bipolar mania: a systematic review and network meta-analysis of double-blind randomized controlled trials. Mol Psychiatry 2022;27(2):1136–44.
57. Kishimoto T, Hagi K, Kurokawa S, et al. Efficacy and safety/tolerability of antipsychotics in the treatment of adult patients with major depressive disorder: a systematic review and meta-analysis. Psychol Med 2022;1–19. https://doi.org/10.1017/S0033291722000745.
58. Maina G, Albert U, Bogetto F. Relapses after discontinuation of drug associated with increased resistance to treatment in obsessive-compulsive disorder. Int Clin Psychopharmacol 2001;16(1):33–8.
59. Pittenger C, Bloch MH, Williams K. Glutamate abnormalities in obsessive compulsive disorder: neurobiology, pathophysiology, and treatment. Pharmacol Ther 2011;132(3):314–32.
60. 2022 Alzheimer's disease facts and figures. Alzheimers Dement 2022;18(4): 700–89.

61. Lu S, Nasrallah HA. The use of memantine in neuropsychiatric disorders: an overview. Ann Clin Psychiatry 2018;30(3):234–48.
62. Modarresi A, Sayyah M, Razooghi S, et al. Memantine augmentation improves symptoms in serotonin reuptake inhibitor-refractory obsessive-compulsive disorder: a randomized controlled trial. Pharmacopsychiatry 2018;51(6):263–9.
63. Andrade C. Augmentation with memantine in obsessive-compulsive disorder. J Clin Psychiatry 2019;80(6):19f13163. https://doi.org/10.4088/JCP.19f13163.
64. de Boer JN, Vingerhoets C, Hirdes M, et al. Efficacy and tolerability of riluzole in psychiatric disorders: a systematic review and preliminary meta-analysis. Psychiatry Res 2019;278:294–302.
65. Pittenger C, Coric V, Banasr M, et al. Riluzole in the treatment of mood and anxiety disorders. CNS Drugs 2008;22(9):761–86.
66. Pittenger C, Kelmendi B, Wasylink S, et al. Riluzole augmentation in treatment-refractory obsessive-compulsive disorder: a series of 13 cases, with long-term follow-up. J Clin Psychopharmacol 2008;28(3):363–7.
67. Coric V, Taskiran S, Pittenger C, et al. Riluzole augmentation in treatment-resistant obsessive-compulsive disorder: an open-label trial. Biol Psychiatry 2005;58(5):424–8.
68. Pittenger C, Bloch MH, Wasylink S, et al. Riluzole augmentation in treatment-refractory obsessive-compulsive disorder: a pilot randomized placebo-controlled trial. J Clin Psychiatry 2015;76(8):1075–84.
69. Emamzadehfard S, Kamaloo A, Paydary K, et al. Riluzole in augmentation of fluvoxamine for moderate to severe obsessive-compulsive disorder: randomized, double-blind, placebo-controlled study. Psychiatry Clin Neurosci 2016;70(8):332–41.
70. Grant PJ, Joseph LA, Farmer CA, et al. 12-week, placebo-controlled trial of add-on riluzole in the treatment of childhood-onset obsessive-compulsive disorder. Neuropsychopharmacology 2014;39(6):1453–9.
71. Bloch MH, Wasylink S, Landeros-Weisenberger A, et al. Effects of ketamine in treatment-refractory obsessive-compulsive disorder. Biol Psychiatry 2012;72(11):964–70.
72. Rodriguez CI, Kegeles LS, Levinson A, et al. Randomized controlled crossover trial of ketamine in obsessive-compulsive disorder: proof-of-concept. Neuropsychopharmacology 2013;38(12):2475–83.
73. Sharma LP, Thamby A, Balachander S, et al. Clinical utility of repeated intravenous ketamine treatment for resistant obsessive-compulsive disorder. Asian J Psychiatr 2020;52:102183.
74. Adams TG, Bloch MH, Pittenger C. Intranasal ketamine and cognitive-behavioral therapy for treatment-refractory obsessive-compulsive disorder. J Clin Psychopharmacol 2017;37(2):269–71.

Neurosurgical Approaches for Treatment-Resistant Obsessive-Compulsive Disorder

Ben Shofty, MD, PHD[a], Ron Gadot, BSC[b], Nicole Provenza, PHD[b],
Eric A. Storch, PHD[c], Wayne K. Goodman, MD[c],
Sameer A. Sheth, MD, PHD[b,d],*

KEYWORDS

- OCD • DBS • Neuromodulation • Neurosurgery

KEY POINTS

- Neurosurgical approaches for trOCD can be highly effective in selected cases.
- DBS of the cortico-striato-thalamo-cortical circuit may lead to ~40% response in 60% to 70% of cases.
- Lesions may be highly effective in cases in which DBS may less appropriate.
- Future therapies will likely incorporate closed-loop stimulation and symptom-based individualization of treatment.

INTRODUCTION

Treatment-resistant obsessive-compulsive disorder (OCD) (trOCD) is a disabling disease, leading to severe quality-of-life impairment and an increased risk of self-harm and suicide.[1] OCD was associated with more disability-adjusted life-years than Parkinson disease and multiple sclerosis combined, according to the World Health Organization assessment.[2] Following exhaustion of multiple noninvasive medical and psychotherapeutic treatment lines, such as serotonin reuptake inhibitors, antipsychotics, exposure and response prevention (ERP), transcranial magnetic stimulation (TMS), and electroconvulsive therapy (ECT), patients may be described as having trOCD.[3] The remaining therapeutic approaches for the ~30% of patients who have trOCD involve ablative or neuromodulatory interventions.[3,4] Patients are generally considered for neurosurgical treatment if they fulfill commonly accepted criteria detailed in **Box 1**.

---

[a] Department of Neurosurgery, University of Utah, 175 North Medical Drive East, 5th Floor, Salt Lake City, UT 84132, USA; [b] Department of Neurosurgery, Baylor College of Medicine, 7200 Cambridge Street Suite 9A, Houston, TX 77030, USA; [c] Menninger Department of Psychiatry and Behavioral Sciences, Baylor College of Medicine, 7200 Cambridge Street, Houston, TX 77030, USA; [d] Department of Psychiatry, Baylor College of Medicine, 7200 Cambridge Street, Houston, TX 77030, USA
* Corresponding author.
E-mail address: sameer.sheth@bcm.edu

Psychiatr Clin N Am 46 (2023) 121–132
https://doi.org/10.1016/j.psc.2022.11.002
0193-953X/23/© 2022 Elsevier Inc. All rights reserved.

Box 1
Criteria for neurosurgical intervention in treatment-resistant obsessive-compulsive disorder and clinical considerations

Criteria	Details
Main diagnosis	OCD is the main psychiatric diagnosis
Chronicity	More than 5 y since initial diagnosis of OCD have passed
Severity	YBOCS score > 28
Drug refractoriness	> 3 appropriate trials of serotonin reuptake inhibitors failed
	Clomipramine trial
	Augmentation therapy
Therapy refractoriness	> 20 h of exposure and response prevention sessions done with an expert therapist
Relative contraindication	
DSM-V section III personality disorder	
Suicidal ideation	
Poor Insight	
Special considerations when choosing a surgical approach	
Body dysmorphic disorder	Wound picking, increased risk for infections
Anorexia/very low body weight	Poor wound healing
Checking compulsion	DBS system may incorporate into OCD rituals

Abbreviations: DBS, deep brain stimulation; DSM-V, *Diagnostic and Statistical Manual of Mental Disorders, Fifth Edition*; YBOCS, Yale-Brown Obsessive Compulsive Scale.

Modern interventions for trOCD have evolved into 2 parallel strategies—lesioning and deep brain stimulation (DBS). Both are aimed at restoring balance to the hyperactive cortico-striato-thalamo-cortical (CSTC) pathway, which connects the medial prefrontal and orbitofrontal cortices to the caudate, subthalamic nucleus, and thalamus.[4] Previous studies have shown that normalization of the activity of this pathway is associated with alleviation of the obsessions and compulsions, as well as improvements in comorbid mood disorders.[5] At present, both strategies have unique advantages and disadvantages and may be performed using multiple approaches aimed at various targets. These developments allow the treating team to tailor therapy to the specific patient while considering the local experience, disease subtype and severity, the patient's background, physical distance from the treating center, and long-term goals. With modern advancements in stereotaxic techniques, the ability to precisely lesion or place an electrode has gradually improved, minimizing the effect on areas outside the CSTC pathway and associated side effects. In addition, advances in imaging technologies and understanding of the pathophysiological circuitry involved in trOCD allow for accurate targeting of involved pathways, maximizing therapeutic yield. This review aims to provide an updated description of recent publications and evidence regarding neurosurgical modulation for trOCD (**Fig. 1**).

Ablations for Treatment-Resistant Obsessive-Compulsive Disorder

White matter thermocoagulation lesioning of the anterior limb of the internal capsule (ALIC) was introduced in the 1950s by Talairach and Leksell[6] and stereotactic cingulotomy was later undertaken by Ballantine and colleagues in 1962[7] (for an extensive review of the history of ablative surgery for psychiatric disorders, see Mustroph and colleagues).[8] Following the emergence from the frontal lobotomy era, cingulotomy

Ablation procedures   **Deep brain stimulation**

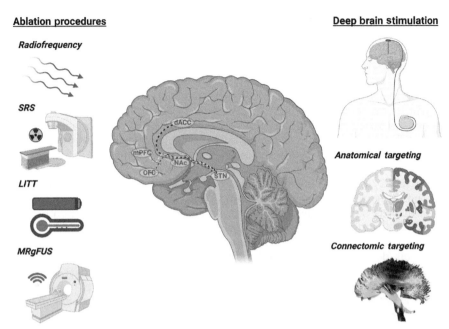

Radiofrequency

SRS

LITT

MRgFUS

Anatomical targeting

Connectomic targeting

Fig. 1. Neurosurgical treatment approaches for trOCD. dACC, dorsal anterior cingulate cortex; LITT, laser interstitial thermal therapy; mPFC, medial prefrontal cortex; MRgFUS, magnetic resonance-guided focused ultrasound; NAc, Nucleus accumbens; OCF, orbito-frontal cortex; SRS, stereotactic radiosurgery; STN, subthalamic nucleus. (Created with biorender. com.)

and subcaudate tractotomy were done separately or combined (complete limbic leucotomy). However, today, most centers concentrate on the cingulate and the ALIC as ablative targets; therefore, this review focuses on these 2 targets.

Anterior Capsulotomy

ALIC ablation or capsulotomy can be performed with thermocoagulation (radiofrequency [RF], laser interstitial thermal therapy [LITT], MRI-guided focused ultrasound [MRgFUS]) or with stereotactic radiosurgery (SRS capsulotomy [SRSc]).

Radiofrequency Capsulotomy

RF capsulotomy is done using a standard stereotactic technique, with the introduction of RF electrodes into the ventral ALIC (vALIC) followed by thermal ablation using fixed lesional parameters. Advantages include short operative time and a relatively uncomplicated procedure, in addition to low procedural cost; however, because it is done blindly, there is no real-time assessment of the lesion created. Several case series describe adequate results with RF capsulotomy.[9–12] In their 2008 publication, Rück and colleagues[11] describe 6 of 11 patients achieving response (>35% YBOCS reduction) with long-term follow-up (>1 year). However, they also describe a significant adverse event (AE) profile with 50% of the patients suffering from at least one side effect, including apathy, sexual disinhibition, weight gain, and urinary incontinence. This side effect profile, which has been replicated in multiple case series,[13,14] as well as the inability to control lesion size, has led to the decline in the use of RF capsulotomy in favor of other, more advanced methods.

Stereotactic Radiosurgery Capsulotomy

SRSc was developed in the late 1980s by Leksell[15] as a noninvasive alternative to RF capsulotomy. The procedure involves externally delivering a high dose of ionizing radiation to a preselected and stetereotically localized and well-circumscribed intracranial volume. Despite the appeal of the noninvasive procedure, the variability in response and significant neuropsychological side effect profile has limited its use.[11] In 2014, Lopes and colleagues[16] published a null result of a double-blind (DB), placebo-controlled, randomized controlled trial. In their trial, 2 of 8 patients who underwent SRSc responded, whereas none of the patients responded in the control group.[16] This trial was terminated earlier than planned as a result of technical difficulties with the SRS cobalt source. Modern, "double shot" SRSc using 2 shots of 140 to 180 Gy to the ventral capsule has been shown to be effective, with a 56% responder rate over a 3-year follow-up period.[17,18] However, several factors diminish the usefulness of this technique. Rasmussen and colleagues[17] describe a gradual treatment effect that takes months to develop, similar to the profile seen in SRSc for other indications. In addition, the side effect profile was nonnegligible, with 9% of patients developing interstitial edema that necessitated outpatient steroid treatment. Brain cysts were a late sequela in 3 patients, with 1 patient becoming severely symptomatic as a result of radionecrosis, concomitant intracranial hypertension, and ultimately requiring multiple surgeries and remaining severely disabled. Importantly, these cysts occurred only with the use of gamma knife model C and not when using model U.[17] The incidence of radionecrotic cysts following SRSc is estimated at 10%,[19] with a direct correlation to radiation dosage of more than 140 Gy.[20]

In a recent cost-effectiveness analysis, Najera and colleagues[21] pooled efficacy results from 158 patients who underwent SRSc and 113 patients who were treated conservatively (treatment as usual [TAU]). The SRSc group had a 63% responder rate with a mean YBOCS reduction of 24 ± 7.6, whereas nonresponders had a mean YBOCS reduction of 9 ± 8.9. In addition, they found that SRSc is a cost-effective procedure when compared with conservative treatment, with a 0.27 quality-adjusted life-year gain over a 3-year horizon.[21] Notably, patients who underwent SRSc also had higher baseline YBOCS scores and comorbid depression when compared with the TAU group, emphasizing the advantage of the intervention from both a clinical and cost-effectiveness perspective.[21]

Laser Interstitial Thermal Therapy Capsulotomy

LITT capsulotomy has become a preferred method of lesioning in recent years. LITT ablation is done under magnetic resonance thermometry, providing a real-time assessment of lesion volume,[22] allowing for precise ablation of ALIC fibers, sparing the surrounding gray matter (Fig. 2).[23,24] In a recent publication by McLaughlin and colleagues,[25] 77.8% of patients who underwent LITT capsulotomy were responders.[25] In another large series, Satzer and colleagues[26] also report favorable outcomes with a 61% responder rate and a 46% ± 32% mean YBOCS reduction. Interestingly, in this series, response correlated with lesion volume and disconnection of the CSTC pathway on tractography.[26] Although no long-term sequelae were evident, 7 patients in this cohort experienced transient apathy. Importantly, when compared with SRSc, response time has been reported to be shorter with a more favorable safety profile.

MRI-Guided Focused Ultrasound Capsulotomy

MRgFUS is a thermal lesioning method that has been extensively used in thalamotomy for essential tremor.[27] The therapy has the advantage of noninvasiveness as well as no

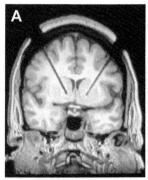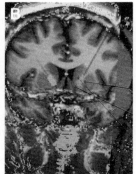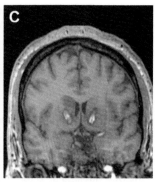

Fig. 2. Example lesion in a patient undergoing LITT capsulotomy for trOCD. (*A*) Coronal T1 MRI demonstrating laser fibers placed in the ALIC bilaterally; (*B*) intraoperative estimation of the thermal lesion (*orange*) and safety marks (*blue crosses*) protecting the caudate, lentiform, and NAc; (*C*) postoperative coronal T1 MRI showing ablation of ventral ALIC fibers.

need for radiation with its associated side effects. Many other emerging indications for MRgFUS are being explored, including lesioning for OCD.[28] The 2 main factors that may preclude the use of MRgFUS are the need for a favorable skull density ratio that will allow the ultrasound waves to be focused and the need to closely shave the head to perform the procedure. Preliminary open-label trials and retrospective case series have demonstrated variable response rates ranging between 30% and 50%.[29,30] Because the size of the lesion created with MRgFUS is somewhat limited, a focused lesion guided by tractography may be a future direction for this therapy.[31]

Cingulotomy

Lesioning of the cingulate gyrus has been used as an ablative option in trOCD since the 1960s. The cingulate cortex is a known hub of intrinsic mood and emotion regulation. Investigators have used each of the above-outlined methods for capsulotomy in cingulotomy for trOCD with varying results.[32–34] In a systematic review of observational studies reporting efficacy and AEs of cingulotomy (n = 2 studies, 81 patients) and capsulotomy (n = 8 studies, 112 patients), Brown and colleagues[35] found that the mean reduction in Y-BOCS scores was 37% in cingulotomy and 55% in anterior capsulotomy procedures. In addition, the rate of transient AEs in cingulotomies and capsulotomies was 14.3% and 56.2%, respectively, whereas the rate of serious or permanent AEs was 5.2% and 21.4%, respectively.[35] Recent studies have found that effective ablation of the cingulum involves more posterior and superior coverage of the ablative lesion along the cingulate sulcus.[36]

Deep Brain Stimulation

Overview

DBS for trOCD has been approved by the US Food and Drug Administration (FDA) under a humanitarian device exemption since 2009 and is a valid approach that has demonstrated superiority to medical treatment.[37] Level I and II evidence supports DBS-based modulation of the CSTC circuit, and it was recently recognized as a medical necessity by some of the major US insurers.[37] DBS can therefore be considered as a well-based, standard-of-care therapy that should be offered to appropriately selected patients suffering from trOCD at specialized centers, much like DBS for movement disorders and advanced neuromodulation for epilepsy. Importantly, restricting access to this therapy is discrimination targeted at a weakened population suffering from severe mental health disabilities and insufficient advocacy.[38]

Targeting

Multiple targets along the CSTC circuit have been investigated in both open-label and randomized trials (**Fig. 3**).[23,24] In a pivotal study by Greenberg and colleagues,[39] the long-term results from 2 multi-institutional studies were published. In addition to the main outcome, which improved with time with outcomes up to 36 months, the investigators also noticed that the outcome further improved with more posterior placement of the leads, with lower stimulation amplitudes. This surprising finding suggested that the optimal average target lies posterior to the anterior commissure (AC) in proximity to the bed nucleus stria terminalis (BNST). Combined results from these studies have led to the FDA approval of ALIC DBS for trOCD on a humanitarian device exemption basis in 2009. Since the FDA approval, multiple studies with various designs have confirmed the efficacy of DBS for trOCD.[40] Small variability in the results of these trials from different countries, designs, and targeting suggests a common OCD pathway that may be manipulated in various locations (for in-depth reviews of surgical DBS targeting, see Refs.[41,42]).

In 2008, Mallet and colleagues[43] published the results of a multicenter, DB randomized controlled crossover trial of STN DBS for trOCD. In that study, 16 patients were implanted with associative/limbic STN DBS and then randomized for either on-off or off-on stimulation. YBOCS scores were significantly lower in the active stimulation

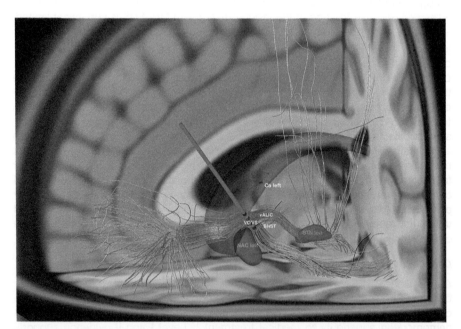

Fig. 3. Regional anatomy and commonly used targets in DBS for trOCD. Commonly used targets have included ventral anterior limb of internal capsule (vALIC, *red fibers*), ventral capsule/ventral striatum (VC/VS), bed nucleus stria terminalis (BNST), subthalamic nucleus (STN), and NAc (nucleus accumbens). Ca = caudate nucleus. Purple fibers demonstrate the anterior commissure. DBS lead in this example is targeting the VC/VS. Figure generated in lead-DBS using the Li and colleagues[23,24] atlas target tract.

period compared with the sham stimulation period (19 ± 8 vs 28 ± 7; $P = 0.01$). Despite these encouraging results, the side effect profile was significant, with 1 intracerebral hemorrhage, 2 infections leading to system removal, and 7 patients experiencing stimulation-related side effects such as hypomania, anxiety, capsular symptoms, and dyskinesias.[43] In 2010, Denys and colleagues[44] published the results from a DB, sham-controlled trial of nucleus accumbens (NAc) stimulation. The investigators reported 56% responders with a mean YBOCS reduction of 46%. Importantly, these results were supported by the sham control phase of the study. In 2016 Luyten and colleagues[45] reported their results from a DB crossover withdrawal study of BNST stimulation, also comparing ALIC (white matter) to BNST (gray matter) stimulation. Again, a 67% response rate was seen in the open-label phase, whereas at last follow-up, 83% response was noted.[45] Two interesting conclusions arose from this study, aside from the recapitulation of VC/VS stimulation efficacy. First, most of the responders were in the BNST group (80%), whereas only 1 patient (16.6%) in the ALIC group responded, suggesting that BNST stimulation (or the white matter fibers surrounding it) might be superior to other targets. Second, individualized stimulation optimization was noted to play a crucial role and may significantly improve outcome, something they noted should be a part of any future trial. In 2021, Mosely and colleagues[46] published another DB sham-controlled BNST stimulation trial, recapitulating the previous results. In their study, patients entered the blinded phase 1 month after surgery, with fixed stimulation parameters centered on the deepest contacts, with increasing amplitude. A significant benefit for active stimulation was evident during the DB phase. At the end of the 1-year open-label phase, 7 of 9 (77%) of patients responded with a mean YBOCS reduction of 16.6 ± 1.9 points. Importantly their trial incorporated a course of ERP during the open-label phase, which showed an additive mean effect of 4.8 ± 3.9 points on the YBOCS. Provenza and colleagues[47] furthered this work by adopting an open-label optimization phase with a cognitive behavioral therapy (CBT) boost component followed by a DB discontinuation phase. Five of 5 patients (100%) in this series achieved full treatment response during the open-label phase with a mean reduction of 55% in Y-BOCS.[47] During the DB discontinuation phase, all 5 patients deteriorated to the point of meeting preset criteria for escape reinitiation of DBS and all experienced a subsequent improvement in their symptoms.

Recently, in their 2020 guidelines, the Congress of Neurological Surgeons summarized current evidence supporting the use of DBS for trOCD and found level 1 evidence for bilateral STN DBS for trOCD, and level 2 evidence for NAc and BNST.[37] In addition, they recommended DBS for OCD over best medical treatment for refractory patients and stated that there is not enough evidence to currently adjudicate between the different targets.[37]

Connectomic

As mentioned, obsessive-compulsive symptoms are now commonly accepted to occur due to dysfunction within the CSTC circuit.[5,48,49] With a variety of surgical targets demonstrating varying degrees of therapeutic success, a connectomic model for neuromodulation in OCD has come to the centerfold.[50] Hartmann and colleagues[51] were among the first to use connectomic modeling using a normative diffusion-weighted MRI (dMRI) brain atlas in patients undergoing ALIC/NAc DBS. The investigators showed that patients in whom activation of white matter fibers reached the right anterior middle frontal gyrus and dorsolateral prefrontal cortex (PFC) demonstrated an optimal clinical response to stimulation.[51]

In a subsequent study, Baldermann and colleagues[52] found that connectivity through a fiber tract within the central and vALIC that passes through the ventral striatum and connects the right medial/lateral middle PFC with the thalamus predicted effective DBS at 1 year. A subsequent landmark study by Li and colleagues[24] showed that a hyperdirect bundle connecting dorsal anterior cingulate and ventrolateral prefrontal cortices to the anteromedial STN explained the positive effects of DBS, which they found involved multiple published gray matter targets clustered around the tract.[24] Still, differences in connectivity profiles and differential cognitive/affective effects of stimulation to different sites (ie, STN vs ALIC) seen in head-to-head studies such as that by Tyagi and colleagues[53] suggest that the modulation of networks interconnected by these sites may address different symptoms within the disease phenotype spectrum. Further study involving a cohort of patients with Tourette syndrome echoes this theory by finding that patients experienced an indirect improvement in OCD symptoms when fibers delineated in Li and colleagues' work were modulated.[54] Furthermore, there is a now established topography within the implicated ALIC bundle, which has been reviewed elsewhere[55] and is crucial to keep in mind when planning electrode targets in this region.

More recent studies have demonstrated that tractography-based targeting in vALIC DBS can result in noninferior outcomes compared with conventional anatomic coordinate-based targeting, with a more favorable side effect profile.[56] The investigators hypothesized that the finding of less hypomanic symptoms with tractography-guided targeting may be due to incidental dorsalization of the deepest contacts such that no contacts ended up in the NAc, a target that has been shown to cause stimulation-induced hypomania.[56] By understanding OCD pathogenesis and stimulation effects through connectomic modeling, patient outcomes can be optimized as this therapy continues to be adopted, and we expect that future targeting will transition to be guided by connectivity and symptoms, rather than by anatomy and intraoperative testing.

Future Directions

The neurosurgical treatments for OCD discussed in this review will continue to be augmented by improved neuroanatomical imaging with higher throughput individual dMRI data along with improved postprocessing tractography pipelines.[57] Importantly, effective tractography for surgical planning must be validated through anatomic studies as both normative and individual tractographic studies continue to be disseminated in the literature.[55]

Some evidence suggests that the clinical benefit associated with successful DBS may be enhanced with targeted psychiatry therapy. Following addition of CBT, Mantione and colleagues[58] showed improved obsessive-compulsive, anxiety, and depressive symptoms in 16 patients (~7 point reduction in YBOCS). When stimulation was discontinued during the DB study phase, obsessive-compulsive, anxiety, and depressive symptoms all significantly worsened and returned to baseline levels. This finding recapitulates the essential role that psychiatrists play in the long-term outcomes of these patients especially following neurosurgical involvement and treatment.

A network-based understanding of different behavioral phenotypes (ie, affective vs cognitive control) will likely be even more precise, leading to patient-specific tailoring of neuromodulatory or ablative strategies.[5,55] Biomarkers for closed-loop neuromodulation informed by long-term neural recordings in native behavioral states[47,59] will lend to expanding noninvasive therapies such as TMS. Furthermore, as the body of evidence supporting neuromodulation for OCD has steadily improved, increased interest in training for psychiatrists and neurosurgeons, as well as access to therapy for patients, will undoubtedly grow.[38]

SUMMARY

Neurosurgical approaches for the treatment of trOCD have expanded since their conception in the mid-twentieth century. Ablative procedures, including capsulotomies and cingulotomies, and neuromodulatory procedures, including DBS, are being increasingly refined to maximize clinical benefit while limiting side effects of therapy. Further study will optimize image-based targeting workflow, identify factors predictive of treatment response, and discover biomarkers for eventual closed-loop and noninvasive neuromodulation for trOCD.

CLINICS CARE POINTS

- For appropriately selected trOCD patients response rate for DBS range between 60-70%.
- In patients where DBS implant is less favorable, lesioning the ALIC provides an adequate alternative.
- Optimizing target selection through intraoperative testing and tractography is advised.

DISCLOSURE

Dr S.A. Sheth is a consultant for Boston Scientific, Neuropace, Abbott, and Zimmer Biomet. All other authors have no relevant disclosures.

REFERENCES

1. Ruscio AM, Stein DJ, Chiu WT, et al. The epidemiology of obsessive-compulsive disorder in the National Comorbidity Survey Replication. Mol Psychiatry 2010; 15(1):53–63.
2. World health organization (WHO). The Global Burden of Disease: 2004 Update. Geneva, Switzerland: World Health Organization; 2008.
3. Hirschtritt ME, Bloch MH, Mathews CA. Obsessive-compulsive disorder: advances in diagnosis and treatment. JAMA 2017;317(13):1358–67.
4. Greenberg BD, Rauch SL, Haber SN. Invasive circuitry-based neurotherapeutics: stereotactic ablation and deep brain stimulation for OCD. Neuropsychopharmacology 2010;35(1):317–36.
5. Bijanki KR, Pathak YJ, Najera RA, et al. Defining functional brain networks underlying obsessive-compulsive disorder (OCD) using treatment-induced neuroimaging changes: a systematic review of the literature. J Neurol Neurosurg Psychiatry 2021;92(7):776–86.
6. Feldman RP, Goodrich JT. Psychosurgery: a historical overview. Neurosurgeryr 2001;48(3):647–57, discussion 657-9.
7. Ballantine HT, Cassidy WL, Flanagan NB, et al. Stereotaxic anterior cingulotomy for neuropsychiatric illness and intractable pain. J Neurosurg 1967;26(5):488–95.
8. Mustroph ML, Cosgrove GR, Williams ZM. The evolution of modern ablative surgery for the treatment of obsessive-compulsive and major depression disorders. Front Integr Neurosci 2022;16:797533.
9. Oliver B, Gascón J, Aparicio A, et al. Bilateral anterior capsulotomy for refractory obsessive-compulsive disorders. Stereotact Funct Neurosurg 2003;81(1–4):90–5.
10. Liu K, Zhang H, Liu C, et al. Stereotactic treatment of refractory obsessive compulsive disorder by bilateral capsulotomy with 3 years follow-up. J Clin Neurosci 2008;15(6):622–9.

11. Rück C, Karlsson A, Steele JD, et al. Capsulotomy for obsessive-compulsive disorder: long-term follow-up of 25 patients. Arch Gen Psychiatry 2008;65(8): 914–21.

12. Csigó K, Harsányi A, Demeter G, et al. Long-term follow-up of patients with obsessive-compulsive disorder treated by anterior capsulotomy: a neuropsychological study. J Affect Disord 2010;126(1–2):198–205.

13. Rück C, Andréewitch S, Flyckt K, et al. Capsulotomy for refractory anxiety disorders: long-term follow-up of 26 patients. Am J Psychiatry 2003;160(3):513–21.

14. Rück C, Edman G, Asberg M, et al. Long-term changes in self-reported personality following capsulotomy in anxiety patients. Nord J Psychiatry 2006;60(6): 486–91.

15. Leksell DG. Stereotactic radiosurgery. Present status and future trends. Neurol Res 1987;9(2):60–8.

16. Lopes AC, Greenberg BD, Pereira CA, et al. Notice of retraction and replacement. lopes et al. gamma ventral capsulotomy for obsessive-compulsive disorder: a randomized clinical trial. JAMA Psychiatry 2014;71(9):1066–76.

17. Rasmussen SA, Noren G, Greenberg BD, et al. Gamma ventral capsulotomy in intractable obsessive-compulsive disorder. Biol Psychiatry 2018;84(5):355–64.

18. Miguel EC, Lopes AC, McLaughlin NCR, et al. Evolution of gamma knife capsulotomy for intractable obsessive-compulsive disorder. Mol Psychiatry 2019;24(2): 218–40.

19. Peker S, Samanci MY, Yilmaz M, et al. Efficacy and safety of gamma ventral capsulotomy for treatment-resistant obsessive-compulsive disorder: a single-center experience. World Neurosurg 2020;141:e941–52.

20. Kasabkojian ST, Dwan AJ, Maziero MP, et al. Delayed brain cyst formation after gamma knife anterior capsulotomy. World Neurosurg 2021;145:298–300.

21. Najera RA, Gregory ST, Shofty B, et al. Cost-effectiveness analysis of radiosurgical capsulotomy versus treatment as usual for treatment-resistant obsessive-compulsive disorder. J Neurosurg 2022;1–11. https://doi.org/10.3171/2022.5. JNS22474.

22. Salem U, Kumar VA, Madewell JE, et al. Neurosurgical applications of MRI guided laser interstitial thermal therapy (LITT). Cancer Imaging 2019;19(1):65.

23. Horn A, Li N, Dembek TA, et al. Lead-DBS v2: Towards a comprehensive pipeline for deep brain stimulation imaging. Neuroimage 2019;184:293–316.

24. Li N, Baldermann JC, Kibleur A, et al. A unified connectomic target for deep brain stimulation in obsessive-compulsive disorder. Nat Commun 2020;11(1):3364.

25. McLaughlin NCR, Lauro PM, Patrick MT, et al. Magnetic resonance imaging-guided laser thermal ventral capsulotomy for intractable obsessive-compulsive disorder. Neurosurgery 2021;88(6):1128–35.

26. Satzer D, Mahavadi A, Lacy M, et al. Interstitial laser anterior capsulotomy for obsessive-compulsive disorder: lesion size and tractography correlate with outcome. J Neurol Neurosurg Psychiatry 2022;93(3):317–23.

27. Agrawal M, Garg K, Samala R, et al. Outcome and complications of MR guided focused ultrasound for essential tremor: a systematic review and meta-analysis. Front Neurol 2021;12:654711.

28. Chang KW, Jung HH, Chang JW. Magnetic resonance-guided focused ultrasound surgery for obsessive-compulsive disorders: potential for use as a novel ablative surgical technique. Front Psychiatry 2021;12:640832.

29. Davidson B, Hamani C, Rabin JS, et al. Magnetic resonance-guided focused ultrasound capsulotomy for refractory obsessive compulsive disorder and major

depressive disorder: clinical and imaging results from two phase I trials. Mol Psychiatry 2020;25(9):1946–57.

30. Kim SJ, Roh D, Jung HH, et al. A study of novel bilateral thermal capsulotomy with focused ultrasound for treatment-refractory obsessive-compulsive disorder: 2-year follow-up. J Psychiatry Neurosci 2018;43(5):327–37.

31. Avecillas-Chasin JM, Hurwitz TA, Bogod NM, et al. An analysis of clinical outcome and tractography following bilateral anterior capsulotomy for depression. Stereotact Funct Neurosurg 2019;97(5–6):369–80.

32. Bourne SK, Sheth SA, Neal J, et al. Beneficial effect of subsequent lesion procedures after nonresponse to initial cingulotomy for severe, treatment-refractory obsessive-compulsive disorder. Neurosurgery 2013;72(2):196–202 ; discussion 202.

33. Sheth SA, Neal J, Tangherlini F, et al. Limbic system surgery for treatment-refractory obsessive-compulsive disorder: a prospective long-term follow-up of 64 patients. J Neurosurg 2013;118(3):491–7.

34. Banks GP, Mikell CB, Youngerman BE, et al. Neuroanatomical characteristics associated with response to dorsal anterior cingulotomy for obsessive-compulsive disorder. JAMA Psychiatry 2015;72(2):127–35.

35. Brown LT, Mikell CB, Youngerman BE, et al. Dorsal anterior cingulotomy and anterior capsulotomy for severe, refractory obsessive-compulsive disorder: a systematic review of observational studies. J Neurosurg 2016;124(1):77–89.

36. Starkweather CK, Bick SK, McHugh JM, et al. Lesion location and outcome following cingulotomy for obsessive-compulsive disorder. J Neurosurg 2022; 136(1):221–30.

37. Staudt MD, Pouratian N, Miller JP, et al. Congress of neurological surgeons systematic review and evidence-based guidelines for deep brain stimulations for obsessive-compulsive disorder: update of the 2014 guidelines. Neurosurgery 2021;88(4):710–2.

38. Visser-Vandewalle V, Andrade P, Mosley PE, et al. Deep brain stimulation for obsessive compulsive disorder: a crisis of access. Nat Med 2022;28(8): 1529–32 (In Press).

39. Greenberg BD, Gabriels LA, Malone DA Jr, et al. Deep brain stimulation of the ventral internal capsule/ventral striatum for obsessive-compulsive disorder: worldwide experience. Mol Psychiatry 2010;15(1):64–79.

40. Gadot R, Najera R, Hirani S, et al. Efficacy of deep brain stimulation for treatment-resistant obsessive-compulsive disorder: systematic review and meta-analysis. J Neurol Neurosurg Psychiatry 2022;jnnp-2021:328738.

41. Karas PJ, Lee S, Jimenez-Shahed J, et al. Deep brain stimulation for obsessive compulsive disorder: evolution of surgical stimulation target parallels changing model of dysfunctional brain circuits. Front Neurosci 2018;12:998.

42. Raviv N, Staudt MD, Rock AK, et al. A systematic review of deep brain stimulation targets for obsessive compulsive disorder. Neurosurgery 2020;87(6):1098–110.

43. Mallet L, Polosan M, Jaafari N, et al. Subthalamic nucleus stimulation in severe obsessive-compulsive disorder. N Engl J Med 2008;359(20):2121–34.

44. Denys D, Mantione M, Figee M, et al. Deep brain stimulation of the nucleus accumbens for treatment-refractory obsessive-compulsive disorder. Arch Gen Psychiatry 2010;67(10):1061–8.

45. Luyten L, Hendrickx S, Raymaekers S, et al. Electrical stimulation in the bed nucleus of the stria terminalis alleviates severe obsessive-compulsive disorder. Mol Psychiatry 2016;21(9):1272–80.

46. Mosley PE, Windels F, Morris J, et al. A randomised, double-blind, sham-controlled trial of deep brain stimulation of the bed nucleus of the stria terminalis for treatment-resistant obsessive-compulsive disorder. Transl Psychiatry 2021; 11(1):190.
47. Provenza NR, Sheth SA, Dastin-van Rijn EM, et al. Long-term ecological assessment of intracranial electrophysiology synchronized to behavioral markers in obsessive-compulsive disorder. Nat Med Dec 2021;27(12):2154–64.
48. Ahmari SE, Spellman T, Douglass NL, et al. Repeated cortico-striatal stimulation generates persistent OCD-like behavior. Science 2013;340(6137):1234–9.
49. Abe Y, Sakai Y, Nishida S, et al. Hyper-influence of the orbitofrontal cortex over the ventral striatum in obsessive-compulsive disorder. Eur Neuropsychopharmacol 2015;25(11):1898–905.
50. Baldermann JC, Schüller T, Kohl S, et al. Connectomic deep brain stimulation for obsessive-compulsive disorder. Biol Psychiatry 2021;90(10):678–88.
51. Hartmann CJ, Lujan JL, Chaturvedi A, et al. Tractography activation patterns in dorsolateral profrontal cortex suggest better clinical responses in OCD DBS. Front Neurosci 2015;9:519.
52. Baldermann JC, Melzer C, Zapf A, et al. Connectivity profile predictive of effective deep brain stimulation in obsessive-compulsive disorder. Biol Psychiatry 2019; 85(9):735–43.
53. Tyagi H, Apergis-Schoute AM, Akram H, et al. A randomized trial directly comparing ventral capsule and anteromedial subthalamic nucleus stimulation in obsessive-compulsive disorder: clinical and imaging evidence for dissociable effects. Biol Psychiatry 2019;85(9):726–34.
54. Johnson KA, Duffley G, Foltynie T, et al. Basal ganglia pathways associated with therapeutic pallidal deep brain stimulation for tourette syndrome. Biol Psychiatry Cogn Neurosci Neuroimaging 2021;6(10):961–72.
55. Haber SN, Yendiki A, Jbabdi S. Four deep brain stimulation targets for obsessive-compulsive disorder: are they different? Biol Psychiatry 2021;90(10):667–77.
56. Graat I, RJT Mocking, Liebrand LC, et al. Tractography-based versus anatomical landmark-based targeting in vALIC deep brain stimulation for refractory obsessive-compulsive disorder. Mol Psychiatry 2022. https://doi.org/10.1038/s41380-022-01760-y.
57. Coenen VA, Reisert M. DTI for brain targeting: Diffusion weighted imaging fiber tractography-Assisted deep brain stimulation. Int Rev Neurobiol 2021;159:47–67.
58. Mantione M, Nieman D, Figee M, et al. The stimulated brain: A psychological perspective on deep brain stimulation for treatment-refractory obsessive-compulsive disorder. 2015.
59. Vissani M, Nanda P, Bush A, et al. Toward closed-loop intracranial neurostimulation in obsessive-compulsive disorder. Biol Psychiatry 2022. https://doi.org/10.1016/j.biopsych.2022.07.003.

Transcranial Magnetic Stimulation in Obsessive-Compulsive Disorder

Tal Harmelech, PhD[a,1], Yiftach Roth, PhD[a,b,1],
Aron Tendler, MD[a,b,2],*

KEYWORDS

• OCD • TMS • H7 Coil • D-B80 coil • Iron core • Figure-8 coil

KEY POINTS

- Converging lines of evidence suggest that OCD involves dysfunction of limbic cortico-striato-thalamo-cortico loops including the orbitofrontal cortex, medial prefrontal cortex (mPFC) and anterior cingulate cortex (ACC).
- The H7 Coil was FDA-cleared for treatment-refractory OCD based on results of two RCTs. Subsequently, a 510K clearance was granted to the D-B80 and iron-core figure-8 coils.
- The physical properties of these coils differ from the H7 Coil, resulting in different functional properties.
- Only the H7 Coil clinical studies follow the FDA-cleared protocol of 20Hz at 100% resting motor threshold of the foot, 4cm anterior to the foot hot spot.
- The H7 Coil studies' point to efficacy of mPFC-ACC stimulation, while no clear target stems from the small heterogenous D-B80 coil and figure-8 coil studies.

INTRODUCTION

Obsessive-compulsive disorder (OCD) is a common, chronic, and oftentimes disabling disorder characterized by unwanted distressing thoughts (obsessions) and repetitive behaviors that the individual feels compelled to perform (compulsions).[1,2] OCD affects 2% to 3% of the US population[3] and is responsible for substantial functional impairment[4,5] and increased risk of early mortality.[6] The only established first-line treatments for OCD are cognitive-behavioral therapy (CBT) with exposure/response prevention (ERP)[7,8] and serotonin reuptake inhibitor medications (SRIs).[8-12] Approximately 25% to 40% of patients fail to respond to either,[13,14] and many patients do not experience remission.[15]

---

[a] BrainsWay Ltd; [b] Department of Life Sciences, Ben Gurion University of the Negev, Israel
[1] Present address: 19 Hartum St, Bynet BuildingHar Hotzvim, Jerusalem 9777518, Israel
[2] Present address: 1 Van de Graaff DriveBurlington, MA 01803, USA
* Corresponding author.
E-mail addresses: aronte@brainsway.com; aron.tendler@gmail.com

Psychiatr Clin N Am 46 (2023) 133–166
https://doi.org/10.1016/j.psc.2022.10.003
0193-953X/23/© 2022 Elsevier Inc. All rights reserved.

Abbreviations	
rTMS	repetitive transcranial magnetic stimulation
OCD	obsessive-compulsive disorder
CSTC	cortico-striato-thalamo-cortical
mPFC	medial prefrontal cortex
dACC	dorsal anterior cingulate cortex
DLPFC	dorsolateral prefrontal cortex
OFC	orbitofrontal cortex
SMA	supplementary motor area
EF	electrical field
Y-BOCS	Yale-Brown obsessive compulsive scale
TBS	theta burst stimulation
HF	high frequency
LF	low frequency
RCT	randomized controlled trial
rMT	resting motor threshold
MOA	mechanism of action
fMRI	functional magnetic resosance imaging
EEG	electroencephalogram
ERN	error-related negativity
PET	positron emission tomography
MDD	major depressive disorder
NMA	network meta-analysis
CBT	cognitive behavioral therapy
ERP	exposure and response prevention
SRI	serotonin reuptake inhibitors

Converging evidence—from studies of brain imaging, cognitive-affective neuroscience, neuromodulation, and animal models—suggest that OCD is a disorder borne of dysfunction within networks of brain regions.[16] One productive way of conceptualizing these networks and studying their dysfunction in OCD is based on the cortico-striato-thalamo-cortical (CSTC) loops and related regions.[17] Using this framework, functional brain imaging studies in OCD have demonstrated consistent results.[17] Positron emission tomography (PET)[18] and functional MRI (fMRI)[19] show increased activation in regions of the orbitofrontal cortex (OFC), dorsal anterior cingulate cortex (dACC), and portions of the basal ganglia in patients compared with healthy controls.[20] These

Iron core figure-8	D-B80	H7-Coil
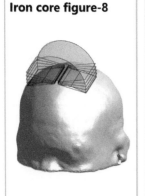	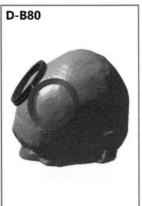	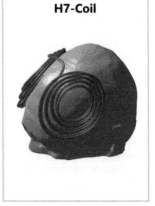

Fig. 1. The Deep TMS H7 Coil, D-B80 coil, and iron core figure-8 coil over a human head.

areas of abnormal activation tend to normalize with successful treatment, whether with medications or ERP.[20-22] Other effective treatment modalities are also associated with reductions in brain activity compared with baseline: deep brain stimulation (DBS),[23,24] neurosurgical lesions,[25,26] and repetitive transcranial magnetic stimulation (rTMS).[27,28]

Hyperactivity of orbitofrontal-subcortical pathways has been found in both human imaging studies in OCD and mouse models of OCD-like behaviors.[29,30] These data provide strong support for the role of OFC hyperactivity in the genesis of abnormal repetitive behaviors. Converging lines of clinical and preclinical evidence suggest that OCD involves dysfunction of limbic CSTC loops that include the OFC, medial prefrontal cortex (mPFC), dACC, and ventral striatum.[31]

In recent years, the FDA cleared 3 different rTMS devices for the treatment of refractory OCD. This review article aims to present and discuss the physical and functional differences between the 3 TMS coils with an emphasis on the current clinical evidence, for a better understanding of the field of TMS for OCD. Sketches of the 3 coils are shown in **Fig. 1**.

Deep Transcranial Magnetic Stimulation H7 Coil

The first TMS device to receive FDA clearance for treatment-refractory OCD was the Deep TMS H7 Coil, which was designed to stimulate primarily the mPFC-dACC (3 cm^3). Additional cortical regions that it stimulates suprathreshold (>100 V/m) include the OFC (8.4 cm^3), dorsolateral prefrontal cortex (DLPFC) (10.5 cm^3), and presupplementary motor area (6.8 cm^3).[32,33] It has 2 layers of 4 elliptically shaped windings one on top of the other, whose major and minor axis ranges are 70 to 130 mm and 55 to 105 mm, respectively. Its subdural depth and volume of stimulation are 3 cm and 40.3 cm^3, respectively.[33] Similar to all other H-Coils, it is flexible and conforms to the shape of the head for maximum magnetic coupling. The experimental system used in the trials that led to the clearance has the sham and active coils in the same helmet; the sham coil does not induce field in the brain but has similar acoustic artifact and scalp sensations as the active coil, to maintain blinding. The system assigns an active or sham coil based on the patient ID.

The safety and efficacy of the H7 Coil in OCD was established in 2 randomized controlled trials (RCT), 4 post hoc analyses, a postmarketing registry study, and a durability study (**Table 1**). The pilot single-center RCT[34] compared 2 different stimulation protocols (20 Hz, 1 Hz) against sham on 41 treatment-resistant patients with OCD. All treatments were administered following personalized symptom provocation and electrophysiological (electroencephalogram [EEG]) recordings were obtained during a Stroop behavioral task to gain insight into the mechanism of action (MOA) of Deep TMS in OCD. Because the interim analysis revealed that only the high-frequency (HF) arm significantly reduced clinical symptoms compared with sham, the low-frequency (LF) arm was discontinued. At the end of the study, the HF group showed significantly greater clinical improvement (reduction in yale-brown obsessive compulsive scale [Y-BOCS]) compared with sham ($P < .01$). No significant adverse events were reported. Following these positive results, a confirmatory multicenter RCT was conducted on 99 patients with OCD from 11 sites.[35] Results revealed a significantly larger reduction in Y-BOCS scores in the active group compared with the sham group (-6.7 vs -3.6, $P = .01$) at the end of treatment- an effect size (Cohen's d) of 0.69. At 1-month follow-up, the average Y-BOCS score decreased by 6.5 points (95% CI: [4.3;8.7]) in the active group versus 4.1 points (95% CI: [1.9;6.2]) in the sham group- an effect size (Cohen's d) of 0.62 ($P = .038$). Thus, the treatment effect was maintained for at least 4 weeks after completion of all treatment sessions.

Table 1
Repetitive transcranial magnetic stimulation studies in obsessive-compulsive disorder

Study #	Reference	Coil Type	Study Type/Design	Sample	Tx Protocol	Target	Stimulation Parameters	Results
On label protocol								
1	Carmi et al,[34] 2017	Deep TMS H7 Coil	Pilot single-site RCT comparing LF, HF, and sham with EEG recording during Stroop task	41 treatment refractory patients with OCD with moderate-severe symptoms (Y-BOCS >20)	5 wk	mPFC and ACC	20 Hz, 100% rMT, 2000 pulses/session	Interim analysis showed only HF significantly reduced clinical symptoms compared with sham—> LF arm discontinued. At the end of the study, HF was superior to sham in Y-BOCS score reduction (P <.01). No significant adverse events were reported. Significant enhancement in ERN following active treatment but not sham (P <.01) that correlated with symptom improvement (P <.01)

#	Study	Device/Coil	Study type	Sample	Duration	Target	Parameters	Results
2	Carmi et al,[35] 2019	Deep TMS H7 Coil	Multicenter RCT. Pivotal	99 patients with moderate-severe OCD with limited response to previous treatments, on maintenance treatment for >2 mo before trial	6 wk	mPFC and ACC	20 Hz, 100% rMT, 2000 pulses/session	Significantly larger reduction in Y-BOCS in active vs sham (effect size 0.69, $P = .01$) that remained significant at 1 mo follow-up (effect size 0.62, $P = .038$). Response rates 38.1% vs 11.1% with active vs sham treatment. NNT 3.7. At 1 mo follow-up, response rates were 45.2% vs 17.8% with active vs sham. NNT 3.64
3	Roth et al,[36] 2021	Deep TMS H7 Coil	Postmarketing registry	22 clinical sites provided data on details of treatment and outcome (Y-BOCS) measures from a total of 219 patients. 167 patients who had at least one postbaseline Y-BOCS measure were	See study 2 above	mPFC and ACC	20 Hz, 100% rMT, 2000 pulses/session	Response rate after 29 Deep TMS treatments was 58%. First response after 18($\pm$9.4) sessions or 28($\pm$22.4) d and sustained response after 19($\pm$9.6) sessions or 30($\pm$24.5) d (faster than the typical 10–13 wk

(continued on next page)

Table 1
(continued)

Study #	Reference	Coil Type	Study Type/Design	Sample	Tx Protocol	Target	Stimulation Parameters	Results
				included in the analyses				with pharmacotherapy/CBT). Continuous gradual reduction in Y-BOCS up to 40 sessions
4	Storch et al,[38] 2021	Deep TMS H7 Coil	Post hoc analysis of data from ref[34]	See study 2 above	See study 2 above	See study 2 above	See study 2 above	Greater treatment benefit was found to be moderated by baseline OCD severity, such that for more severe patients (Y-BOCS >28) Deep TMS showed stronger efficacy relative to sham at posttreatment and follow-up
5	Roth et al,[39] 2020	Deep TMS H7 Coil	Post hoc analysis of data from ref[34]	See study 2 above	See study 2 above	See study 2 above	See study 2 above	Significantly higher response rate at posttreatment with Deep TMS vs sham for patients who had insufficient response to 3+ meds (41.4% vs 8.3%, $P = .0109$)

and prior CBT (33.3% vs 3.3%, $P = .0041$). Deep TMS is an effective treatment option, regardless of prior nonresponse to pharmacotherapy or CBT (likely different MOA)

No.	Study	Coil	Design	Population				Results
6	Harmelech et al,[40] 2020	Deep TMS H7 Coil	Post hoc analysis of data from ref[34]	Subset of patients with OCD with MDD comorbidity (Y-BOCS >20; HDRS21 > 16) from the active Deep TMS (N = 9) and sham (N = 10) groups in the pivotal trial (Carmi et al. 2019)	See study 2 above	See study 2 above	See study 2 above	Response rate of 44.4% posttreatment and 55.6% at 1 mo follow-up vs 10% and 30% with active vs sham treatment, respectively
7	Tendler et al,[41] 2021	Deep TMS H7 Coil	Post hoc analysis of data from ref[35]	Subset of patients with OCD with MDD comorbidity (Y-BOCS >20; HDRS-21 > 16/PHQ-9>10/BDI-II >20/IDS-SR >24; N = 59) from the OCD postmarketing data (Roth et al. 2020)	See study 6 above	See study 6 above	See study 6 above	Significant decrease in MDD symptoms following 5 Deep TMS sessions and at any point beyond that. Most patients demonstrated benefit from treatment in both disorders after 30 sessions, with an

(continued on next page)

Table 1
(continued)

Study #	Reference	Coil Type	Study Type/Design	Sample	Tx Protocol	Target	Stimulation Parameters	Results
								average decrease of 30% in Y-BOCS scores and an average decrease of 38% in MDD scores
8	Alyagon et al,[42] 2021	Deep TMS H7 Coil	Post hoc analysis of behavioral data from ref[33]	Pretreatment and Posttreatment Stroop data was available for 12 patients of the active group and 10 patients of the sham group from the feasibility study (Carmi et al. 2017)	See study 1 above	See study 1 above	See study 1 above	Significant reduction in PES following Deep TMS but not sham ($P < .05$). PEA reduction regardless of condition. Correlation between PES and PEA changes following active but not sham. Shorter PES following active treatment was associated with reduced PEA, as seen in healthy population, suggesting treatment-induced normalization of the speed-accuracy trade-off

9	Harmelech et al,[44] 2022	Deep TMS H7 Coil	Longitudinal follow-up on responders from refs[34,35]	7 sites provided durability data on 60 responders. 28 of those had functional disability data as well	See study 2 above	See study 2 above	See study 2 above	13.3% had durability of <1 y, 86.7% had durability of >1 y, and 43.3% had durability of >2 y. The average durability of Deep TMS for OCD was >1.98(±0.13) y. Importantly, 62% of patients were still considered to have Deep TMS durability at the time of the survey

Off label protocols

10	Nauczyciel et al,[28] 2014	D-B80 coil	Double-blind crossover study with PET imaging on subgroup	19 treatment-resistant patients with OCD; only comorbidities allowed were depressive/anxious disorders; not allowed to change meds during trial	Two 1-wk treatment periods (2 sessions per day; 10 sessions total per treatment condition) separated by 1 wk washout period	right OFC	1Hz, 120% rMT, 1200 pulses/session	NS (Significant decrease from baseline Y-BOCS in both active and sham). Active vs sham PET results relate stimulation to bilateral decrease in OFC metabolism

(continued on next page)

Table 1
(continued)

Study #	Reference	Coil Type	Study Type/Design	Sample	Tx Protocol	Target	Stimulation Parameters	Results
11	Modirrousta et al,[45] 2015	D-B80 coil	Open-label study	10 patients with moderate-severe OCD (all but 1 with baseline Y-BOCS >20); axis I comorbidities excluded; taking 1 SSRI/SNRI or no medications; not allowed to change meds during trial (from 2 wk before to 4 wk post)	10 d (10 sessions, 1/d)	mPFC	1Hz, 110% rMT, 1200 pulses/session	39% reduction in Y-BOCS score from baseline ($P < .001$) that persisted for 1 mo following the last session
12	Dunlop et al,[27] 2016	D-B80 coil	Predictors of response to rTMS in OCD (Open label), nonremitters offered extension to 30 sessions	20 patients with OCD with limited response to previous treatments, on maintenance treatment for >4 wk before study	4-6 wk (20-30 sessions, 5/wk)	Left, then right mPFC	10 Hz, 120% rMT, 3000 pulses/ hemisphere/ session	50% response rate. Responders had higher mPFC-ventral striatal connectivity. The extent of reduction in connectivity correlated with extent of reduction in Y-BOCS
13	Greenberg et al,[49] 1997	Figure-8 coil	Randomized controlled study (comparing right DLPFC, left DLPFC,	12 patients with OCD on stable medication regimens	1 session	Right DLPFC	20 Hz, 80% rMT	Compulsive urges (on a modified NIMH self-rating scale) decreased

#	Study	Coil	Design	Patients	Schedule	Site	Parameters	Results
				midoccipital/control)	for >8 wk before trial			significantly for 8 h after right DLPFC stimulation, nonsignificantly after stimulation of left DLPFC and midoccipital site. Mood (on VAS) improved during and 30 min after right DLPFC stimulation
14	Mansur et al,[50] 2011	Figure-8 coil	RCT, clinicians administering treatment not blind to group assignment	30 treatment-refractory patients with OCD (scoring ≤30% on the Y-BOCS after ≥3 complete courses of SRIs (including clomipramine) and 20 h of CBT or intolerance to either)	6 wk (30 sessions, 5/wk)	Right DLPFC	10 Hz, 110% rMT, 60,000 pulses/session	NS (One patient in each group showed a positive response. For Y-BOCS score, there was significant effect of time but no significant group effect or group × time interaction)
15	Elbeh et al,[51] 2016	Figure-8 coil	RCT comparing LF, HF, and sham with a 3-mo follow-up	45 patients with OCD with no psychiatric comorbidities; on stable medication regimens for the duration of the study	2 wk (10 sessions, 5/wk)	right DLPFC	1 Hz/10 Hz, 100% rMT, 2000 pulses/session	There was a significant time × group interaction for 1 Hz vs sham but not for 10 Hz vs sham. 1 Hz vs 10 Hz groups

(continued on next page)

Table 1
(continued)

Study #	Reference	Coil Type	Study Type/Design	Sample	Tx Protocol	Target	Stimulation Parameters	Results
								showed a significant interaction for Y-BOCS and HAM-A (P = .001 and .0001, respectively). 1 Hz rTMS has a greater clinical benefit than 10 Hz or Sham. There was also a significantly larger percentage change in GCI-S in the 1 Hz group vs either 10 Hz or sham
16	Seo et al,[52] 2016	Figure-8 coil	RCT, clinicians administering treatment not blind to group assignment	27 patients with OCD with residual moderate–severe symptoms (baseline Y-BOCS ≥16) despite 2 medication trials; on stable medication regimens for the duration of the study	3 wk, (15 sessions, 5/wk)	Right DLPFC	1Hz, 100% rMT, 1200 pulses/session	Significant reduction in Y-BOCS after 3 wk in active vs sham. Significant effect of time and time × group interaction on HDRS and CGI-S. No reports of any serious adverse effects following

17	Prasko et al,[53] 2006	Figure-8 coil	RCT, clinicians administering treatment not blind to group assignment	33 patients with OCD with prior nonresponse to 8 wk of SRIs; MDD and substance use comorbidities excluded	2 wk (10 sessions, 5/wk)	Left DLPFC	1 Hz, 110% rMT, 1800 pulses/session	NS (Both groups improved during the study period but the treatment effect did not differ between them in any of the assessments active and sham rTMS treatments.
18	Sachdev et al,[54] 2007	Figure-8 coil	RCT with an open extension up to 20 sessions, clinicians administering treatment not blind to group assignment	18 treatment-resistant (have failed ≥2 adequate trials of medications and CBT); psychiatric comorbidities excluded	2 wk (10 sessions, 5/wk)	Left DLPFC	10 Hz, 110% rMT, 1500 pulses/session	NS (The 2 groups did not differ on change in Y-BOCS or Maudsley Obsessive-Compulsive Inventory during 10 sessions, with/without correction for depression ratings. During 20 sessions, there was a significant reduction in total Y-BOCS scores but not after controlling for depression.)
19	Haghighi et al,[55] 2015	Figure-8 coil	Single-blind crossover	21 patients with treatment-refractory (no response in the	2 wk (10 sessions, 5/wk)	Sequential bilateral DLPFC (left, then right).	20 Hz, 100% rMT, 750 pulses/session	According to both Y-BOCS and CGI, symptom severity reduced in the

(continued on next page)

Table 1
(continued)

Study #	Reference	Coil Type	Study Type/Design	Sample	Tx Protocol	Target	Stimulation Parameters	Results
				last 10 wk to ≥3 antidepressant trials of sufficient dose (including clomipramine) and CBT), moderate-severe symptoms (baseline Y-BOCS >17); psychiatric comorbidities excluded; 1 wk before its start and throughout the study patients were treated with a standard SSRI/clomipramine at therapeutic dosages and CBT for ≥10 consecutive weeks		Targeting followed the "5-cm method" (ie, 5 cm anterior to motor area along a parasagital line)		active as compared with the sham condition. Full and partial responses were observed with active but not with sham stimulation
20	Jahangard et al,[56] 2016	Figure-8 coil	Single-blind crossover design, examining effect on symptom severity and	10 patients; see inclusion/ exclusion criteria in study 19 above	2 wk (10 sessions, 5/wk)	Sequential bilateral DLPFC (left, then right). Targeting followed	20 Hz, 100% rMT, 750 pulses/session	Reduction in symptom severity only after active rTMS and a parallel improvement in

#	Coil	Design	Sample	Duration	Target	Parameters	Results
		cognitive performance			the "5-cm method" (ie, 5 cm anterior to motor area)		cognitive performance (auditory and visual perception, short-term memory, and processing speed)
21	Shayganfard et al,[57] 2016	Figure-8 coil	Single-blind crossover design, examining effect on symptom severity and executive functions	See study 20 above	2 wk (10 sessions, 5/wk)	Sequential bilateral DLPFC (left, then right). Targeting followed the "5-cm method" (ie, 5 cm anterior to motor area)	20 Hz, 100% rMT, 750 pulses/session	Reduction in symptom severity only after active rTMS. Continuous improvement in executive functions (Wisconsin Card Sorting Test) but unrelated to treatment condition
22	Ruffini et al,[58] 2009	Figure-8 coil	RCT with 3 mo follow-up, clinicians administering treatment not blind to group assignment	23 treatment-resistant patients with OCD (failed ≥2 adequate trials of 12 wk max dosage medications and CBT; moderate–severe symptoms (baseline Y-BOCS ≥16); axis I comorbidities excluded	3 wk (15 sessions, 5/wk)	Left OFC	1 Hz, 80% rMT	Significant reduction of Y-BOCS scores in active vs sham immediately after rTMS (19.7% vs 6.7%) that remained significant for 10 wk follow-up with loss of significance after 12 wk (14.7% vs 5.7%)

(continued on next page)

Table 1
(continued)

Study #	Reference	Coil Type	Study Type/Design	Sample	Tx Protocol	Target	Stimulation Parameters	Results
23	Mantovani et al,[59] 2010	Figure-8 coil	RCT, clinicians administering treatment not blind to group assignment; nonresponders to sham and responders to active/sham offered 4 wk extension (open label); responders followed-up at 3 mo	18 patients with OCD with residual moderate-severe symptoms (baseline Y-BOCS ≥16) despite an adequate trial of SRI and CBT; severe MDD, substance use comorbidities excluded	4-8 wk (20-40 sessions, 5/wk)	Bilateral pre-SMA	1 Hz, 100% rMT, 1200 pulses/session	NS (Y-BOCS decreased significantly ($P < .001$) in both the active group (6 points, 25.4%) and the sham group (3.2 points, 12%) without significant difference between the 2 treatment conditions)
26	Arumugham et al,[60] 2015	Figure-8 coil	RCT, clinicians administering treatment not blind to group assignment	36 patients with moderate-severe OCD (Y-BOCS ≥16) with partial/poor response to adequate SRI trial; psychotic, bipolar and severe MDD comorbidities excluded; on stable medications regimens throughout the study	18 sessions over 3 wk	Bilateral pre-SMA	1 Hz, 100% rMT, 1200 pulses/session	NS (there were no significant differences between the groups after 3 wk of treatment in Y-BOCS, response rates, depressive and anxiety symptoms)

27	Pelissolo et al,[61] 2016	Figure-8 coil	RCT, clinicians administering treatment not blind to group assignment	36 patients with moderate–severe OCD (baseline Y-BOCS >15) with ≥8-wk adequate SSRI trials without satisfying results	4 wk (20 sessions, 5/wk)	Bilateral pre-SMA	1 Hz, 100% rMT, 1500 pulses/session	NS (no significant difference between the 2 groups in Y-BOCS change from baseline to 4 wk. Responder rates at week 4 were not different between groups (10.5% in active vs 20% in sham, $P = .63$)
25	Gomes et al,[62] 2012	Figure-8 coil	RCT with 3 mo follow-up; clinicians administering treatment not blind to group assignment	22 patients with moderate–severe OCD (baseline Y-BOCS ≥16); failed ≥2 medication trials; psychiatric comorbidities (except MDD) excluded; medication regimens unchanged for the duration of the study	2 wk (10 sessions, 5/wk)	Bilateral pre-SMA	1 Hz, 100% rMT, 1200 pulses/session	At the end of treatment, the response rate was 42% with active and 12% with sham treatment ($P < .001$). After 14 wk, the response rate was 35% with active and 6.02% with sham ($P < .001$)
24	Kang et al,[63] 2009	Figure-8 coil	RCT, clinicians administering treatment not blind to group assignment	20 treatment-resistant patients with OCD	10 d (10 sessions, 1/d)	Right DLPFC and SMA sequentially	1 Hz, 110% rMT, 1200 pulses/target/session	NS (Similar improvements in OCD and depressive symptoms were observed for

(continued on next page)

Table 1
(continued)

Study #	Reference	Coil Type	Study Type/Design	Sample	Tx Protocol	Target	Stimulation Parameters	Results
								active and sham rTMS at 2 wk after the end of treatment. Y-BOCS reductions were 2.9 points (10.9%) and 3.4 (12.9%) for active and sham rTMS, respectively)

Abbreviations: MDD, major depressive disorder

Posttreatment, the response rate (defined as $\geq$30% reduction in Y-BOCS from base-line) in the active group was 38.1% versus 11.1% in the sham group (P = .0033), trans-lating to a number needed to treat (NNT) of 3.7. The partial response rate (defined as $\geq$20% reduction in Y-BOCS score from baseline) in the active group was 54.8% versus 26.7% in the sham group (P = .0076). At 1-month follow-up, the response rate was 45.2% in the active group compared with 17.8% in the sham group (P = .0057) with NNT of 3.64.

Real-world data on 219 patients with OCD was obtained from 22 clinical sites with the H7 Coil.[36] 167 patients with at least 1 postbaseline Y-BOCS were included in the analysis. Response rate after 29 treatments was 58%—higher than reported in the multicenter trial.[33] Interestingly, patients responded within a shorter time-frame (4 weeks on average) than typical for psychotherapy or pharmacotherapy (10–13 weeks[37]). Additionally, a continuous gradual reduction in Y-BOCS was evident up to 40 treatments.[36]

The H7 Coil's efficacy in OCD was further explored by post hoc analyses demon-strating: (1) greater treatment benefit relative to sham for more severe patients (base-line Y-BOCS>28)[38]; (2) significant efficacy regardless of prior nonresponse to pharmacotherapy or CBT[39]; and (3) significant improvement in depressive symptoms for OCD-MDD comorbid patients.[40,41] Because Deep TMS is effective even for pa-tients who failed to respond to pharmacotherapy/CBT, as well as demonstrating response in a shorter timeframe, it seems that it exerts its effect via a different MOA. The hypothesized underlying mechanism of Deep TMS in OCD is direct modu-lation of the CSTC circuitry. EEG and behavioral analyses of the pilot study data as well as a separate magnetic resonance spectroscopy (MRS) study addressed the question of the H7 Coil's MOA in OCD. First, electrophysiological recordings in the pilot study revealed a significant enhancement of the error-related negativity (ERN)—a signal, occurring when a behavioral error was made, that is attributed to the dACC (the treat-ment stimulation target)—following active but not sham treatment. This ERN enhance-ment was correlated with symptom improvement.[34] Second, analysis of behavioral data from the Stroop task performed in the pilot study demonstrated that posttreat-ment patients reduced their posterror slowing, sacrificing accuracy, similarly to healthy individuals (i.e., normalization of the speed–accuracy trade-off).[42] Third, a ^{1}H MRS study[43] found significant increases in levels of Naphthaleneacetic acid (NAA), choline, and creatine in the dACC following Deep TMS with the H7 Coil in pa-tients with OCD, indicating direct neural stimulation in this region.

Finally, the question of response durability was explored by surveying responders from the multicenter RCT and the postmarketing registry.[44] The average durability of Deep TMS for OCD was found to be 1.98($\pm$0.13) years or greater (62% of patients were still considered to have durability at the time of the survey). Durability was not assessed using symptomatic ratings but pragmatically defined as the elapsed time from the end of Deep TMS treatment until a change in treatment was necessary. None-theless, the findings shed light on how durable the treatment is.

D-B80 (Double-Cone) Coil

In 2020, the FDA granted a 510(k) clearance, or statement of substantial equivalence, of a cooled 120° bent figure-8 coil, the D-B80 coil, based on electric field (EF) modeling.

The D-B80 coil and the Deep TMS H7 Coil differ in diameter of their circular wings and distance between the 2 wings. D-B80 has an outer diameter of 95 mm and in-ner diameter of 67 mm, whereas the H7 Coil has major and minor axis ranges of 70 to 130 mm and 55 to 105 mm, respectively. The density of the windings in each

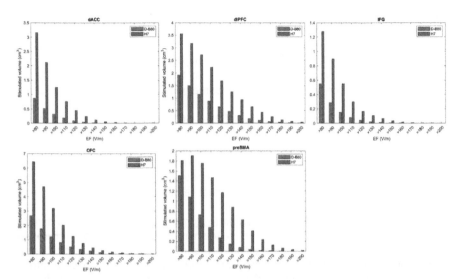

Fig. 2. Distribution of values of electric field intensity within specific brain regions. Histograms of distribution of the volume in cubic centimeter according to the induced electric field range for the Deep TMS H7 Coil and the D-B80 coil are plotted for 5 brain regions (dACC, dlPFC, IFG, OFC, and pre-SMA). Field columns are in bins of 10 V/m. Shown are the averaged results of 22 simulated head models (reproduced from ref[33]).

circular coil is also different (D-B80 has 2 layers, 3 windings on top and 4 beneath. H7 has 2 layers of 4 windings each). Additionally, the D-B80 has a rigid fixed 120° angle between the 2 wings while the H7 has flexible windings that conform to the subject's head. Tzirini and colleagues[32,33] performed a comprehensive analysis of the EF distributions of the 2 coils over the mPFC (OCD treatment location) using both phantom field measurements and 22 head models simulations. The H7 was found to induce significantly higher maximal EFs ($P < .0001$) and to stimulate 2 to 5 times larger volumes in the brain ($P < .0001$). The distribution of field values is significantly different between the coils in specific CSTC regions implicated in OCD (including dACC, dorsolateral prefrontal cortex (DLPFC), OFC, inferior frontal gyrus (IFG), and pre-SMA, **Fig. 2**), where the H7 induces significantly higher intensities in broader volumes. For example, the H7 induced EF greater than 80 V/m in 15% of the dACC compared with 1.3% with the D-B80. Due to the substantial differences between the coils, the clinical efficacy of the D-B80 for OCD should be independently investigated in an appropriately powered RCT.

Three published studies on the use of the D-B80 coil for the treatment of OCD currently exist (see **Table 1**). However, the stimulation protocols applied in these studies differ from the current FDA-cleared protocol of 20 Hz stimulation at 100% of foot resting motor threshold (rMT), 4 cm anterior to the foot hotspot and they would be considered off label.

The first pilot study[28] included 19 patients, aiming to assess the coil's efficacy using LF stimulation over OFC. A randomized, double-blind, crossover design was implemented with two 1-week treatment periods (active stimulation vs sham stimulation) separated by a 1-month washout period. Concomitantly, a subgroup of patients underwent a PET scan after each stimulation sequence. At day 7, a significant decrease from baseline in Y-BOCS scores was observed after both active ($P < .01$) and sham stimulation ($P = .02$). This decrease tended to be larger after active compared with sham stimulation: − 6 (−29, 0) points versus − 2 (−20, 4) points (P = .07). Active versus sham PET scan contrasts showed that stimulation was related to bilateral decrease in OFC metabolism. Although these results might hint at a potentially efficacious target and treatment protocol, this study suffered from low power and needs confirmation in an extended study with a larger sample of patients. Second, there were substantial (and statistically significant) responses in the sham condition group. This may have been, in part, due to the crossover design that is more prone to unblinding as noticeable differences between the sham and active coils exist.

The next study[45] used the D-B80 coil, in an open-label design, to target with LF the mPFC of 10 patients with OCD for 10 days. Results showed a 39% reduction in Y-BOCS score from baseline ($P < .001$) that persisted for 1 month following treatment. Although this is a positive result, this study is limited by its open-label nature in addition to its small sample size. Thus, confirmatory RCTs are warranted.

Finally, a study of predictors of response to the D-B80 coil was conducted on 20 patients with OCD.[27] Resting-state fMRI was used to identify neural correlates of response to 20 to 30 sessions of 10 Hz stimulation over mPFC. A region of interest in mPFC was used to generate whole brain functional connectivity maps pretreatment

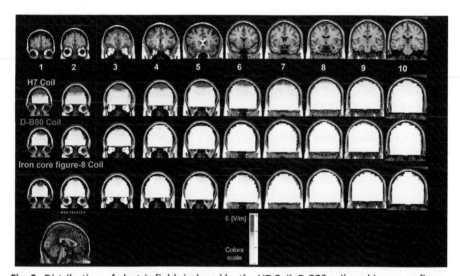

Fig. 3. Distribution of electric fields induced by the H7 Coil, D-B80 coil, and iron core figure-8 coil. The electric field distribution was measured in a phantom model of the human head (15 cm × 13 cm × 18 cm), filled with physiologic saline solution. The colored field maps indicate the electrical field absolute magnitude in each pixel, for 10 coronal slices, 1 cm apart, along with the appropriate MRI coronal images. The colored regions on the anatomic MR coronal slices on the top row represent the brain regions (OFC: Brodmann area [BA] 10-*yellow*, BA11-*brown*, BA47-*medium blue*; IFG: BA45-*turquise*; DLPFC: BA9-*green*, BA46-*sky blue*; dACC: BA32-*green*; pre-SMA: BA8-*dark blue*) associated with the pathophysiology of OCD. The coils were placed over the theoretic frontal cortex of the head model and the field in each pixel was measured using a "pick-up" dipole probe, attached to an oscilloscope. The red colors indicate field magnitude above the threshold for neuronal activation, which was set to 100 V/m based on the average threshold for motor activation of the foot. The field maps are adjusted for 100% of the foot motor threshold (100 V/m), in accordance with the FDA-cleared protocol.

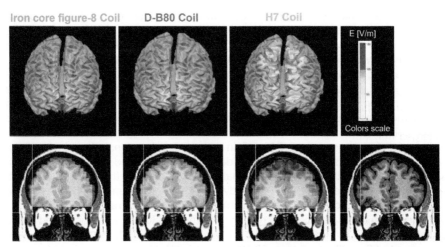

Fig. 4. Top panel: Surface plots of the electric field distribution induced by the H7 Coil, D-B80 coil, and iron core figure-8 coil, based on phantom head model field measurements. Bottom panel: Electric field maps at a coronal slice 3 cm from the nasion, which includes part of the dACC (indicated in brown on the bottom right image). The color maps are partially transparent to make the dACC visible.

and posttreatment. Half of the patients met response criteria ($\geq$50% reduction in Y-BOCS from baseline). Responders had higher mPFC-ventral-striatal connectivity at baseline and the extent of its reduction from pretreatment to posttreatment correlated with the extent of Y-BOCS reduction. This is consistent with previous fMRI studies of DBS in OCD[46] but opposite to reports on mechanisms of mPFC-rTMS in MDD.[47] fMRI could prove useful in predicting response to mPFC-rTMS in OCD. Nevertheless, it should be noted that this study suffers from similar limitations of an open-label design as well as small sample size.

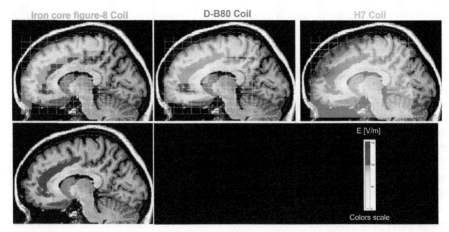

Fig. 5. Electric field maps for the H7 Coil, D-B80 coil, and iron core figure-8 coil at a midsagittal slice 1 cm from the midline. The anterior cingulate cortex (ACC) is indicated in blue. The color maps are partially transparent to make the ACC visible.

Iron Core (Figure-8) Coil

In 2022, the FDA granted a 510(k) clearance to a third rTMS coil, the iron core figure-8 coil. The iron core figure-8 coil is made of 2 mm laminated 3% grain-oriented silicon steel.[48] Due to winding limitations, a modified figure-8 coil fits into the center and side spaces of the core. This coil is designed to reduce power requirements and heat generation, while improving penetration of the magnetic field.[49] To better understand the comparative capabilities of the iron core figure-8 coil, its EF distribution was measured. Maps of EF distribution of the 3 coils are shown in **Fig. 3**. Surface plots and enlarged maps of a coronal slice 3 cm from the nasion, which includes part of the dACC, are shown in **Fig. 4**. Maps over a midsagittal slice 1 cm from the midline are shown in **Fig. 5**. Red pixels indicate EF values greater than 100 V/m, which is the threshold for motor activation. Orange pixels indicate EF values of between 80 and 100 V/m. Although 80 to 100 V/m is insufficient to recruit neurons for a visible motor response over the motor cortex, it still stimulates millions of neurons beneath the coil. It is evident that the H7 Coil induces much broader and deeper stimulation compared with the 2 other coils. Only the H7 Coil induces suprathreshold EF, which stimulates structures in the dACC.

Because clinical evidence of the efficacy of the iron core figure-8 coil in OCD is lacking, we will present the available evidence for the figure-8 coil to which its configuration is most similar. However, none of the studies using the figure-8 coil in OCD followed the current FDA-cleared protocol and are therefore considered off-label.

Although most studies of rTMS in OCD since 1997 have been done using a figure-8 coil, due to a large variability in targets and protocols, it is difficult to draw definitive conclusions on its efficacy.

Of the 15 studies conducted to date (see **Table 1**), 6 different targets were explored (right DLPFC, left DLPFC, bilateral DLPFC, OFC, pre-SMA, SMA). Beyond differing in stimulation target, the studies also differ in stimulation parameters and protocols, making it challenging to combine findings and determine the efficacy of the figure-8 coil in OCD.

Of the 4 studies examining the right DLPFC target,[49–52] the 2 that used LF stimulation[51,52] reported positive results; however, both had small sample sizes and were not properly blinded. Two studies examined the left DLPFC target and had negative results[53,54] and 3 crossover RCTs from the same group examined HF sequential bilateral DLPFC stimulation and reported improvement in OCD symptom severity[55–57] as well as in cognitive performance[56] but not in executive functions.[57] These studies also had small samples and were only single-blinded (i.e., the clinician administering the treatment was aware of treatment condition). Only one (single-blinded) study used the figure-8 coil to explore the efficacy of LF OFC stimulation and reported significant reduction in symptom severity lasting 10 weeks after the end of treatment and losing significance at 12 weeks posttreatment.[58]

The efficacy of LF pre-SMA stimulation was investigated in 4 RCTs, 3 of which[59–61] failed to find superiority over sham. The fourth[62] reported positive results with superiority over sham lasting for 14 weeks posttreatment. The results of this study are limited, however, by the small sample size and the noticeable differences between the active and sham procedures. Finally, one study with negative results was published on the efficacy of sequential LF stimulation of the right DLPFC and SMA in OCD.[63]

Theta Burst Stimulation

In 2005, Huang and colleagues[64] developed a paradigm of theta burst stimulation (TBS) —low-intensity bursts of rTMS at 50 Hz—as a safer, more controllable, more

Table 2
TBS studies in obsessive-compulsive disorder

Study #	Reference	Coil Type	Study Type/ Design	Sample Size	Tx Protocol	Target	Stimulation Parameters	Results
1	Wu et al,[65] 2010	Figure-8 coil	Case report	1	10 sessions of cTBS followed by 10 iTBS sessions	Sequential bilateral DLPFC (right followed by left)	50 HZ bursts repeated at 5 Hz, 80% rMT, 1200 pulses per session	Patient responded dramatically (Y-BOCS 19->8, HDRS 49->29->15). Improvement in OCD symptoms was associated with a marked reduction in right DLPFC activity on fMRI acquired during symptom provocation
2	Naro et al,[66] 2019	Figure-8 coil	Randomized crossover study with EEG recording	10	5 sessions of iTBS	Left DLPFC	50HZ bursts repeated at 5 Hz, 80% rMT, 600 pulses per session	All patients improved in OCD symptomatology up to 1 mo following active iTBS (≥25% reduction in Y-BOCS score), although 4 among them improved up to 3 mo follow-up. These patients were those showing a more extensive reshape of frontal areas phase synchronization and frontoparietal coherence compared with the other participants

#	Study	Coil	Design	N	Protocol	Target	Parameters	Results
3	Harika-Germaneau et al,[67] 2019	Figure-8 coil	RCT	30	6 wk of cTBS	Pre-SMA	50 Hz bursts repeated at 5 Hz, 70% rMT, 600 pulses/session	NS (there was no significant difference between active and sham cTBS groups in treatment efficacy)
4	Syed et al,[68] 2021	D-B80 coil	Open label case series	12	Average of 16.5(5.8) sessions of iTBS	Sequential bilateral mPFC-ACC	50 Hz bursts at 5 Hz, 90%–100% rTMS, 600 pulses/hemisphere/session	There was a statistically significant decrease in Y-BOCS scores [31.4(6.6) vs 23.3 (9.9), t(11) = 3.53 $P < .005$)] with a mean decrease of 25.44%. Five of the 12 patients (41.67%) met criteria for response (>35% reduction in Y-BOCS scores). 2 patients dropped out citing poor tolerability
5	Williams et al,[70] 2021	Figure-8 coil	Open label case series	7	5 consecutive days of accelerated cTBSmod (10 sessions/d). Localite Neuronavigation System was used to position the TMS coil over	Right frontal pole	Each session composed 1800 pulses, delivered in a continuous train of 600 bursts. Each burst contained 3 pulses at 30 Hz, repeated at 6 Hz (18,000 pulses/d, hourly; 90,000 total)	Response rate at day 14 (primary endpoint) was 57%, and overall response rate at ≥ 1 time point was 71%. Statistically significant Y-BOCS score reduction from baseline to

(continued on next page)

Table 2
(continued)

Study #	Reference	Coil Type	Study Type/ Design	Sample Size	Tx Protocol	Target	Stimulation Parameters	Results
					the individualized stimulation target		pulses). Stimulation was delivered at 90% rMT	Day 14 (P = .018). At Day 14, 3 participants no longer met diagnostic criteria for OCD Responders showed greater decrease in bilateral DLPFC activation compared with nonresponders (P = .05) during inhibitory cognitive control activation (go/no-go task) Only minimal side effects were experienced
6	Dutta et al,[71] 2021	Figure-8 coil	RCT	33	2 sessions a day for 5 d a wk (10 sessions in total) of cTBS	OFC	50HZ bursts repeated at 5 Hz, 80% rMT, 1200 pulses per day	Significant improvement only in anxiety symptoms and global severity

consistent, and longer-lasting rTMS. The continuous TBS (cTBS) inhibits, whereas the intermittent TBS (iTBS) enhances excitability in the motor cortex, although this rule is not generalizable across all neurons. Six studies of TBS in OCD have been published to date, 5 using the figure-8 coil and 1 using the D-B80 coil (**Table 2**). The first application of TBS to the treatment of psychiatric disorders was a case report[65] of a patient with comorbid OCD-MDD who responded dramatically to treatment with cTBS over right DLPFC followed by iTBS over left DLPFC. OCD symptom improvement was associated with reduction in right DLPFC activity on fMRI acquired during symptom provocation.

A randomized crossover pilot study followed[66] with 10 patients undergoing 1 month of active or sham iTBS over left DLPFC. Results showed that all the patients improved in OCD symptomatology up to 1 month following active iTBS, whereas 4 of them improved up to 3 months follow-up. These patients were those showing a more extensive reshape of frontal areas phase synchronization and frontoparietal coherence compared with the other participants, suggesting that iTBS efficacy depends on the extent of frontal and frontoparietal connectivity modulation.

An RCT that evaluated the efficacy and tolerability of 6 weeks of cTBS over SMA in 30 patients with OCD failed to demonstrate superiority over sham.[67] Although it is possible that the lack of effect in this study was a result of understimulation (concerning both intensity and number of pulses), broader and deeper stimulation target regions should be explored before dismissing cTBS as a protocol.

More recently, Syed and colleagues[68] reported on their experience treating 12 OCD patients with an average of 16.5($\pm$5.8) iTBS sessions over bilateral mPFC-dACC. A statistically significant mean decrease of 25.44% in Y-BOCS scores ($P < .005$) was found. Five of the 12 patients (41.67%) met criteria for response (>35% reduction in Y-BOCS scores). Considering the shorter stimulation duration and lower intensity of intervention, iTBS may be a promising protocol for deep rTMS in treatment-resistant OCD. Although the D-B80 coil has been shown to be capable of stimulating deeper cortical structures like mPFC,[27] it may require higher stimulation intensities due to dispersion of magnetic flux as the depth of target region increases,[69] lowering its tolerability. In line with this, 2 subjects dropped out citing poor tolerability (i.e., headache and scalp discomfort). Interestingly, 2 out of 3 subjects in whom symptom provocation was attempted had shown substantial decline in the Y-BOCS score (53.5% and 44.7%). Interpretation is limited because this is an open-labeled case-series and assessments were unblinded. This report provides preliminary evidence in support of efficacy of iTBS in treatment-resistant OCD; however, the protocol needs to be evaluated in sham-controlled trials to establish its efficacy and tolerability.

Another open-label case-series on 7 treatment-resistant moderate OCD patients applied accelerated (10 sessions/d) modified cTBS to their right frontal pole.[70] Following treatment, at the primary outcome timepoint (Day 14), a statistically significant reduction in Y-BOCS ($P = .018$) was found with a 57% response rate. At Day 14, 3 participants no longer met diagnostic criteria for OCD. Responders showed a greater decrease in bilateral DLPFC activation than nonresponders ($P = .05$) during inhibitory cognitive control in the go/no-go task-based fMRI.

Finally, 33 patients were randomized to receive active or sham cTBS over OFC for 2 sessions a day for 5 days a week (10 sessions in total).[71] Y-BOCS, depression and anxiety, and global severity scales were assessed at baseline, immediately following treatment, and 2 weeks posttreatment. Results revealed significant improvement only in anxiety symptoms and global severity.

DISCUSSION

Since OCD is quite common and debilitating, there has been focus on finding alternative effective therapies.

In 2018, the first rTMS device, Deep TMS H7 Coil, was cleared by the FDA for the treatment of OCD based on the positive results of a pilot study and multicenter RCT that followed. Two additional coils, the D-B80 coil and the iron core figure-8 coil, have been granted 510(k) clearance by the FDA (based on substantial equivalence without clinical data submission) in 2020 and 2022, respectively. However, the physical properties of these coils differ from the H7 Coil, resulting (as evident from EF distribution measurements) in different functional properties. Therefore, the purpose of this review was to compare the 3 coils on their physical properties and the functional/clinical implications. We also presented the data for non-FDA approved protocols and targets, with the available clinical evidence for the D-B80 and figure-8 coils over different regions than the mPFC. Our hope is that this review will aid in a clearer view of a changing treatment landscape and as such, might serve as a reference guide for rTMS in OCD.

During the past decade, 10 reviews and meta-analyses of rTMS in OCD have been published.[72–81] Although relevant in generating information on promising rTMS targets and stimulation parameters, combined effect results have limitations in enhancing our understanding of clinical predictors (e.g., age, duration/severity of OCD, prior treatment resistance) and stimulation-relevant factors (e.g., target, stimulation frequency, number of pulses) that are potentially associated with positive treatment outcomes. Although the Deep TMS H7 Coil studies' results point to efficacy of the mPFC-dACC, no clear target stems from the small heterogenous D-B80 and figure-8 coil studies. The modest number of studies, clinical heterogeneity, as well as different protocols and sham conditions, among studies call for careful interpretation. Meta-analyses that attempted to combine these heterogenous studies fell short in guiding clinical practice.

Most recently, a network meta-analysis (NMA) was the first to compare available treatments for OCD across modalities.[81] Unlike pairwise meta-analysis, NMA allows data synthesis from multiple trials with different interventions and enables direct and indirect comparisons using a common comparator.[82] Fifty-five RCTs examining 19 treatments or placebo involving 2011 participants were included in the NMA. Ondansetron [standardized mean difference −2.01 (95% CI: −3.19, −0.83)], Deep TMS [−1.95 (−3.25, −0.65)], therapist administered CBT [−1.46 (−2.93, 0.01)], and aripiprazole [−1.36 (−2.56, −0.17)] were ranked as the best 4 treatments on using surface under the cumulative ranking percentage values (85.4%, 83.2%, 80.3%, 67.9%, respectively). In sensitivity analyses, Deep TMS was ranked as the best treatment strategy for SRI-resistant OCD. rTMS (excluding Deep TMS) was not significant in this NMA.

A recent cost-effectiveness analysis of Deep TMS relative to other established treatment options for OCD, demonstrated that it is more cost-effective than antipsychotics and intensive, facilities-based ERP approaches.[83] Hence, it may be an incremental strategy to use before sending patients to higher levels of care, and it is reasonable to implement even before routine outpatient ERP if there is a waiting list.

Areas that should be further explored in the field of TMS for OCD in the hopes of improving its efficacy are (1) personalization of treatment, building on the promising evidence for predictors and moderators of response to mPFC-dACC stimulation,[38,27] (2) response durability[44] and (3) accelerated and patterned stimulation paradigms such as iTBS (over mPFC-dACC), and (4) use of rotational field Deep TMS H-Coils[84] to engage more neurons in the CSTC.

CLINICS CARE POINTS

- Before starting Deep TMS treatment, conduct a detailed clinician interview with the YBOCS symptom checklist, calculate the YBOCS severity score, and create a hierarchy of individualized OCD provocations for the TMS technician to use daily. Review the patient's specific OCD with the TMS technician and track the patients progress using the YBOCS severity score on a weekly basis.

- After placing the coil in the treatment position but before treating with the Deep TMS coil over the CSTC, the TMS technician must provoke the patient's OCD to a moderately-severe level of distress while preventing the patient from engaging in compulsions during the treatment session.

- The CSTC is stimulated with Deep TMS at 100% of the resting motor threshold of the anterior tibialis, to ensure neural activation at depth. The motor threshold intensity must be rechecked at least weekly for efficacy and safety purposes.

- During treatment patients may become more difficult to provoke due to improvement or due to a change in OCD symptoms. Patients may utilize more avoidance behaviors. The usual reduction in the YBOCS with deep TMS is gradual and continuous. A precipitous drop in the YBOCS, or a plateau for more than two weeks, warrants a detailed clinician review of the patient's OCD.

DISCLOSURE

A. Tendler and Y. Roth have a financial interest in BrainsWay. Y. Roth and T. Harmelech are employed by BrainsWay.

REFERENCES

1. American Psychiatric Association. Diagnostic and statistical manual of mental disorders. 5th edition. Washington, DC: American Psychiatric Association; 2013.
2. Rasmussen SA, Eisen JL. The epidemiology and clinical features of obsessive compulsive disorder. Psychiatr Clin North Am 1992;15:743–58.
3. Ruscio AM, Stein DJ, Chiu WT, et al. The epidemiology of obsessive-compulsive disorder in the National Comorbidity Survey Replication. Mol Psychiatry 2010;15: 53–63.
4. Norberg MM, Calamari JE, Cohen RJ, et al. Quality of life in obsessive-compulsive disorder: an evaluation of impairment and a preliminary analysis of the ameliorating effects of treatment. Depress Anxiety 2008;25:248–59.
5. Adam Y, Meinlschmidt G, Gloster AT, et al. obsessive-compulsive disorder in the community: 12-month prevalence, comorbidity and impairment. Soc Psychiatry Psychiatr Epidemiol 2012;47:339–49.
6. Meier SM, Mattheisen M, Mors O, et al. Mortality among persons with obsessive-compulsive disorder in Denmark. JAMA Psychiatry 2016;73:268–74.
7. Deacon BJ, Abramowitz JS. Cognitive and behavioral treatments for anxiety disorders: a review of meta-analytic findings. J Clin Psychol 2004;60:429–41.
8. Koran LM, Hanna GL, Hollander E, et al. Practice guideline for the treatment of patients with obsessive-compulsive disorder. Am J Psychiatry 2007; 164(Suppl):5–53.
9. Goodman WK, Price LH, Delgado PL, et al. Specificity of serotonin reuptake inhibitors in the treatment of obsessive-compulsive disorder. Comparison of fluvoxamine and desipramine. Arch Gen Psychiatry 1990;47:577–85.
10. Pittenger C, Bloch MH. Pharmacological treatment of obsessive-compulsive disorder. Psychiatr Clin North Am 2014;37:375–91.

11. Pigott TA, Seay SM. A review of the efficacy of selective serotonin reuptake inhibitors in obsessive-compulsive disorder. J Clin Psychiatry 1999;60:101–6.

12. Ackerman DL, Greenland S. Multivariate meta-analysis of controlled drug studies for obsessive-compulsive disorder. J Clin Psychopharmacol 2002;22:309–17.

13. Romanelli RJ, Wu FM, Gamba R, et al. Behavioral therapy and serotonin reuptake inhibitor pharmacotherapy in the treatment of obsessive-compulsive disorder: a systematic review and meta-analysis of head-to-head randomized controlled trials. Depress Anxiety 2014;31:641–52.

14. Öst LG, Havnen A, Hansen B, et al. Cognitive behavioral treatments of obsessive-compulsive disorder. A systematic review and meta-analysis of studies published 1993-2014. Clin Psychol Rev 2015;40:156–69.

15. Simpson HB, Huppert JD, Petkova E, et al. Response versus remission in obsessive-compulsive disorder. J Clin Psychiatry 2006;67:269–76.

16. Yuste R. From the neuron doctrine to neural networks. Nat Rev Neurosci 2015;16:487–97.

17. Milad MR, Rauch SL. Obsessive-compulsive disorder: beyond segregated cortico-striatal pathways. Trends Cogn Sci 2012;16:43–51.

18. Baxter LR Jr, Schwartz JM, Mazziotta JC, et al. Cerebral glucose metabolic rates in nondepressed patients with obsessive-compulsive disorder. Am J Psychiatry 1988;145:1560–3.

19. Breiter HC, Rauch SL, Kwong KK, et al. Functional magnetic resonance imaging of symptom provocation in obsessive-compulsive disorder. Arch Gen Psychiatry 1996;53:595–606.

20. Saxena S, Rauch SL. Functional neuroimaging and the neuroanatomy of obsessive-compulsive disorder. Psychiatr Clin North Am 2000;23:563–86.

21. Schwartz JM, Stoessel PW, Baxter LR Jr, et al. Systematic changes in cerebral glucose metabolic rate after successful behavior modification treatment of obsessive-compulsive disorder. Arch Gen Psychiatry 1996;53:109–13.

22. Benkelfat C, Nordahl TE, Semple WE, et al. Local cerebral glucose metabolic rates in obsessive-compulsive disorder. Patients treated with clomipramine. Arch Gen Psychiatry 1990;47:840–8.

23. Park HR, Kim IH, Kang H, et al. Electrophysiological and imaging evidence of sustained inhibition in limbic and frontal networks following deep brain stimulation for treatment refractory obsessive compulsive disorder. PLoS One 2019;14:e0219578.

24. Le Jeune F, Vérin M, N'Diaye K, et al. Decrease of prefrontal metabolism after subthalamic stimulation in obsessive-compulsive disorder: a positron emission tomography study. Biol Psychiatry 2010;68:1016–22.

25. Zuo C, Ma Y, Sun B, et al. Metabolic imaging of bilateral anterior capsulotomy in refractory obsessive compulsive disorder: an FDG PET study. J Cereb Blood Flow Metab 2013;33:880–7.

26. Yin D, Zhang C, Lv Q, et al. Dissociable frontostriatal connectivity: mechanism and predictor of the clinical efficacy of capsulotomy in obsessive-compulsive disorder. Biol Psychiatry 2018;84:926–36.

27. Dunlop K, Woodside B, Olmsted M, et al. Reductions in cortico-striatal hyperconnectivity accompany successful treatment of obsessive-compulsive disorder with dorsomedial prefrontal rTMS. Neuropsychopharmacology 2016;41:1395–403.

28. Nauczyciel C, Le Jeune F, Naudet F, et al. Repetitive transcranial magnetic stimulation over the orbitofrontal cortex for obsessive-compulsive disorder: a double-blind, crossover study. Transl Psychiatry 2014;4:e436.

29. Ting JT, Feng G. Neurobiology of obsessive-compulsive disorder: insights into neural circuitry dysfunction through mouse genetics. Curr Opin Neurobiol 2011; 21:842–8.

30. Ahmari SE, Spellman T, Douglass NL, et al. Repeated cortico-striatal stimulation generates persistent OCD-like behavior. Science 2013;340:1234–9.

31. Greenberg BD, Rauch SL, Haber SN. Invasive circuitry-based neurotherapeutics: stereotactic ablation and deep brain stimulation for OCD. Neuropsychopharmacology 2010;35:317–36.

32. Tzirini M, Roth Y, Harmelech T, et al. Electrical field measurements and simulation of the H7 and D-B80 coils: Non-equivalence of the TMS coils for obsessive compulsive disorder. Brain Stimul 2021;14(6):1525–7.

33. Tzirini M, Roth Y, Harmelech T, et al. Measurements and simulations of electric field distribution of two TMS coils cleared for obsessive compulsive disorder. PLoS ONE 2022;17(8):e0263145.

34. Carmi L, Alyagon U, Barnea-Ygael N, et al. Clinical and electrophysiological outcomes of deep TMS over the medial prefrontal and anterior cortices in OCD patients. Brain Stimulation 2018;11:158–65.

35. Carmi L, Tendler A, Bystritsky A, et al. Efficacy and safety of deep transcranial magnetic stimulation for obsessive-compulsive disorder: a prospective multicenter randomized double-blind placebo-controlled trial. Am J Psychiatry 2019; 176:931–8.

36. Roth Y, Tendler A, Arikan MK, et al. Real-world efficacy of deep TMS for obsessive-compulsive disorder: Post-marketing data collected from twenty-two clinical sites. J Psychiatr Res 2021;137:667–72.

37. Soomro GM, Altman D, Rajagopal S, et al. Selective serotonin re-uptake inhibitors (SSRIs) versus placebo for obsessive compulsive disorder (OCD). Cochrane Database Syst Rev 2008;1:CD001765.

38. Storch EA, Tendler A, Schneider SC, et al. Moderators and predictors of response to deep transcranial magnetic stimulation for obsessive-compulsive disorder. J Psychiatry Res 2021;136:508–14.

39. Roth Y, Barnea-Ygael N, Carmi L, et al. Deep transcranial magnetic stimulation for obsessive-compulsive disorder is efficacious even in patients who failed multiple medications and CBT. Psychiatry Res 2020;290:113179.

40. Harmelech T, Tendler A, Roth Y, et al. Do comorbid OCD-MDD patients need two separate dTMS protocols? Brain Stimul 2020;13:1000–1.

41. Tendler A, Roth Y, Harmelech T. Deep repetitive TMS with the H7 coil is sufficient to treat comorbid MDD and OCD. Brain Stimul 2021;14:658–61.

42. Alyagon U, Barnea-Ygael N, Carmi A, et al. Modifications of cognitive performance in the Stroop task following deep rTMS treatment course in OCD patients. Brain Stimul 2021;14:48–50.

43. Reddy S, Goyal N, Shreekantiah U. Adjunctive deep transcranial magnetic stimulation (dTMS) in obsessive compulsive disorder: Findings from 1H magnetic resonance spectroscopy. Asian J Psychiatry 2021;62:102721.

44. Harmelech T, Tendler A, Arikan MK, et al. Long-term outcomes of a course of deep TMS for treatment-resistant OCD. Brain Stimul 2022;15:226–8.

45. Modirrousta M, Shams E, Katz C, et al. The efficacy of deep repetitive transcranial magnetic stimulation over the medial prefrontal cortex in obsessive compulsive disorder: results from an open-label study. Depress Anxiety 2015;32:445–50.

46. Figee M, Luigjes J, Smolders R, et al. Deep brain stimulation restores frontostriatal network activity in obsessive-compulsive disorder. Nat Neurosci 2013;16: 386–7.

47. Salomons TV, Dunlop K, Kennedy SH, et al. Resting-state cortico-thalamic-striatal connectivity predicts response to dorsomedial prefrontal rTMS in major depressive disorder. Neuropsychopharmacology 2014;39:488–98.
48. Epstein CM, Davey KR. Iron-Core Coils for Transcranial Magnetic Stimulation. J Clin Neurophysiol 2002;19(4):376–81.
49. Greenberg BD, George MS, Martin JD, et al. Effect of prefrontal repetitive transcranial magnetic stimulation in obsessive-compulsive disorder: a preliminary study. Am J Psychiatry 1997;154(6):867–9.
50. Mansur CG, Myczkowki ML, de Barros Cabral S, et al. Placebo effect after prefrontal magnetic stimulation in the treatment of resistant obsessive-compulsive disorder: a randomized controlled trial. Int J Neuropsychopharmacol 2011; 14(10):1389–97.
51. Elbeh KA, Elserogy YM, Khalifa HE, et al. Repetitive transcranial magnetic stimulation in the treatment of obsessive–compulsive disorders: double blind randomized clinical trial. Psychiatry Res 2016;238:264–9.
52. Seo HJ, Jung YE, Lim HK, et al. Adjunctive low-frequency repetitive transcranial magnetic stimulation over the right dorsolateral prefrontal cortex in patients with treatment-resistant obsessive-compulsive disorder: A randomized controlled trial. Clin Psychopharmacol Neurosci 2016;14(2):153–60.
53. Prasko J, Pasková B, Zálesky R, et al. The effect of repetitive transcranial magnetic stimulation (rTMS) on symptoms in obsessive compulsive disorder. a randomized, double-blind, sham controlled study. Neuro Endocrinol Lett 2006; 27(3):327–32.
54. Sachdev PS, Loo CK, Mitchell PB, et al. Repetitive transcranial magnetic stimulation for the treatment of obsessive-compulsive disorder: a double-blind controlled investigation. Psychol Med 2007;37(11):1645–9.
55. Haghighi M, Shayganfard M, Jahangard L, et al. Repetitive transcranial magnetic stimulation (rTMS) improves symptoms and reduced clinical illness in patients suffering from OCD—Results from a single-blind, randomized clinical trial with sham cross-over condition. J Psychiatr Res 2015;68:238–44.
56. Jahangard L, Haghighi M, Shayganfard M, et al. Repetitive transcranial magnetic stimulation improved symptoms of obsessive-compulsive disorder, but also cognitive performance: Results from a randomized clinical trial with a crossover design and sham condition. Neuropsychobiology 2016;73:224–32.
57. Shayganfard M, Jahangard L, Nazaribadie M, et al. Repetitive transcranial magnetic stimulation improved symptoms of obsessive-compulsive disorders but not executive functions: Results from a randomized clinical trial with crossover design and sham condition. Neuropsychobiology 2016;74:115–24.
58. Ruffini C, Locatelli M, Lucca A, et al. Augmentation effect of repetitive transcranial magnetic stimulation over the orbitofrontal cortex in drug-resistant obsessive–compulsive disorder patients: a controlled investigation. Prim Care Companion J Clin Psychiatry 2009;11(5):226–30.
59. Mantovani A, Simpson HB, Fallon BA, et al. Randomized sham-controlled trial of repetitive transcranial magnetic stimulation in treatment-resistant obsessive-compulsive disorder. Int J Neuropsychopharmacol 2010;13(2):217–27.
60. Arumugham SS, Subhasini VS, Madhuri HN, et al. Augmentation effect of low frequency-repetitive transcranial magnetic stimulation over pre-supplementary motor area in obsessive compulsive disorder: a randomized controlled trial. Brain Stimul 2015;8(2):391.
61. Pelissolo A, Harika-Germaneau G, Rachid F, et al. Repetitive transcranial magnetic stimulation to supplementary motor area in refractory obsessive-

compulsive disorder treatment: a sham-controlled trial. Int J Neuropsychopharmacol 2016;19(8):pyw025.

62. Gomes PV, Brasil-Neto JP, Allam N, et al. A randomized, double-blind trial of repetitive transcranial magnetic stimulation in obsessive–compulsive disorder with three-month follow-up. J Neuropsychiatry Clin Neurosci 2012;24(4):437–43.

63. Kang JI, Kim CH, Namkoong K, et al. A randomized controlled study of sequentially applied repetitive transcranial magnetic stimulation in obsessive-compulsive disorder. J Clin Psychiatry 2009;70(12):1645–51.

64. Huang YZ, Edwards MJ, Rounis E, et al. Theta burst stimulation of the human motor cortex. Neuron 2005;45:201–6.

65. Wu CC, Tsai CH, Lu MK, et al. Theta-burst repetitive transcranial magnetic stimulation for treatment-resistant obsessive-compulsive disorder with concomitant depression. J Clin Psychiatry 2010;71:504–6.

66. Naro A, Billeri L, Cannavò A, et al. Theta burst stimulation for the treatment of obsessive–compulsive disorder: a pilot study. J Neural Transm 2019;126: 1667–77.

67. Harika-Germaneau G, Rachid F, Chatard A, et al. Continuous theta burst stimulation over the supplementary motor area in refractory obsessive-compulsive disorder treatment: A randomized sham-controlled trial. Brain Stimul 2019;12(6): 1565–71.

68. Syed FA, Naik SS, Arumugham SS, et al. Adjuvant intermittent theta burst stimulation over dorsomedial prefrontal cortex in treatment-resistant obsessive-compulsive disorder type: Letter to the editor. Brain Stimul 2021;14(1):74–6.

69. Deng ZD, Lisanby SH, Peterchev AV. Electric field depth–focality tradeoff in transcranial magnetic stimulation: simulation comparison of 50 coil designs. Brain Stimul 2013;6:1–13.

70. Williams NR, Sudheimer KD, Cole EJ, et al. Accelerated neuromodulation therapy for Obsessive Compulsive Disorder. Brain Stimul 2021;14(2):435–7.

71. Dutta P, Dhyani M, Garg S, et al. Efficacy of intensive orbitofrontal continuous theta burst stimulation (iOFcTBS) in obsessive compulsive disorder: A randomized placebo controlled study. Psychiatry Res 2021;298:113784.

72. Slotema CW, Blom JD, Hoek HW, et al. Should we expand the toolbox of psychiatric treatment methods to include repetitive transcranial magnetic stimulation (rTMS)? A meta-analysis of the efficacy of rTMS in psychiatric disorders. J Clin Psychiatry 2010;71(7):873–84.

73. Blom RM, Figee M, Vulink N, et al. Update on repetitive transcranial magnetic stimulation in obsessive–compulsive disorder: different targets. Curr Psychiatry Rep 2011;13(4):289–94.

74. Jaafari N, Rachid F, Rotge JY, et al. Safety and efficacy of repetitive transcranial magnetic stimulation in the treatment of obsessive–compulsive disorder: a review. World J Biol Psychaitry 2012;13(3):164–77.

75. Berlim MT, Neufeld NH, van den Eynde F. Repetitive transcranial magnetic stimulation (rTMS) for obsessive–compulsive disorder (OCD): an exploratory meta-analysis of randomized and sham-controlled trials. J Psychiatr Res 2013;47(8): 999–1006.

76. Ma ZR, Shi LJ. Repetitive transcranial magnetic stimulation (rTMS) augmentation of selective serotonin reuptake inhibitors (SSRIs) for SSRI-resistant obsessive-compulsive disorder (OCD): a meta-analysis of randomized controlled trials. Int J Clin Exp Med 2014;7(12):4897–905.

77. Trevizol AP, Shiozawa P, Cook IA, et al. Transcranial magnetic stimulation for obsessive–compulsive disorder: an updated systematic review and meta-analysis. J ECT 2016;32(4):262–6.
78. Zhou DD, Wang W, Wang GM, et al. An updated meta-analysis: short-term therapeutic effects of repeated transcranial magnetic stimulation in treating obsessive-compulsive disorder. J Affect Disord 2017;215:187–96.
79. Lusicic A, Schruers KRJ, Pallanti S, et al. Transcranial magnetic stimulation in the treatment of obsessive-compulsive disorder: current perspectives. Neuropsychiatr Dis Treat 2018;14:1721–36.
80. McCathern AG, Mathai DS, Cho RY, et al. Deep transcranial magnetic stimulation for obsessive compulsive disorder. Expert Rev Neurother 2020;20:1029–36.
81. Suhas S, Kumar Malo P, Kumar V, et al. Treatment strategies for serotonin reuptake inhibitor-resistant obsessive-compulsive disorder: A network meta-analysis of randomized controlled trials. World J Biol Psychiatry 2022. https://doi.org/10.1080/15622975.2022.2082525.
82. Li T, Puhan MA, Vedula SS, et al. Network meta-analysis - highly attractive but more methodological research is needed. BMC Med 2011;9:79.
83. Gregory ST, Goodman WK, Kay B, et al. Cost-effectiveness analysis of deep transcranial magnetic stimulation relative to evidence-based strategies for treatment-refractory obsessive-compulsive disorder. J Psychiatr Res 2022;146:50–4.
84. Roth Y, Pell GS, Barnea-Ygael N, et al. Rotational field TMS: Comparison with conventional TMS based on motor evoked potentials and thresholds in the hand and leg motor cortices. Brain Stimul 2020;13:900–7.

Cognitive-Behavioral Therapy for Obsessive-Compulsive Disorder

Samuel D. Spencer, MA[a],*, Jordan T. Stiede, MS[a],
Andrew D. Wiese, PhD[a], Wayne K. Goodman, MD[a],
Andrew G. Guzick, PhD[a], Eric A. Storch, PhD[b]

KEYWORDS

- Obsessive-compulsive disorder • OCD • Cognitive behavioral therapy • CBT
- Exposure and response prevention • Case vignette

KEY POINTS

- Cognitive-behavioral therapy (CBT) is an empirically supported psychotherapeutic treatment of obsessive-compulsive disorder (OCD).
- Exposure and response/ritual prevention (E/RP) is the active component underlying the efficacy of CBT for OCD.
- Practice guidelines for clinicians using CBT for OCD include thorough assessment and case conceptualization, effective implementation of E/RP with fidelity to the underlying model, and flexible, idiosyncratic adaptation of treatment for diverse patients.

COGNITIVE-BEHAVIORAL THERAPY FOR OBSESSIVE-COMPULSIVE DISORDER

Obsessive-compulsive disorder (OCD) is characterized by the presence of obsessions (ie, unwanted and intrusive thoughts, images, or impulses that lead to anxiety and distress) and compulsions (ie, repetitive behaviors or mental acts in response to obsessions that serve to reduce distress or prevent feared outcomes).[1] OCD has an estimated lifetime prevalence of approximately 1% to 3%,[2–4] and most individuals are also diagnosed with comorbid conditions.[5–7] The Yale-Brown Obsessive-Compulsive Scale (Y-BOCS)[8] and its revised version (Y-BOCS-II)[9] are considered the gold standard instruments for assessing the presence and severity of OCD symptoms in adults. A corresponding pediatric version of the YBOCS-II has also been developed (ie, CY-BOCS-II).[10] Individuals with OCD often experience significant functional impairment in social, occupational, and familial domains, which leads to decreased quality of life.[11–13] OCD is also associated with interpersonal relationship difficulties, loss of

[a] Baylor College of Medicine, One Baylor Plaza, MS:350, Houston, TX 77030, USA; [b] One Baylor Plaza, MS:350, 1977 Butler Boulevard, Houston, TX 77030, USA
* Corresponding author.
E-mail address: samuel.spencer@bcm.edu

Psychiatr Clin N Am 46 (2023) 167–180
https://doi.org/10.1016/j.psc.2022.10.004
0193-953X/23/© 2022 Elsevier Inc. All rights reserved.

work, and increased family burden.[12] The substantial impairment in functioning, restricted autonomy, and significant distress experienced by individuals with OCD necessitates the importance of developing efficacious treatments. As articulated below, cognitive-behavioral therapy (CBT) is the front-line psychotherapeutic treatment of OCD supported by a substantial body of theoretical and empirical support.

THEORETIC FOUNDATIONS

Within CBT, several empirically supported conceptual and applied models of OCD exist that share an emphasis on the role of cognitive processes and behavioral learning principles in the etiology, maintenance, and treatment of OCD. These include the *cognitive model*,[14] which lays the foundation for modern CBT approaches for OCD and provides a theoretical explanation for the emergence and maintenance of OCD symptoms. Additional models include *emotional processing theory*,[15] and the *inhibitory learning model*,[16] which offer direct implications for treatment by explicating the mechanisms underlying exposure and response/ritual prevention (E/RP), the active ingredient of CBT treatment for OCD.

Cognitive Model

Consistent with traditional Beckian cognitive therapy,[17] the *cognitive model of OCD* posits maladaptive beliefs and distorted interpretations concerning intrusive mental content (ie, obsessions) as critical maintenance factors.[18] According to this perspective, it is not the inherent *presence* of unwanted intrusive thoughts per se that is problematic (survey research has indicated that intrusive, unwanted thoughts are ubiquitous in individuals with and without OCD).[19] Rather, it is the *interpretation* of such threatening thoughts as excessively salient (ie, automatic negative thoughts about intrusions), along with the equation of such intrusive thoughts with the actual behavior being enacted (ie, thought–action fusion) and an excessive need for certainty concerning the feared content of obsessive thoughts (ie, intolerance of uncertainty) that are at the core of OCD from a cognitive perspective.[14,20] Additional dysfunctional biases or assumptions within the cognitive model include (a) failure to prevent harm to self or others is equivalent to having actually caused harm, (b) failure to neutralize intrusive thoughts through rituals is equivalent to desiring the worst-case scenario specified in the intrusive thought to actually occur, and (c) that one should be able to exert continuous control over one's thoughts.[20] Treatment of OCD from this perspective involves restructuring or modifying automatic negative thoughts (ie, interpretations) related to the intrusive obsessive content, along with a similar focus on modifying the core beliefs/dysfunctional cognitive biases mentioned above.[21] In cognitively specialized CBT for OCD, cognitive exercises are focused on challenging these underlying beliefs rather than the rationality of specific obsessive thoughts, which can actually be harmful for individuals with OCD, to the extent that these exercises lead to compulsive self-reassurance or thought-stopping.[22]

Behavioral models

Behavioral learning principles have been used to conceptualize OCD and offer key treatment implications in terms of explaining the mechanism of action in E/RP—the active ingredient in CBT for OCD. From this perspective, classic conditioning processes explain how a neutral stimulus (intrusive thoughts) becomes paired with a heightened anxiety/fear response. Operant learning principles suggest that compulsive behaviors, which function to attenuate or neutralize anxious distress from the obsessive thoughts, are negatively reinforced and thus more likely to occur in the future in the presence of obsessions.[23] Passive and active avoidance of obsessive triggers are also negatively reinforced via reduced frequency of OCD-related distress. Both compulsions and avoidance behaviors narrow adaptive behavioral repertoires and contribute to the functional impairment associated with OCD.[24] Although these negatively reinforced behaviors result in fleeting relief from obsessions, this behavioral process paradoxically strengthens the salience of intrusive thoughts (ie, fear networks), denies an opportunity for corrective learning about obsessive fears, and perpetuates the OCD cycle.

Based on these behavioral accounts, Foa and Kozak developed *emotional processing theory* to explain the mechanism of change within E/RP treatment for OCD.[25] The process of exposure to obsessive content while simultaneously refraining from engaging in compulsive behavior/avoidance (ie, response prevention) allows for (a) extinction of the classically conditioned relationship between obsessive stimuli and the anxiety/distress response (ie, habituation), (b) attenuation of the negative reinforcement cycle (ie, functional link between obsessions and compulsions) via response prevention, and (c) new learning concerning the disconfirmation of OCD beliefs (ie, worst-case scenario did not, or does not have to, materialize).

Recent research on fear conditioning and extinction has revealed some novel intricacies within the extinction learning process underlying exposure,[26] which has led to the development of the *inhibitory learning model*. This model posits that deficits in extinction learning processes in individuals with OCD and anxiety disorders mean that exposure operates via the development of two meaning systems—the original fear-based one, plus an additional inhibitory one that develops during exposure (ie, obsessional stimuli no longer associated with fear response). This points to the possibility that habituation may not necessarily be required for exposure to be effective.[16] Rather than solely relying on extinguishing the original fear-based system, this model suggests a central mechanism of strengthening the inhibitory learning system involves maximizing expectancy violations, generalizing exposure efforts to a wide variety of situations (increase retrievability of inhibitory learning), and increasing distress tolerance skills and acceptance of variability in habituation.[27]

Core Treatment Elements

The following sections describe core components of the CBT treatment model for OCD, with deliberate focus on E/RP, which is considered a gold-standard treatment of OCD. Although space limitations preclude a detailed (ie, session-by-session) explication of the CBT for OCD protocol,[23] the following sections offer an overview of core treatment elements. Most CBT protocols used in randomized trials include approximately 14 to 20 twice weekly or weekly sessions.[28]

Information-gathering, psychoeducation, goal setting

Initial sessions involve integrating assessment data into an individualized case formulation of the patient's presenting concerns, often conceptualized within the context of specific OCD subtypes. This is done through ongoing assessment of the content of obsessive thoughts, obsessive triggers, and manifestations of compulsive behaviors and avoidance and their functional link to the obsessive content. Probing for subtle compulsions (eg, mental rituals) and (active and passive) avoidance behaviors is also important because overlooked rituals or other safety behaviors can interfere with effective E/RP. This information-gathering process can also be facilitated by patient self-monitoring and tracking of triggers, obsessions, and compulsions, along with informant input (eg, parents, partner). Additionally, patients receive psychoeducation about OCD, the rationale for E/RP treatment, and the components/course of treatment. These initial discussions also allow therapists to explicate treatment goals, set treatment expectations, socialize the patient to the CBT approach, and instill hope for improvement in terms of increased flexibility in behavioral repertoires of daily living (rather than rigid governance by obsessive thoughts).

Exposure and response/ritual prevention

E/RP posits that by exposing patients to the feared content (obsessions) while instructing them to refrain from engaging in the compulsive behavior, new learning occurs, thus leading to a decrease in the salience (and frequency) of obsessive content along with decreases in the frequency of compulsions.[23] This process unfolds in practice through in vivo and imaginal exposure exercises that are conducted in session and assigned as out-of-session homework. In vivo exposures involve patients exposing themselves to the actual triggering stimuli (eg, touching a toilet seat for contamination-related OCD, holding a knife for harm-related OCD), whereas imaginal exposures consist of patients vividly imagining themselves in triggering situations—often through utilization of a written or recorded script that is read or listened to repeatedly—while refraining from engaging in rituals or compulsive behaviors. Imaginal exposures are often used in situations where in vivo exposures are either logically or ethically impossible, such as handling needles due to concern of contracting HIV/AIDS, or fear of harm coming to oneself while playing baseball. Importantly, both modalities seem effective in addressing OCD specific symptoms.[29]

In practice, E/RP work begins by providing a clear rationale for the importance of frequent and repeated practice of exposure exercises to affect symptom reduction. Highlighting the collaborative nature of E/RP, patients are informed that they will never be forced to engage in exposure exercises without their consent, but will be encouraged to vigorously pursue exposures, because greater magnitude of immersion within E/RP leads to better treatment outcomes.[24] Subsequently, therapist and patient work to develop an exposure hierarchy, which accounts for all of the patient's OCD-related triggers and feared situations. Trigger situations are then arranged from least to most distressing, and exposure exercises are often structured in a way that works to sequentially proceed with exposures of greater difficulty until all items on the hierarchy are mastered.[23] Contemporary models of exposure encourage flexible progression along this exposure list based on the patient's willingness rather than rigid adherence to the originally outlined hierarchy (ie, beginning with least distressing, then trying the second-least distressing) because increased variability in distress during exposure can enhance learning generalization.[27]

In practice, exposure exercises typically involve the patient fully exposing to a trigger situation and tracking subjective units of discomfort (SUDs; eg, rated 0–100, with 0 being perfectly relaxed and 100 being the most intolerable distress ever) before, during, and after the exposure exercise. Careful tracking of SUDs ratings during exposure exercises allows patients to experientially contact the process of habituation during exposure, and highlights possible violations of expectancy (ie, by comparing preexposure estimated peak SUDs to actual SUDs). Consistent with the cognitive model of OCD, postexposure processing (and review of homework) often consists of emphasizing new learning from exposure and targeting beliefs about uncertainty and inflated sense of responsibility.

Maintenance, termination, and sustaining remission

As therapy progresses and patients become more adept at independently designing and implementing exposures in the context of their daily lives, focus shifts toward maintaining gains made during treatment and planning for eventual termination. Implementation of less frequent maintenance and booster sessions, along with the development of a detailed relapse prevention plan, are additional components that can facilitate successful termination.

Throughout this process, overarching themes and insights gleaned from treatment are highlighted and integrated into the patient's life context, especially because they relate to the patient autonomously integrating E/RP principles into their day-to-day life. In essence, patients learn to *live a life of exposure* and move toward what matters to them without being held back by OCD. As such, this final phase of treatment focuses on fostering patient rehabilitation and promoting expansion of adaptive behavioral repertoires to numerous life domains previously constricted by OCD. This can include pursuing hobbies, recreation, employment, and relationships with a newfound sense of flexibility and autonomy.

Research Support

CBT (ie, E/RP) has established a very strong evidence base in the treatment of children, adolescents, and adults with OCD, delivered both in-person and via telehealth.[30] This is reflected in its superiority to psychological and pill placebo controls as well as serotonin reuptake inhibitors (SRIs) in numerous randomized controlled trials,[31-33] large effect sizes of treatment identified by multiple meta-analyses,[34-36] and consistent recommendations as an evidence-based treatment in practice guidelines and reviews.[37-39]

Specifically, recent meta-analyses have demonstrated large effect sizes of E/RP for OCD relative to waitlist and placebo controls, as well as significant superiority to antidepressant medication in both youth and adults.[34-36] Estimates of effect sizes from these meta-analyses relative to active control conditions (eg, relaxation-based therapy) range from $d = .21$ to 1.13, and nonactive controls (eg, waitlist, placebo) from $d = 1.27$ to 1.53. E/RP has also demonstrated modest but significant superiority to SRIs, with meta-analytic effect size ranging from .22 to .36.[34-36] Treatment response rates are estimated to be 65% to 70% after a course of E/RP, remission rates as high as 57%,[34-36] and dropout rates are also consistently low compared with other treatments.[37,40]

In terms of practice guidelines, the American Psychological Association Society of Clinical Psychology provided a "strong recommendation" (ie, second-highest ranking level) for E/RP in 2015 based on universally strong superiority to control conditions identified in systematic reviews and meta-analyses.[41] Since then, several additional RCTs have been published,[42] which likely will lead to future revision of the strength of support to a "very strong recommendation." Similarly, family-based E/RP for youth with OCD has earned a designation as a "well-established" treatment by the Society for Clinical Child and Adolescent Psychology,[38] reflecting the highest standard of evidence for psychological therapy. This recommendation was based on multiple randomized controlled trials demonstrating the superiority of these therapies relative to active comparison conditions.[43] The American Psychiatric Association and American Academy of Child and Adolescent Psychiatry provide similar recommendations, with E/RP (or SRIs) being described as a first-line treatment of adults,[44] and as the first-line treatment alone for youth with mild-to-moderate OCD, or in combination with an SRI in the case of moderate-to-severe OCD.[39]

Limitations of this research should be noted, however, because most of the evidence base that supports E/RP has been conducted with White, middle-class individuals in specialty research settings. Although efforts have been made to increase the diversity of OCD study participants, more research is needed in real-world settings with more culturally diverse populations because there is only preliminary support in these settings.[41,45]

Case Vignettes[a]

Pediatric obsessive-compulsive disorder case example

Noah was a 10-year-old boy who presented for treatment with his mother (Jill) because of struggles with frequent, intrusive, and distressing thoughts about harming his parents, along with compulsive reassurance-seeking and active avoidance of certain objects and places (eg, the kitchen when knives are out, keeping his hands in his pockets whenever he is in the same room as a sharp object). He also endorsed intrusive thoughts about his parents being harmed when separated from them and engagement in reassurance-seeking behaviors (eg, repeated text-messages). Noah and Jill also reported a nightly ritual in which they say "I love you" four times in a row before bed. Additionally, Noah indicated struggling with things being "just-right," including tying both shoes a similar tightness, wearing socks the same length, and brushing his teeth evenly on both sides. He reported time-consuming, repetitive per-formance of such behaviors until it feels symmetric. Because of this, he has been late to school almost every day this year. His score on the CY-BOCS-II was 28 (moderate-to-severe range).

A family-based E/RP treatment plan included an initial assessment of obsessions and compulsions, OCD-related functional impairment, and family accommodation. During the initial session, Noah and Jill were provided with psychoeducation about OCD, in which intrusive thoughts and rituals were normalized, and the development and maintenance of OCD was explained as a process in which people pay excessive attention to intrusive thoughts and spend excessive time responding to them. This initial session also involved identifying the different domains of Noah's life affected by OCD. Additionally, the rationale for E/RP was provided using developmentally appropriate language, describing the goal of E/RP to help with new learning about obsessive fears and increase the amount of time Noah spends in other fun activities and hobbies, rather than stuck within OCD cycles. Finally, Noah and Jill were encour-aged to think of a funny name for Noah's OCD to "externalize" OCD. This exercise helped Noah and his mother psychologically distance from OCD, which had become entangled with their daily lives and relationship, and gave them a common focus to address during therapy.

In subsequent sessions, Noah and Jill developed a treatment hierarchy with their therapist, which included a list of potential E/RP exercises that Noah rated using a SUDS rating scale of 0 to 10. This collaborative process facilitated building a flexible roadmap for treatment that was revisited in subsequent sessions. Noah's therapist proposed E/RP exercises he hoped Noah would find fun or enjoyable to facilitate engagement, like having a 3-legged race with his mom with uneven socks to challenge just-not-right experiences or eating his favorite candy after first "stabbing it" with a knife. See **Table 1** for Noah's hierarchy.

Most of subsequent sessions involved the following format: first, his therapist checked in on "wins" from the previous week, or E/RP homework in which he approached feared situations and/or resisted compulsions. Next, they completed in-session E/RP, which sometimes involved out-of-office exercises (eg, to the bath-room to challenge his teeth-brushing ritual). Jill would join sessions to facilitate gener-alization of E/RP to Noah's family context. During E/RP, the therapist routinely encouraged Noah to maintain focus on the feared situation. They also carefully

---

[a] The following cases are based on an integration of several individuals with OCD who have been treated in our clinical work and are intended to illustrate E/RP as it is done in practice. They are not meant to reflect any one individual person.

Table 1
Sample exposure and response prevention hierarchy for a 10-year-old boy with obsessive-compulsive symptoms related to symmetry and harm

Exposure Challenge	0–10 Rating
Pressing a sharp knife against mom's neck without asking her questions about her safety/pain	10
Holding a sharp knife against mom's skin without asking her questions about her safety/pain	10
Pressing a dinner knife against mom's neck without asking her questions about her safety/pain	9
Holding a dinner knife against mom's skin without asking her questions about her safety/pain	9
Wear different length socks and shoes tied unevenly for a whole school day	9
Writing a story or drawing a picture about harming someone by accident	8
"Stabbing" favorite candy with a knife and eating it	7
Go to bed without saying "I love you"	7
Brush teeth on only one side of mouth	7
Drawing a picture with a knife with finger paint	6
Wear different socks (long and short)	6
Eating a favorite meal using a knife	5
Go to bed, only say "I love you" once	5
Spending the whole day at school without checking on parents' safety and GPS location	4
Brush teeth only once	4
Three-legged uneven race with mom	3
Stand in the kitchen with knives out with hands out of pockets	3
Have mom tie shoes different tightness	2
Saying the word "Stab"	1

monitored overt and subtle compulsions during exposure to minimize them as much as possible. Over time, the therapist encouraged Jill to take the lead in E/RP coaching to prepare them for at-home exercises, and to identify ways she accommodates at home (eg, engaging in bedtime rituals, responding to text-messages about her safety), and resisting these urges.

Throughout the course of treatment, obsessional distress gradually reduced, and time spent engaging in compulsive rituals dramatically decreased, which resulted in increased adaptive behavioral functioning in key life domains (family, school, relationships), reduced OCD-related impairment, and more time engaging in hobbies/fun activities. To quantitatively assess progress, the therapist readministered the CY-BOCS-II, which fell in the nonclinical range (total score of 8). After spacing the last 2 sessions out during 2 to 3 weeks, therapy concluded with a "relapse prevention" session in which Noah and Jill were encouraged to reflect on what had been most beneficial and how to prepare for the future if OCD symptoms reemerge.

Adult obsessive-compulsive disorder case example
Steven was a 26-year-old man who presented with long-standing OCD symptoms specific to contamination involving bodily fluids, and compulsions surrounding avoidance of objects perceived to be contaminated, use of barriers, and excessive and

ritualistic handwashing/bathing. His intake assessment yielded a diagnosis of OCD along with a YBOCS-II score of 24 (moderate–severe range).

During the first E/RP session, psychoeducation concerning OCD and CBT (ie, E/RP) was provided. Steven was encouraged to apply this content to his personal experience with OCD and was able to identify how obsessive thoughts related to contamination caused anxiety, and in turn facilitated avoidance and compulsive behaviors. Additionally, he identified successful (albeit inadvertent) instances of habituation to anxiety, including an occasion where he was unable to bathe immediately following exercise, and recognized how this could be applied to E/RP treatment. An exposure hierarchy was developed, and initial exercises were added and assigned in the first session; Steven agreed to continue developing his hierarchy and track symptoms on an ongoing basis throughout treatment.

Steven's second session was used to finish developing his hierarchy; initial exposure exercises were practiced in-session with Steven agreeing to handle doorknobs in the clinic without washing. After the exercise, Steven and the therapist discussed what occurred and how his anxiety eventually habituated in the absence of handwashing rituals. Steven also noted there was no evidence supporting predictions that he would become sick from touching the doorknob. His therapist pointed out that neither of them could be 100% certain, however, that he would not get sick from the doorknob, an observation intended to help Steven challenge a need for certainty over his feared outcomes. For homework, Steven agreed to practice this exercise 3 times daily before the next session.

The third session started with a review of exposure homework. Much like the exposure practice during his previous visit, Steven's exposure tracking documents provided evidence of habituation during exposures. Additionally, habituation occurred more quickly during successive trials, and peak SUDs ratings reduced across trials. Steven further explained that while intrusive thoughts specific to contamination were still present while handling doorknobs, the urge to wash was less pronounced and he felt confident in resisting washing. Cognitive therapy techniques were also used to maximize inhibitory learning from exposures in terms of highlighting the discrepancy between the expectancy of feared outcome before ERP and the actual outcome.[46] The third visit concluded with Steven selecting exposures from his hierarchy to practice in-session (handling doorknob without washing and cross-contaminating his face). Steven agreed to practice and record this exercise 3 times daily before next session.

Sessions 4 through 12 proceeded in a similar manner, with the agenda including a review of homework assigned, identification of in-session exposures, and planning subsequent exposure homework. After the 12th session, Steven's score on the YBOCS-II was 13 (mild range). Additionally, Steven completed all exposure exercises on his hierarchy. From there, Steven and the therapist met for 4 additional sessions every 2 weeks to allow additional time for independent exposure practice. During these booster sessions, Steven took a more active role in integrating E/RP principles into his day-to-day lived experiences. The final maintenance visit included development of a symptom relapse prevention plan. A follow-up YBOCS-II measure yielded a score of 12 (mild range). Steven and the therapist agreed to discontinue treatment due to symptom reduction and his ongoing ability to independently maintain treatment progress.

DISCUSSION

Prognosis and outcomes for children and adults suffering from OCD have improved greatly during the last 40 years due to advances in CBT (ie, E/RP) and SRI treatments,[24] which both possess a strong evidence base supporting their efficacy. These treatments are often combined in practice (especially for more severe presentations) and have demonstrated robust efficacy based on a large body of research and associated practice guidelines.[38,39,41,43,44] E/RP consistently demonstrates sustained benefits following active treatment, greater remission rates relative to SRIs, and has shown to be effective for individuals who may not respond to (or prefer) SRIs.[42,47] As such, CBT, with an emphasis on E/RP, should be a core component of treatment for individuals with OCD.[38,41] As demonstrated in the series of case vignettes presented here, cognitive and behavioral models of OCD—with an emphasis on E/RP—are broad in scope yet offer potential for individualized care. This section discusses several key issues germane to clinicians delivering CBT for OCD and offers recommendations for overcoming some of the challenges and pitfalls that may arise in practice.

Exposure and Response/Ritual Prevention: Challenges and Opportunities

As described earlier, E/RP is the active ingredient of successful CBT treatment of OCD.[27,48] Despite the repeated demonstrations of E/RP's efficacy, survey studies indicate that individuals treated for OCD do not always receive E/RP.[49] Reasons for therapist hesitancy in delivering E/RP with fidelity include negative beliefs about the safety of the approach, patient's ability to tolerate exposures, and faulty perceptions of E/RP as nonessential in the treatment of OCD.[50] These beliefs are oftentimes unfounded, however (eg, survey research reveals that serious negative consequences of E/RP are extremely rare).[51] Fortunately, such clinician beliefs have been shown to be amenable to modification, which further underscores the importance of increasing promotion of E/RP through clear articulation of the rationale for, and safety of, E/RP to patients and other professionals.

Additionally, when E/RP is deliberately targeted in treatment, there are several pitfalls that can—and indeed often do—result in reduced efficacy of treatment and an unfortunate prolonging of OCD symptoms. These include (a) only engaging in mild-to-moderate difficulty exposures and leaving more challenging ones untouched, (b) failing to notice subtle patient safety behaviors or inadvertently providing reassurance during exposures, (c) designing exposure exercises that are less relevant to the patient's lived experience or failing to promote generalization of in vivo exposures to the patient's life context, and (d) focusing on challenging the rationality of obsessive thoughts as is done in traditional cognitively focused CBT.[50,52] Fortunately, awareness of these common pitfalls can assist therapists in conducting E/RP with fidelity and designing exposures with the greatest likelihood of having a positive impact in the patient's day-to-day life.

Addressing Clinical Complexities

Comorbid psychiatric conditions in individuals with OCD presenting for treatment often seems to be the rule, rather than the exception. Commonly encountered comorbid conditions include generalized anxiety disorder, major depressive disorder, obsessive-compulsive personality disorder, chronic tic disorders (especially in youth), and attention deficit-hyperactivity disorder, to name a few.[4-7] Because such comorbidities can present additional complexities and challenges, thorough assessment, case conceptualization, and treatment planning are essential for optimal care. Additional considerations involve whether to treat comorbid conditions simultaneously or sequentially in the context of OCD and evaluating the impact of comorbidities on successful implementation of E/RP. To the extent that comorbid conditions dramatically interfere with E/RP progress, addressing the comorbid concern *before* beginning a course of CBT for OCD may be indicated.[23] However, in many cases, E/RP can be tailored to address comorbid conditions without affecting response.[53] Further, data suggest that many comorbid conditions (eg, depression, anxiety) improve following successful E/RP.[54,55] Distinguishing closely related clinical concerns (eg, ruminative anxiety, patterns of repetitive behaviors in trichotillomania and excoriation disorders) from independent OCD symptomology is another important consideration. Additional areas of clinical complexity include presentations of OCD with low levels of insight, comorbid disorganized or tangential thought processes (including psychotic spectrum disorders), substance abuse, and treatment planning for more severe cases in which a higher level of care (eg, residential, partial hospitalization) may be warranted.

Recommendations and Clinical Care Points for Clinicians

CBT—specifically E/RP—represents a well-established, cost-effective, evidence-based approach for treating OCD with potential for alleviating symptomology and improving quality of life. Based on the cognitive and behavioral models of OCD presented above, the following recommendations for clinicians treating patients with OCD are proffered:

- Implement a deliberate focus on thorough assessment, case formulation, and treatment planning idiographically tailored to fit the needs of diverse patients.
- Use an E/RP framework to design and carry out relevant exposure exercises tailored to patients' unique lived experiences that lead to resounding improvement in patient adaptive behavioral functioning.
- Consider possible complex clinical presentations (ie, comorbidities, severe symptomology) when personalizing CBT for OCD.

CLINICS CARE POINTS

- Implement a deliberate focus on thorough assessment, case formulation, and treatment planning idiographically tailored to fit the needs of diverse patients.
- Use an E/RP framework to design and carry out relevant exposure exercises tailored to patients' unique lived experiences that lead to resounding improvement in patient adaptive behavioral functioning.
- Consider possible complex clinical presentations (ie, comorbidities, severe symptomology) when personalizing CBT for OCD.

DISCLOSURE

Production of this article was supported by a grant from the Eunice Kennedy Shriver National Institute of Child Health and Human Development of the National Institutes of Health under Award Number P50HD103555 for use of the Clinical and Translational Core facilities. The content is solely the responsibility of the authors and does not necessarily represent the official views of the National Institutes of Health.

REFERENCES

1. American Psychiatric Association. Diagnostic and statistical manual of mental disorders. 5th edition, Text revision. American Journal of Psychiatry; 2022.

2. Kessler RC, Berglund P, Demler O, et al. Lifetime prevalence and age-of-onset distributions of DSM-IV disorders in the National Comorbidity Survey Replication. Arch Gen Psychiatry 2005;62(6):593–602.
3. Ruscio AM, Stein DJ, Chiu WT, et al. The epidemiology of obsessive-compulsive disorder in the National Comorbidity Survey Replication. Mol Psychiatry 2010; 15(1):53.
4. Torres AR, Prince MJ, Bebbington PE, et al. Obsessive-compulsive disorder: Prevalence, comorbidity, impact, and help-seeking in the British National Psychiatric Morbidity Survey of 2000. Am J Psychiatry 2006;163(11):1978–85.
5. Brakoulias V, Starcevic V, Belloch A, et al. Comorbidity, age of onset and suicidality in obsessive-compulsive disorder (OCD): An international collaboration. Compr Psychiatry 2017;76:79–86.
6. de Mathis MA, Diniz JB, Hounie AG, et al. Trajectory in obsessive-compulsive disorder comorbidities. Eur Neuropsychopharmacol 2010;23(7):594–601.
7. Pallanti S, Grassi G, Sarrecchia ED, et al. Obsessive-compulsive disorder comorbidity: Clinical assessment and therapeutic implications. Front Psychiatry 2011; 2:1–11.
8. Goodman WK, Price LH, Rasmussen SA, et al. The Yale-Brown Obsessive Compulsive Scale: I. development, use, and reliability. Arch Gen Psychiatry 1989;46:1006–11.
9. Storch EA, Rasmussen SA, Price LH, et al. Development and psychometric evaluation of the Yale-Brown Obsessive Compulsive Scale-Second Edition. Psychol Assess 2010;22:223–32.
10. Storch EA, McGuire JF, Wu MS, et al. Development and psychometric evaluation of the Children's Yale-Brown Obsessive-Compulsive Scale Second Edition. J Am Acad Child Adolesc Psychiatry 2019;58(1):92–8.
11. Asnaani A, Kaczkurkin AN, Alpert E, et al. The effect of treatment on quality of life and functioning in OCD. Compr Psychiatry 2017;73:7–14.
12. Hollander E, Stein DJ, Fineberg NA, et al. Quality of life outcomes in patients with obsessive-compulsive disorder: Relationship to treatment response and symptom relapse. J Clin Psychiatry 2010;71(6):784–92.
13. Huppert JD, Simpson HB, Nissenson KJ, et al. Quality of life and functional impairment in obsessive-compulsive disorder: a comparison of patients with and without comorbidity, patients in remission, and healthy controls. Depress Anxiety 2009;26(1):39–45.
14. Rachman S. A cognitive theory of obsessions: Elaborations. Behav Res Ther 1998;36(4):385–401.
15. Foa EB, McLean CP. (2016). The efficacy of exposure therapy for anxiety-related disorders and its underlying mechanisms: The case of OCD and PTSD. Annu Rev Clin Psychol 2016;12:1–18.
16. Craske M, Liao B, Brown L, et al. The role of inhibition in exposure therapy. J Exp Psychopathol 2012;3(3):322–45.
17. Beck AT, Rush A, Shaw B, et al. Cognitive therapy of depression. New York: The Guilford Press; 1979.
18. Berman NC, Schwartz R, Park J. Psychological models and treatments of OCD for adults. In: Abramowitz JS, McKay D, Storch EA, editors. The wiley handbook of obsessive compulsive disorders. John Wiley & Sons; 2017. Incorporated.
19. Radomsky AS, Alcolado GM, Abramowitz JS, et al. Part 1- you can run but you can't hide: Intrusive thoughts on six continents. J Obsessive Compuls Relat Disord 2014;3(3):269–79.

20. Salkovskis PM. Obsessional-compulsive problems: A cognitive-behavioural analysis. Behav Res Ther 1985;23:571–84.
21. Wilhelm S, Steketee GS. Cognitive therapy for obsessive compulsive disorder: a guide for professionals. Oakland, CA: New Harbinger; 2006.
22. McKay D, Abramowitz JS, Storch EA. Mechanisms of harmful treatments for obsessive-compulsive disorder. Clin Psychol Sci Pract 2021;28(1):52–9.
23. Foa EB, Yadin E, Lichner TK. Exposure and response (ritual) prevention for obsessive-compulsive disorder. 2nd Edition. Oxford University Press; 2012.
24. Franklin ME, Foa EB. Obsessive-compulsive disorder. In: Barlow DH, editor. Clinical handbook of psychological disorders. Sixth Edition. Guilford Press; 2021. p. 133–78.
25. Foa EB, Kozak MJ. Emotional processing of fear: Exposure to corrective information. Psychol Bull 1986;99(1):20–35.
26. Craske MG, Kircanski K, Zelikowsky M, et al. Optimizing inhibitory learning during exposure therapy. Behav Res Ther 2008;46(1):5–27.
27. Abramowitz JS, Arch JJ. Strategies for improving long-term outcomes in cognitive behavioral therapy for obsessive-compulsive disorder: Insights from learning theory. Cogn Behav Pract 2014;21(1):30–1.
28. Simpson HB, Foa EB, Liebowitz MR, et al. Cognitive-behavioral therapy vs. risperidone for augmenting serotonin reuptake inhibitors in obsessive-compulsive disorder. JAMA Psychiatry 2013;70(11):1190–9.
29. Foa EB, Steketee G, Grayson JB. Imaginal and in vivo exposure: A comparison with obsessive-compulsive checkers. Behav Ther 1985;16(3):292–302.
30. Dèttore D, Pozza A, Andersson G. Efficacy of technology-delivered cognitive behavioural therapy for OCD versus control conditions, and in comparison with therapist administered CBT: Meta-analysis of randomized controlled trials. Cogn Behav Ther 2015;44(3):190–211.
31. Foa EB, Liebowitz MR, Kozak MJ, et al. Randomized, placebo-controlled trial of exposure and ritual prevention, clomipramine, and their combination in the treatment of obsessive-compulsive disorder. AJP 2005;162(1):151–61.
32. Freeman J, Sapyta J, Garcia A, et al. Family-based treatment of early childhood obsessive-compulsive disorder: The pediatric obsessive-compulsive disorder treatment study for young children (POTS Jr) - A randomized clinical trial. JAMA Psychiatry 2014;71(6):689–98.
33. The Pediatric OCD Treatment Study (POTS) Team. Cognitive-behavior therapy, sertraline, and their combination for children and adolescents with obsessive-compulsive disorder – The pediatric OCD treatment study (POTS) randomized controlled trial. JAMA Psychiatry 2004;292(16):1969–76.
34. Ost LG, Havnen A, Hansen B, et al. Cognitive behavioral treatments of obsessive-compulsive disorder. A systematic review and meta-analysis of studies published 1993-2014. Clin Psychol Rev 2015;40:156–69.
35. McGuire JF, Piacentini J, Lewin AB, et al. A meta-analysis of cognitive behavior therapy and medication for child obsessive-compulsive disorder: Moderators of treatment efficacy, response, and remission. Depress Anxiety 2015;32(8):580–93.
36. Ost LG, Riise EN, Wergeland GJ, et al. Cognitive behavioral and pharmacological treatments of OCD in children: A systematic review and meta-analysis. J Anxiety Disord 2016;43:58–69.
37. Ong CW, Clyde JW, Bluett EJ, et al. Dropout rates in exposure with response prevention for obsessive-compulsive disorder: What do the data really say? J Anxiety Disord 2016 May;40:8–17.

38. Freeman J, Benito K, Herren J, et al. Evidence base update of psychosocial treatments for pediatric obsessive-compulsive disorder: Evaluating, improving, and transporting what works. J Clin Child Adolesc Psychol 2018;47(5):669–98.
39. Geller DA, March J. Practice parameter for the assessment and treatment of children and adolescents with obsessive-compulsive disorder. J Am Acad Child Adolesc Psychiatry 2012;51(1):98–113.
40. Johnco C, McGuire JF, Roper T, et al. A meta-analysis of dropout rates from exposure with response prevention and pharmacological treatment for youth with obsessive compulsive disorder. Depress Anxiety 2020 May;37(5):407–17.
41. Tolin D, Melnyk T, Marx B. Exposure and response prevention for obsessive-compulsive disorder: empirically supported treatment report. Society of Clinical Psychology, American Psychological Association 2015. https://doi.org/10.1037/e675592012-001.
42. Foa EB, Simpson HB, Gallagher T, et al. Maintenance of wellness in patients with obsessive-compulsive disorder who discontinue medication after exposure/response prevention augmentation: A randomized clinical trial. JAMA Psychiatry 2022;79(3):193–200.
43. Southam-Gerow MA, Prinstein MJ. Evidence base updates: The evolution of the evaluation of psychological treatments for children and adolescents. J Clin Child Adolesc Psychol 2014;43(1):1–6.
44. Koran LM, Simpson HB. Guideline watch (march 2013): practice guideline for the treatment of patients with obsessive-compulsive disorder. American Psychiatric Association; 2013. https://doi.org/10.1176/appibooks.9780890423363.149114.
45. Mancebo MC, Steketee G, Muroff J, et al. Behavioral therapy teams for adults with OCD in a community mental health center: An open trial. J Obsessive Compuls Relat Disord 2017;13:18–23.
46. McGuire JF, Storch EA. An inhibitory learning approach to cognitive-behavioral therapy for children and adolescents. Cogn Behav Pract 2019;26(1):214–24.
47. Tolin DF, Maltby N, Diefenbach GJ, et al. Cognitive-behavioral therapy for medication nonresponders with obsessive-compulsive disorder: A wait-list-controlled open trial. J Clin Psychiatry 2004;65(7):922–31.
48. Foa EB, McNally RJ. Mechanisms of change in exposure therapy. In: Rapee RM, editor. Current controversies in the anxiety disorders. New York: Guilford; 1996. p. 329–43.
49. Keleher J, Jassi A, Krebs G. Clinician-reported barriers to using exposure with response prevention in the treatment of pediatric obsessive-compulsive disorder. J Obsessive Compuls Relat Disord 2020;24. https://doi.org/10.1016/j.jocrd.2019.100498.
50. Deacon BJ, Farrell NR, Kemp JJ, et al. Assessing therapist reservations about exposure therapy for anxiety disorders: The Therapist Beliefs about Exposure Scale. J Anxiety Disord 2013;27(8):772–80.
51. Schneider SC, Knott L, Cepeda SL, et al. Serious negative consequences associated with exposure and response prevention for obsessive-compulsive disorder: A survey of therapist attitudes and experiences. Depress Anxiety 2020;37(5):418–28.
52. Moritz S, Kulz A, Voderholzer U, et al. Phobie a deux" and other reasons why clinicians do not apply exposure with response prevention in patients with obsessive-compulsive disorder. Cogn Behav Ther 2019;48(2):162–76.
53. Storch EA, Merlo LJ, Larson MJ, et al. Impact of comorbidity on cognitive-behavioral therapy response in pediatric obsessive-compulsive disorder. J Am Acad Child Adolesc Psychiatry 2008;47(5):583–92.

54. Zandberg LJ, Zang Y, McLean CP, et al. Change in obsessive-compulsive symptoms mediates subsequent change in depressive symptoms during exposure and response prevention. Behav Res Ther 2015;68:76–81.
55. Bakhshaie J, Geller DA, Wilhelm S, et al. Temporal precedence of the change in obsessive-compulsive symptoms and change in depressive symptoms during exposure and response prevention for pediatric obsessive-compulsive disorders. Behav Res Ther 2020;133:103697.

Hoarding Disorder
The Current Evidence in Conceptualization, Intervention, and Evaluation

Nancy Lin, MSW, RSW[a], Lindsay Bacala, MSW[b], Spenser Martin, BA[c],
Christiana Bratiotis, PhD, MSW[a], Jordana Muroff, PhD, MSW[d],*

KEYWORDS

- Hoarding disorder • Clinical treatment • Medication • Special populations
- Community-based response • CBT

KEY POINTS

- Hoarding disorder is a distinct diagnosis in the DSM-5, characterized by excessive acquisition, saving, and difficulty discarding.
- Various models have been proposed to explain hoarding behaviors, including cognitive-behavioral, attachment, neurobiological, and animal.
- Validated measures have been developed for assessment. Best practice recommends the combined use of patient self-report, external collaterals, and behavioral testing.
- Psychotherapeutic treatments such as CBT adapted for hoarding have the best evidentiary support. Complementary approaches that address community-based risks such as harm reduction and case management are increasingly used in practice.
- Vulnerable populations such as older adults, children, and involuntary clients require specialized support to mitigate higher risk potential.

Hoarding is characterized as a condition involving extreme accumulation of objects in the home, as well as an associated difficulty with discarding possessions that others would generally not keep.[1] This current conceptualization is based on Frost and Hartl's 1996 definition,[2] which detailed 3 major characteristics:

acquisition of, and failure to discard, a large number of possessions that appear to be useless or of limited value; living spaces sufficiently cluttered so as to preclude activities for which those spaces were designed; and significant distress or impairment in functioning caused by the hoarding.

The authors report no financial relationships with commercial interests.
[a] University of British Columbia, School of Social Work, Jack Bell Building, 2080 West Mall, Vancouver, British Columbia V6T 1Z2, Canada; [b] University of Manitoba, Faculty of Social Work, 521 Tier Building, 173 Dafoe Road West, Winnipeg, Manitoba R3J 2N2, Canada; [c] Canadian Mental Health Association, 930 Portage Avenue, Winnipeg, Manitoba R3G 0P8, Canada; [d] Boston University, School of Social Work, 264 Bay State Road, Boston, MA 02215, USA
* Corresponding author.
E-mail address: jmuroff@bu.edu

Psychiatr Clin N Am 46 (2023) 181–196
https://doi.org/10.1016/j.psc.2022.10.007
0193-953X/23/© 2023 Elsevier Inc. All rights reserved.

Historically, hoarding was considered a subtype of obsessive-compulsive disorder (OCD). However, in 2013, the American Psychiatric Association recognized hoarding disorder (HD) as a distinct condition with its own diagnostic criteria including the following: (1) "persistent difficulty discarding or parting with possessions, regardless of their actual value", (2) "due to a perceived need to save the items and to the distress associated with discarding them", (3) that "results in the accumulation of possessions that congest and clutter active living areas and substantially compromises their intended use", and (4) "causes clinically significant distress or impairment in social, occupational, or other important areas of functioning" (p. 247).[3] The diagnostic criteria also include specifiers for excessive acquisition and level of insight. The adult prevalence of HD in the United States and parts of Europe and Australia is approximately 2% to 6%,[4–6] with similar rates across sexes. The mean age of hoarding symptoms onset is 16.7 years.[6] Hazardous home environments caused by hoarding affect all socioeconomic groups.[7] Rates of comorbidity in hoarding are high: approximately 60% of individuals with HD also meet the diagnostic criteria for at least one other psychiatric condition.[8] Most commonly, hoarding has been found to co-occur with major depressive disorder (50%–52%), generalized anxiety disorder (24%), and social phobia (23%).[9] One out of four individuals with HD has attempted suicide in their lifetime.[10] This clinical complexity makes it difficult to differentiate hoarding from other psychiatric conditions[11] and complicates targeting the treatment of hoarding specifically.

Significant clutter in the home impairs completion of activities of daily living[12] and has been associated with increased social isolation.[13] Hoarding environments increase the risk of accidental death[7] and self-reported cardiovascular disease, chronic pain, and sleep apnea.[14] HD also creates risks for cooccupants and shared-wall neighbors.[15] Fire risks increase when combustible items are stored near heat sources and exposed electrical wiring. Blocked exits caused by high clutter volumes create safety hazards for both occupants and emergency responders.[12] Neglect of regular home maintenance leads to degradation of the home, poor sanitation, pest infestation, and structural damage.[12] Legal consequences include the risk of eviction, as well as the potential involvement of child protection, adult guardianship, and animal welfare services.[1,16]

ASSESSMENTS FOR HOARDING BEHAVIORS

HD's complex presentation necessitates a comprehensive assessment to identify relevant hoarding-specific features and establish targeted treatment plans. A detailed hoarding interview collects information on the severity of hoarding symptoms, general life circumstances, housing conditions, and social supports, which can then be used to conceptualize the individual's hoarding presentation and establish a starting point for intervention.[17]

The most common and validated hoarding assessment instruments are described in **Table 1**.[18–30] In addition to these measures that primarily assess symptom severity and clutter, there are additional tools that examine the home environments, including the HOMES Multidisciplinary Risk Assessment,[27] Environmental Cleanliness and Clutter Scale,[31] and Home Environment Index.[32] There has also been increasing research on adapting existing hoarding measures into non-English languages.[33] However, a recent psychometric evaluation of self-report measures for hoarding behavior found that most received a rating of *inadequate* utilizing formal criteria (with the exception of the Saving Inventory-Revised), noting the need to improve the measures' psychometric properties.[34] In contrast to self-report measures, behavioral measures do not rely on patients' variable levels of insight. Behavioral measures include tasks to assess specific hoarding behaviors, including simulated acquiring and discarding

Table 1
Hoarding assessment instruments

Hoarding Assessment	Subscales and/or Areas	Description and Scoring
Structured Interview for Hoarding Disorder (SIHD)[18]	• DSM-5 diagnostic criteria for hoarding • Acquisition • Insight specifiers	• Semistructured interview guide • Clinician-administered
UCLA Hoarding Severity Scale (UHSS)[19]	• Clutter • Acquisition levels • Difficulty discarding • Functional impairment • Indecisiveness • Perfectionism • Task prolongation • Procrastination	• 10-item scale • Semistructured, clinician-administered interview • Includes patient and informant input • Final scoring (maximum score of 40) dependent on the clinical judgement of the interviewer
The Hoarding Rating Scale (HRS)[20,21]	• Severity of clutter • Difficulty discarding possessions • Excessiveness of acquisition • Levels of hoarding-related distress • Functional impairment	• 5-item scale • Completed by clinicians, patients, or family members • Items are rated on a 9-point scale, 0 (none/not at all) to 8 (extreme) • Total score ranges from 0 to 40 • Higher scores indicating greater hoarding disorder severity • Cutoff score of 14 or higher indicates a clinical level of hoarding
Saving Inventory-Revised (SI-R)[22,23]	• Acquiring • Clutter • Difficulty discarding	• 23-item self-report • Items rated 0 (none/not at all) to 4 (All/Extreme) • Score of 41 and above distinguishes clinical hoarding from normative behavior[24] • Cutoff scores for each subscale also available[77]
Savings Cognition Inventory (SCI)[25]	• Emotional attachment • Concerns about memory • Control over possessions • Responsibility towards possessions	• 24-item self-report • Each item is rated on a 7-point scale, 0 (not at all) to 7 (very much) • Maximum score is 168 • The average total scores for individuals with HD is 95.9, and 42.2 for those without[26] • Specific cutoff scores for each subscale are also available[77]

(continued on next page)

Table 1
(continued)

Hoarding Assessment	Subscales and/or Areas	Description and Scoring
Activities of Daily Living for Hoarding (ADL-H)[28]	• Ability to complete everyday activities (eg, cooking, sleeping, bathing) and exit the home quickly	• 15-item self-report • Scale from 1 (none) to 5 (severe) • Averaged scores of 2.2 and higher are typical of clinical levels of Hoarding
Hoarding Disorder-Dimensional Scale (HD-D)[29]	• Difficulty discarding • Distress • Clutter levels • Avoidance • Interference	• 5-item self-report • Each item is rated from 0 (none) to 4 (extreme) • Total scores range from 0 to 20 • Higher scores reflect greater symptom severity
Clutter Image Rating (CIR)[30]	• Clutter severity	• Pictorial scale including a set of 9 photos with increasing levels of clutter for each of 3 rooms living room, kitchen, and bedroom • Completed by self, practitioners, service providers, and/or family/friends • Scale from 1 (no clutter) to 9 (severe clutter) • Mean composite score" across 3 rooms • Scores of 4 or higher for a room indicate clutter is clinically significant
Child Saving Inventory (CSI)–Parent Report[104]	• Acquiring • Clutter • Difficulty/discarding • Distress/impairment	• 20-item parent-report • Scale from 0 (none/not at all) to 4 (all/extreme) • Total score 0–80 • Higher score reflect greater symptom severity
HOMES Multidisciplinary Risk Assessment[27]	• Health • Obstacles • Mental Health • Endangerment • Structure & Safety	• Completed by practitioner, service provider, family/friends
Environmental Cleanliness and Clutter Scale (ECCS)[31]	• Squalor, clutter, and cleanliness	• 10 items • Completed by practitioners and service providers • Scale 0 to 3 with specific anchors • Total score 0–30 • Scores greater than 12 may indicate moderate or severe squalor • Higher score reflect more severe conditions

(continued on next page)

Table 1 (continued)		
Hoarding Assessment	**Subscales and/or Areas**	**Description and Scoring**
Home Environment Index (HEI)[32]	• Squalor (eg, domestic and personal, impact)	• 15 items self-report • Scale from 0 (none) to 3 (severe) • Total score 0–45 • Greater score reflect more severe conditions

tasks,[35] item categorization tasks,[36] and interpretive bias tasks.[37] Thus, they can be limited by the situation and context within which they are implemented.

MODELS AND MECHANISMS FOR HOARDING
Animal Models

There has been limited, preliminary research on using animal models to conceptualize hoarding behaviors in humans. Rat models seem to be the most applicable to human hoarding, as hoarding behaviors in both species increased with age and abnormalities were exhibited in the same brain regions.[38]

Neurobiological and Genetic

Neuroimaging studies using functional MRI have found neurological abnormalities in people who hoard. Participants with hoarding exhibited an impulsive response pattern with shorter reaction times and increased commission errors.[39] Participants who underwent discarding exercises were found to have abnormal functional connectivity in key frontal and emotional processing regions of the brain.[40,41] Participants with hoarding also performed worse in neuropsychological tasks involving visual perception compared with controls, and showed inefficient visual processing.[42] Researchers reported various abnormalities in the frontal white matter tracts related to hoarding symptom severity.[43] Neurological findings further indicate that people with HD may experience cognitive impairments, including difficulties with working memory,[44] attention,[45] self-control,[46] decision-making,[47] and categorization.[31] Despite these impairments, some found that baseline neurocognitive functioning did not have a significant effect on hoarding treatment outcomes.[48]

Adult twin studies' estimates of heritability for hoarding are 35% to 51%[49,50] and heritability estimates at age 15 are 33% for boys and 17% for girls.[51] Another study suggests higher estimates for the heritability of the hoarding trait dimension among youth.[52] Greater hoarding symptoms have been associated with having a parent with hoarding behaviors.[53]

In a pediatric sample, specific serotonin gene variants were associated with hoarding traits without accompanying OCD symptoms.[5] The L_G + S variant of 5-HTTLPR was significantly associated with hoarding in men, whereas a variation downstream of HTR1B may be linked with hoarding in women.[5] Both T-allele carriers and Val-allele carriers have been associated with hoarding.[54,55] A large-scale genome-wide association study found no evidence to support genome-wide linkages with hoarding.[56] However, 2 genomic loci on chromosomes 5 and 6 did show potential association with hoarding traits.[56] Preliminary evidence exists to suggest a link between the glutamatergic system and hoarding.[57] Further investigation on the genetic basis of HD is needed to determine genetic risk factors, enhance understandings of underlying biological mechanisms, and develop new animal and cellular models for therapeutic testing purposes.[57]

Attachment and Identity

A growing body of literature centralizes attachment theory to explain people who hoard's significant connection to objects.[58] The attachment theory model hypothesizes that individuals who hoard have unmet interpersonal needs stemming from adverse early life experiences,[59] and subsequently form primary, secure attachments with their possessions as a compensatory response.[60] Possessions serve to regulate difficult emotions,[61] may take on human-like attributes,[58] and can be physical extensions of self-identity.[35] Object attachment has been suggested as a form of loss aversion,[35] and a tendency to maximize in decision-making has been significantly correlated with hoarding symptoms.[62] A recent study found that participants with HD symptoms had mixed emotions toward their sentimental objects, including feelings of disgust, anxiety, and anger.[63]

HD has also been associated with personality disorder traits[64,65] and poor social cognition.[66] The incongruence between high emotional empathy (ie, sharing the emotions of another person) and poor cognitive empathy (ie, understanding the thoughts and emotions of another person) exhibited by people who hoard was proposed as a reason for poor interpersonal functioning.[67] Further research is needed to better understand the association between social cognition and HD.[66]

Cognitive and Behavioral

The cognitive-behavioral model of hoarding posits that HD develops from a combination of life course vulnerabilities, information processing impairments, thoughts and beliefs about possessions, and emotional dysregulation.[25] Among the tested elements of the cognitive-behavioral model are emotional awareness and acceptance, emotional reactivity,[68] impulsivity,[69] intolerance of uncertainty,[70] anxiety sensitivity,[70] catastrophizing the potential consequences of forgetting,[71] planning and problem-solving challenges,[71] cognitive inflexibility,[72] and challenges with using emotion regulation strategies.[73]

Insight and Motivation

People who hoard often have limited insight into the severity of their accumulation and the varied consequences that may result from it.[74] Decreased insight is related to increased health and safety risks, interpersonal conflict, and higher rates of involuntary service involvement.[27] Family participants reported significantly higher hoarding severity ratings compared with what they thought the affected person would rate themselves.[74] Research also suggests that people with hoarding have low motivation to address the problem.[75] As such, individuals with poor insight often avoid help and resist intervention efforts.[76]

INTERVENTIONS
Cognitive-Behavioral Therapy

Cognitive-behavioral therapy (CBT) for hoarding has been manualized and updated,[17,77] extensively tested,[78] and is presently considered the gold standard[79] treatment of HD. CBT for hoarding is a time-limited therapy involving cognitive restructuring, emotion modification, sorting and discarding exercises, organization training, exposure to nonacquiring activities, and motivational interviewing.[17] It has been delivered in individual, group, and peer-led formats (eg, Buried in Treasures),[80,81] with the latter found to be as effective as clinician-led group treatment.[82] CBT has been found to improve outcomes in discarding, clutter reduction, and acquisition behaviors, regardless of modality.[78,79] However, limited patient compliance has been reported[83] and the accessibility of this highly specialized therapy is limited due to a shortage of trained providers.[1]

Compassion-Focused Therapy

An emerging psychotherapeutic treatment of HD under study is compassion-focused therapy (CFT). CFT emphasizes the use of emotional regulation strategies such as mindfulness exercises to enhance self-compassion, shift self-blame, and cope with negative emotions.[84] A pilot study found that CBT that incorporated CFT techniques produced greater treatment effects than CBT alone.[84] Despite these promising early findings, further research is needed to assess CFT efficacy, particularly because it has shown limited effectiveness at addressing attachment-related concerns and hoarding thoughts.

Virtual and Blended Therapies

From as early as 1998, those with hoarding have sought support for their hoarding using web-based interventions. There has been increasing interest in the use of technology-based hoarding interventions such as web-based self-help platforms,[85] video-teleconferencing,[86–88] and "blended" approaches involving both in-person and virtual assistance[89] delivered individually and in groups.[86] This modality provides a multitude of benefits including enhanced flexibility, treatment personalization, accessibility to trained providers, and cost-effectiveness.[86] Overall, virtual and blended therapies have demonstrated effectiveness in increasing treatment completion rates, reducing treatment duration, and achieving high patient satisfaction ratings.[86,88] A related emerging area with a limited but growing body of literature is the use of virtual reality (VR) for hoarding treatment. VR has been used to simulate hoarding environments,[90] which is particularly beneficial for patients who have difficulty engaging in mental imagery tasks, and can act as an alternative to in-person home visits.[91]

Coordinated Community Interventions

The significant public health and safety concerns caused by severe hoarding behavior necessitates the involvement of diverse sectors, including fire prevention, sanitation, child and adult protective services, legal services, health, and mental health.[12,92] Beyond individual practitioners' interventions, many cities across North America have developed approaches to coordinate interdisciplinary responses through community-level task forces.[76] The aims of these initiatives typically include risk mitigation for severe hoarding, enhancing physical and mental health, community functioning, and preserving housing.[27]

Case management is an approach that has been commonly implemented in these community-level responses, and includes interventions such as client identification, assessment, goal setting, service planning, supportive counselling, service plan implementation, monitoring, and evaluation.[12] The wraparound support that case management provides is well suited to the complex needs of marginalized populations such as people who hoard.[12] However, recent research suggests the need for complementary approaches beyond case management alone to meaningfully alleviate eviction risk caused by severe hoarding.[93]

Harm Reduction

The use of involuntary clean-outs is not advised due to both its traumatic nature for the person who hoards and long-term ineffectiveness with associated high-recidivism rates.[76] If it is the sole option in a severe case, then mental health care would be crucial to mitigate harm.[76] An alternate approach is a harm-reduction approach for hoarding, where the goal of intervention is to mitigate risks associated with the problematic behavior, as opposed to eliminating the symptoms and behavior.[94] Harm-reduction interventions may include assistance to reduce clutter volume, and/or reorganizing belongings into safer configurations (eg, away from heat sources), instead of removal.[76] Clinical training is not required. Increasingly used by community-based providers, harm reduction necessitates the person who hoards to engage actively in decision-making processes and the establishment of a nonjudgmental individual-provider collaboration.

Medication

Pharmacotherapy research for HD has been limited by small sample sizes, open label designs, sampling patients with OCD who have hoarding symptoms instead of a primary HD diagnosis, use of nonspecific or nonvalidated hoarding measures, and minimal replication.[95,96] Thus far, the evidence for the effectiveness of serotonergic drugs has been mixed, with some studies reporting improved hoarding symptoms,[19] whereas others have found no significant effect.[97,98] Examination of other categories of drugs, including norepinephrine reuptake inhibitors, such as atomoxetine, were found to decrease hoarding severity by targeting inattention and impulsivity symptoms.[97] A review of second-generation antipsychotics such as quetiapine and risperidone found no evidence of effectiveness at treating hoarding symptoms.[99] Further research is needed to examine the potential of pharmacotherapy as a hoarding intervention, either as a standalone treatment or in combination with CBTs.

SPECIAL POPULATIONS
Children and Adolescents

Research on pediatric presentations of hoarding is limited, with much of the extant knowledge borrowed from literature on children with OCD.[100] The incidence of hoarding in youth is estimated to be between 2% and 3% of the adolescent population.[101,102] Children are rarely able to accumulate items to the same severity as adults, as authority figures such as parents can often control the child's ability to obtain more objects.[103] Acquisition usually presents alongside extreme care about the location and condition of the collected objects, and possessions can become part of the child's identity, resulting in possibly traumatic discarding attempts.[102] Similar to adults, children who hoard also exhibit associated cognitive deficits such as affected insight, indecision, inattention, poor memory, problem-solving and planning problems, increased avoidance, and psychiatric comorbidities.[103] Social challenges such as decreased social networks, risk of being bullied, and increased family strain have also been documented among youth who hoard.[102]

Standardized hoarding assessments that have been validated for use with children are the Child Saving Inventory[104] and the Hoarding Rating Scale.[20,21,102] With respect to treatment, there is early evidence to suggest the effectiveness of CBT with pediatric samples.[102] Further research is needed to assess the appropriateness and efficacy of pharmacological treatments for this population.

Older Adults

Hoarding among older adults is estimated to be 3 times higher than the general population[105] and becomes more severe with age.[53] Older adults experience worse consequences and functional impairment due to the hoarding.[106] The accumulation of clutter can pose higher risks for fire endangerment, falls hazards, medication misman-agement, inadequate nutrition, poor sanitation, social isolation, and difficulty completing activities of daily living.[23,107] Sleep disturbance was also associated with increased hoarding severity.[108] Cognitive difficulties with functions such as plan-ning, problem-solving, and memory are prevalent among older adults who hoard, and complicate assessment and intervention.

Although assessments validated for the general adult population are generally suit-able for this population, it is recommended that self-reports be comprehensively corroborated through clinician home visits, social support collateral, neurocognitive assessment, and evaluation of functional abilities.[109] Thus far, cognitive rehabilitation and exposure-sorting therapy, which combines cognitive training with behavioral exposure, has produced clinically significant improvements in symptom severity for older adults who hoard.[110,111] This is despite recent research, which suggested that older adults actually experience less distress when exposed to discarding than younger samples.[112] A recent study examining the efficacy of CBT combined with in-home support found high attrition rates among older adult patients with low social support, highlighting the importance of social connectedness for this population.[113] Further research is required to understand the therapeutic mechanisms underlying effective hoarding treatments.

Nonvoluntary Clients

As previously described, people who hoard may have limited insight into the severity of their behaviors and the associated consequences. Most people who hoard do not voluntarily seek assistance without insistence from support persons or the wider com-munity.[114] Therefore, hoarding-related problems are commonly externally identified through routine building or fire inspections.[76] Emotional attachment to possessions can lead to avoidance of the issue, manifesting in rejections of offers to help, cancel-ling or missing appointments, not responding to service provider contact attempts, and withdrawing previously provided consent to engage in treatment.[76] The combina-tion of such chronic avoidance and heightened safety risk can result in the application of legal sanctions for forced compliance.[76,114]

Family

Family members of people who hoard are exposed to the same health and safety risks that the person themselves experience, including the loss of functional living space, poor sanitation, social isolation, financial challenges, and family strain.[115,116] Children, in particular, have been documented as vulnerable to the effects of hoard-ing, with feelings of grief, loss, and anger toward their parent who hoards lasting into adulthood.[116] The degree of caregiver burden experienced by those caring for a person who hoards has been found to be equal to or greater than that of peo-ple with dementia.[117] In response to the person who hoard's poor insight, treatment ambivalence, and risk of harm, family members experience increased frustration, hopelessness, and distress.[115–117] Feelings of shame and embarrassment can result in the isolation or outright rejection of the person who hoards by their family.[115,116]

Interventions targeting family members of people who hoard have been developed, and typically include components such as hoarding psychoeducation, harm reduction strategies, communication training, and self-care techniques.[115] Family-focused inter-ventions have been found to decrease caregiver burden, improve family relationships, and encourage the person who hoards to accept treatment.[94,115]

SUMMARY

In the 26 years since Frost and Hartl's seminal article,[2] research on hoarding has predominantly focused on differentiating HD from OCD by delineating its distinct symptoms. This line of inquiry has led to developments in various models to conceptualize hoarding and has clarified key components for hoarding assessment, treatment planning, and outcome evaluation. More research is needed to enhance understandings of how hoarding is impacted by cognitive and affective decision-making, and a greater appreciation of the neurobiological underpinnings of the disorder may lead to further innovations in the identification and selection of treatment targets.

Regarding intervention, the current evidence base strongly supports the standard use of CBTs adapted for hoarding populations. Opportunities exist to better assess and engage those with hoarding, improve interventions and access, and maximize outcomes. Technology-based treatments, cognitive rehabilitation, CFT, and harm reduction have demonstrated early promise, and warrant further examination to expand intervention options. Future pharmacotherapy research needs to apply more robust experimental designs, include participants with a primary diagnosis of HD, and examine the combined effect of psychotherapy with medication. Further adaptations of validated assessments and evidence-based treatments are necessary to ensure their efficacy and relevance to varying age, cultural, and language groups. Beyond the numerous advances made during the past few decades, many opportunities remain for new discoveries and innovations in the study of hoarding.

CLINICS CARE POINTS

- Hoarding is a distinct psychiatric diagnosis that poses significant risk to personal health and community safety.
- Assessment should entail complementary use of standardized measures including client self-report, family and/or assessor completed assessments, practitioner-led interviews, social support collateral, and behavioral assessments.
- CBT adapted for hoarding is the gold standard psychotherapeutic treatment. Case management and harm-reduction approaches are indicated to address community-based risks.
- Populations such as older adults, children, and involuntary clients are particularly vulnerable and require specialized attention to address higher risk of harm.

REFERENCES

1. Bratiotis C, Woody SR. What's so complicated about hoarding? A view from the nexus of psychology and social work. J Obsessive-Compulsive Relat Disord 2020;24. https://doi.org/10.1016/j.jocrd.2019.100496.
2. Frost RO, Hartl TL. A cognitive-behavioral model of compulsive hoarding. Behav Res Ther 1996;34(4):341–50.
3. Association AP. Diagnostic and Statistical manual of mental disorders (DSM-5®). Am Psychiatr Publishing 2013.
4. Postlethwaite A, Kellett S, Simmonds-Buckley N. Exploring emotions and cognitions in hoarding: a Q-methodology analysis. Behav Cogn Psychother 2020; 48(6):672–87.

5. Sinopoli VM, Erdman L, Burton CL, et al. Serotonin system genes and hoarding with and without other obsessive-compulsive traits in a population-based, pediatric sample: a genetic association study. Depress Anxiety 2020;37(8):760–70.

6. Zaboski BA, Merritt OA, Schrack AP, et al. Hoarding: a meta-analysis of age of onset. Depress Anxiety 2019;36(6):552–64.

7. Waters DM, Eckhardt M, Eason EA. Characteristics of deaths with evidence of pathological hoarding in cook county 2017 to 2018. Am J Forensic Med Pathol 2022;43(1):2–6.

8. Timpano KR, Bainter SA, Goodman ZT, et al. A network analysis of hoarding symptoms, Saving and acquiring motives, and comorbidity. J Obsessive-Compulsive Relat Disord 2020;25. https://doi.org/10.1016/j.jocrd.2020.100520.

9. Frost RO, Steketee G, Tolin DF. Comorbidity in hoarding disorder. Depress Anxiety 2011;28(10):876–84.

10. Pellegrini L, Maietti E, Rucci P, et al. Suicidality in patients with obsessive-compulsive and related disorders (OCRDs): a meta-analysis. Compr Psychiatry 2021;108:152246.

11. Pertusa A, Frost RO, Mataix-Cols D. When hoarding is a symptom of OCD: a case series and implications for DSM-V. Behav Res Ther 2010;48(10):1012–20.

12. Bratiotis C, Woody S, Lauster N. Coordinated Community-Based Hoarding Interventions: Evidence of Case Management Practices. Families Soc 2019;100(1): 93–105.

13. Woody SR, Lenkic P, Bratiotis C, et al. How well do hoarding research samples represent cases that rise to community attention? Behav Res Ther 2020;126: 103555.

14. Nutley SK, Camacho MR, Eichenbaum J, et al. Hoarding disorder is associated with self-reported cardiovascular/metabolic dysfunction, chronic pain, and sleep apnea. J Psychiatr Res 2021;134:15–21.

15. Lucini G, Monk I, Szlatenyi C. An analysis of fire incidents involving hoarding households. Worcester, MA: Worcester Polytechnic Institute; 2009. Available at: http://web.cs.wpi.edu/~rek/Projects/MFB_D09.pdf.

16. Bratiotis C. Community-based interventions for hoarding: impacts on children, youth and families. Child Aust 2020;45(3):193–5.

17. Steketee G, Frost RO. Compulsive hoarding and acquiring: therapist guide. New York, NY: Oxford University Press; 2007.

18. Nordsletten AE, Fernández de la Cruz L, Pertusa A, et al. The structured interview for hoarding disorder (SIHD): development, usage and further validation. J Obsessive-Compulsive Relat Disord 2013;2(3):346–50.

19. Saxena S, Sumner J. Venlafaxine extended-release treatment of hoarding disorder. Int Clin Psychopharmacol 2014;29(5):266–73.

20. Tolin DF, Gilliam CM, Davis E, et al. Psychometric properties of the Hoarding Rating Scale-Interview. J Obsessive-Compulsive Relat Disord 2018;16:76–80.

21. Tolin DF, Frost RO, Steketee G. A brief interview for assessing compulsive hoarding: the Hoarding Rating Scale-Interview. Psychiatry Res 2009;178(1): 147–52.

22. Frost RO, Steketee G, Grisham J. Measurement of compulsive hoarding: saving inventory-revised. Behav Res Ther 2004;42(10):1163–82.

23. Ayers CR, Dozier ME, Mayes TL. Psychometric evaluation of the saving inventory-revised in older adults. Clin Gerontologist 2017;40(3):191–6.

24. Tolin DF, Meunier SA, Frost RO, et al. Hoarding among patients seeking treatment for anxiety disorders. J Anxiety Disord 2010;25(1):43–8.

25. Steketee G, Frost RO, Kyrios M. Cognitive aspects of compulsive hoarding. Cogn Ther Res 2003;27(4):463–79.
26. Muroff J, Steketee G, Frost RO, et al. Cognitive behavior therapy for hoarding disorder: follow-up findings and predictors of outcome. Depress Anxiety 2014;31(12):964–71.
27. Bratiotis C, Schmalisch CS, Steketee G. The hoarding handbook: a guide for human service professionals. New York, NY: Oxford University Press; 2011.
28. Frost RO, Hristova V, Steketee G, et al. Activities of daily living scale in hoarding disorder. J Obsessive-Compulsive Relat Disord 2012;2(2):85–90.
29. Carey EA, del Pozo de Bolger A, Wootton BM. Psychometric properties of the Hoarding Disorder-Dimensional Scale. J Obsessive-Compulsive Relat Disord 2019;21:91–6.
30. Frost RO, Steketee G, Tolin DF, et al. Development and validation of the Clutter Image Rating. J Psychopathology Behav Assess 2007;30(3):193–203.
31. Halliday G, Snowdon J. The environmental cleanliness and clutter scale (ECCS). Int psychogeriatrics 2009;21(6):1041–50.
32. Rasmussen JL, Steketee G, Frost RO, et al. Assessing squalor in hoarding: the home environment index. Community Ment Health J 2013;50(5):591–6.
33. Stamatis CA, Muroff J, Bocanegra ES, et al. A spanish translation of the hoarding rating scale: differential item functioning and convergent validity. J Psychopathol Behav Assess 2021;43(4):946–59.
34. Ong CW, Krafft J, Levin ME, et al. A systematic review and psychometric evaluation of self-report measures for hoarding disorder. J Affect Disord 2021;290:136–48.
35. Preston SD, MacMillan-Ladd AD. Object attachment and decision-making. Curr Opin Psychol 2021;39:31–7.
36. Grisham JR, Norberg MM, Williams AD, et al. Categorization and cognitive deficits in compulsive hoarding. Behav Res Ther 2010;48(9):866–72.
37. David J, Baldwin PA, Grisham JR. To save or not to save: the use of cognitive bias modification in a high-hoarding sample. J Obsessive-Compulsive Relat Disord 2019;23:100457.
38. Andrews-McClymont JG, Lilienfeld SO, Duke MP. Evaluating an animal model of compulsive hoarding in humans. Rev Gen Psychol 2013;17(4):399–419.
39. Suñol M, Martínez-Zalacaín I, Picó-Pérez M, et al. Differential patterns of brain activation between hoarding disorder and obsessive-compulsive disorder during executive performance. Psychol Med 2020;50(4):666–73.
40. Stevens MC, Levy HC, Hallion LS, et al. Functional neuroimaging test of an emerging neurobiological model of hoarding disorder. Biol Psychiatry Cogn Neurosci Neuroimaging 2020;5(1):68–75.
41. Levy HC, Poppe A, Hiser J, et al. An examination of the association between subjective distress and functional connectivity during discarding decisions in hoarding disorder. Biol Psychiatry Cogn Neurosci Neuroimaging 2021;6(10):1013–22.
42. Liu N, Zakrzewski JJ, Mathews CA, et al. Electrophysiological dynamics of visuocortical processing in hoarding disorder. Psychophysiology 2021;58(2):e13711.
43. Mizobe T, Ikari K, Tomiyama H, et al. Abnormal white matter structure in hoarding disorder. J Psychiatr Res 2022;148:1–8.
44. Grisham JR, Brown TA, Savage CR, et al. Neuropsychological impairment associated with compulsive hoarding. Behav Res Ther 2007;45(7):1471–83.

45. Hartl TL, Duffany SR, Allen GJ, et al. Relationships among compulsive hoarding, trauma, and attention-deficit/hyperactivity disorder. Behav Res Ther 2005;43(2): 269–76.

46. Mischel W, Ayduk O, Berman MG, et al. Willpower' over the life span: decomposing self-regulation. Social Cogn Affective Neurosci 2011;6(2):252–6.

47. Lawrence NS, Wooderson S, Mataix-Cols D, et al. Decision making and set shifting impairments are associated with distinct symptom dimensions in obsessive-compulsive disorder. Neuropsychology 2006;20(4):409–19.

48. J Zakrzewski J, A Gillett D, R Vigil O, et al. Visually mediated functioning improves following treatment of hoarding disorder. J Affect Disord 2020;264: 310–7.

49. Mathews CA, Delucchi K, Cath DC, et al. Partitioning the etiology of hoarding and obsessive-compulsive symptoms. Psychol Med 2014;44(13):2867–76.

50. Monzani B, Rijsdijk F, Harris J, et al. The structure of genetic and environmental risk factors for dimensional representations of DSM-5 Obsessive-Compulsive spectrum disorders. JAMA Psychiatry (Chicago, Ill 2014;71(2):182–9.

51. Ivanov VZ, Nordsletten A, Mataix-Cols D, et al. Heritability of hoarding symptoms across adolescence and young adulthood: a longitudinal twin study. PloS one 2017;12(6):e0179541.

52. Burton CL, Park LS, Corfield EC, et al. Heritability of obsessive-compulsive trait dimensions in youth from the general population. Transl Psychiatry 2018; 8(1):191.

53. Dozier ME, Porter B, Ayers CR. Age of onset and progression of hoarding symptoms in older adults with hoarding disorder. Aging Ment Health 2016;20(7): 736–42.

54. Alonso P, Gratacòs M, Menchón JM, et al. Genetic susceptibility to obsessive-compulsive hoarding: the contribution of neurotrophic tyrosine kinase receptor type 3 gene. Genes, Brain Behav 2008;7(7):778–85.

55. Timpano KR, Schmidt NB, Wheaton MG, et al. Consideration of the BDNF gene in relation to two phenotypes: hoarding and obesity. J Abnorm Psychol (1965) 2011;120(3):700.

56. Perroud N, Guipponi M, Pertusa A, et al. Genome-wide association study of hoarding traits. Am J Med Genet B, Neuropsychiatr Genet 2011;156B(2):240–2.

57. Grünblatt E. Genetics of OCD and related disorders; Searching for shared factors. Curr Top Behav Neurosci 2021;49:1–16.

58. Mathes BM, Timpano KR, Raines AM, et al. Attachment theory and hoarding disorder: a review and theoretical integration. Behav Res Ther 2020;125:103549.

59. Chia K, Pasalich DS, Fassnacht DB, et al. Interpersonal attachment, early family environment, and trauma in hoarding: a systematic review. Clin Psychol Rev 2021;90:102096.

60. Yap K, Grisham JR. Object attachment in hoarding disorder and its role in a compensatory process. Curr Opin Psychol 2021;39:76–81.

61. Timpano KR, Port JH. Object attachment and emotion (Dys)regulation across development and clinical populations. Curr Opin Psychol 2021;39:109–14.

62. Wheaton MG, Topilow K. Maximizing decision-making style and hoarding disorder symptoms. Compr Psychiatry 2020;101:152187.

63. Yap K, Grisham JR. Object attachment and emotions in hoarding disorder. Compr Psychiatry 2020;100:152179.

64. Dozier ME, DeShong HL. The association between personality traits and hoarding behaviors. Curr Opin Psychiatry 2022;35(1):53–8.

65. Chan J, Powell C, Collett J. Profiling hoarding within the five-factor Model of personality and self-determination theory. Behav Ther 2022;53(3):546–59.

66. Stumpf BP, de Souza LC, Mourão MSF, et al. Cognitive impairment in hoarding disorder: a systematic review. CNS Spectr 2022;1–13. https://doi.org/10.1017/S1092852922000153.

67. Chen W, McDonald S, Wearne T, et al. Investigating associations between hoarding symptoms and affective and cognitive empathy. Br J Clin Psychol 2021;60(2):177–93.

68. Krafft J, Ong CW, Cruz RA, et al. An ecological momentary assessment study investigating the function of hoarding. Behav Ther 2020;51(5):715–27.

69. Siev J, Darst-Campbell M, Rouder IC, et al. Grit predicts less severe hoarding symptoms among patients seeking treatment at an anxiety disorders clinic. Bull Menninger Clin 2022;86(1):20–34.

70. Hillman SR, Lomax CL, Khaleel N, et al. The roles of intolerance of uncertainty, anxiety sensitivity and distress tolerance in hoarding disorder compared with OCD and healthy controls. Behav Cogn Psychother 2022;50(4):392–403.

71. Mataix-Cols D, Pertusa A, Snowdon J. Neuropsychological and neural correlates of hoarding: a practice-friendly review. J Clin Psychol 2011;67(5):467–76.

72. Chamberlain SR, Solly JE, Hook RW, et al. Cognitive Inflexibility in OCD and Related Disorders. Curr Top Behav Neurosci 2021;49:125–45.

73. Akbari M, Seydavi M, Mohammadkhani S, et al. Emotion dysregulation and hoarding symptoms: a systematic review and meta-analysis. J Clin Psychol 2022;78(7):1341–53.

74. Tolin DF, Fitch KE, Frost RO, et al. Family informants' perceptions of insight in compulsive hoarding. Cogn Ther Res 2008;34(1):69–81.

75. Frost RO, Tolin DF, Maltby N. Insight-related challenges in the treatment of hoarding. Cogn Behav Pract 2010;17(4):404–13.

76. Kysow K, Bratiotis C, Lauster N, et al. How can cities tackle hoarding? Examining an intervention program bringing together fire and health authorities in Vancouver. Health Soc Care Community 2020;28(4):1160–9.

77. Steketee G, Frost RO. Treatment for hoarding disorder: therapist guide. 2nd edition. New York, NY: Oxford University Press; 2014.

78. Tolin DF, Frost RO, Steketee G, et al. Cognitive behavioral therapy for hoarding disorder: a meta-analysis. Focus (Am Psychiatr Publ) 2021;19(4):468–76.

79. Rodgers N, McDonald S, Wootton BM. Cognitive behavioral therapy for hoarding disorder: An updated meta-analysis. J Affect Disord 2021;290:128–35.

80. Bodryzlova Y, Audet JS, Bergeron K, et al. Group cognitive-behavioural therapy for hoarding disorder: systematic review and meta-analysis. Health Soc Care Community 2019;27(3):517–30.

81. Linkovski O, Zwerling J, Cordell E, et al. Augmenting Buried in Treasures with in-home uncluttering practice: pilot study in hoarding disorder. J Psychiatr Res 2018;107:145–50.

82. Mathews CA, Mackin RS, Chou CY, et al. Randomised clinical trial of community-based peer-led and psychologist-led group treatment for hoarding disorder. BJPsych Open 2018;4(4):285–93.

83. Wootton BM, Bragdon LB, Worden BL, et al. Measuring within-session and between-session compliance in hoarding disorder: a preliminary investigation of the psychometric properties of the CBT compliance measure (CCM) and patient exposure/response prevention adherence scale for hoarding (PEAS-H). Assessment 2021;28(6):1694–707.

84. Chou CY, Tsoh JY, Shumway M, et al. Treating hoarding disorder with compassion-focused therapy: a pilot study examining treatment feasibility, acceptability, and exploring treatment effects. Br J Clin Psychol 2020; 59(1):1–21.

85. Muroff J, Steketee G, Himle J, et al. Delivery of internet treatment for compulsive hoarding (D.I.T.C.H.). Behav Res Ther 2010;48(1):79–85.

86. Muroff J, Otte S. Innovations in CBT treatment for hoarding: Transcending office walls. J Obsessive-Compulsive Relat Disord 2019;23:100471.

87. Yap K, Chen W, Wong SF, et al. Is it as good as being in person? The effectiveness of a modified clinician facilitated buried in treasures group for hoarding disorder using video teleconferencing. Psychiatry Res 2022;314:114631.

88. Muroff J, Steketee G. Pilot trial of cognitive and behavioral treatment for hoarding disorder delivered via webcam: feasibility and preliminary outcomes. J Obsessive-Compulsive Relat Disord 2018;18:18–24.

89. Fitzpatrick M, Nedeljkovic M, Abbott J-A, et al. Blended" therapy: The development and pilot evaluation of an internet-facilitated cognitive behavioral intervention to supplement face-to-face therapy for hoarding disorder. Internet Interventions 2018;12:16–25.

90. McCabe-Bennett H, Lachman R, Girard TA, et al. A virtual reality study of the relationships between hoarding, clutter, and claustrophobia. Cyberpsychol Behav Soc Netw 2020;23(2):83–9.

91. St-Pierre-Delorme M-E, O'Connor K. Using virtual reality in the inference-based treatment of compulsive hoarding. Front Public Health 2016;4:149.

92. Gleason A, Perkes D, Wand AP. Managing hoarding and squalor. Aust Prescr 2021;44(3):79–84.

93. Millen AM, Levinson A, Linkovski O, et al. Pilot study evaluating critical time intervention for individuals with hoarding disorder at risk for eviction. Psychiatr Serv 2020;71(4):405–8.

94. Tompkins MA, Hartl TL. Digging out: helping your loved one manage clutter, hoarding & compulsive acquiring. Oakland, CA: New Harbinger Publications; 2009.

95. Brakoulias V, Eslick GD, Starcevic V. A meta-analysis of the response of pathological hoarding to pharmacotherapy. Psychiatry Res 2015;229(1):272–6.

96. Piacentino D, Pasquini M, Cappelletti S, et al. Pharmacotherapy for hoarding disorder: how did the picture change since its excision from OCD? Curr Neuropharmacology 2019;17(8):808–15.

97. Grassi G, Albani G, Terenzi F, et al. New pharmacological and neuromodulation approaches for impulsive-compulsive behaviors in Parkinson's disease. Neurol Sci 2021;42(7):2673–82.

98. Amiaz R, Fostick L, Gershon A, et al. Naltrexone augmentation in OCD: a double-blind placebo-controlled cross-over study. Eur Neuropsychopharmacol 2008;18(6):455–61.

99. Kim D, Ryba NL, Kalabalik J, et al. Critical review of the use of second-generation antipsychotics in obsessive-compulsive and related disorders. Drugs R D 2018;18(3):167–89.

100. Rozenman M, McGuire J, Wu M, et al. Hoarding symptoms in children and adolescents with obsessive-compulsive disorder: clinical features and response to cognitive-behavioral therapy. J Am Acad Child Adolesc Psychiatry 2019;58(8): 799–805.

101. Akıncı MA, Turan B, Esin İ, et al. Prevalence and correlates of hoarding behavior and hoarding disorder in children and adolescents. Eur Child Adolesc Psychiatry 2021. https://doi.org/10.1007/s00787-021-01847-x.
102. Carnevale T. Identifying adolescents with hoarding disorder. J Child Adolesc Psychiatr Nurs 2021;34(2):120–4.
103. Hojgaard D, Skarphedinsson G, Ivarsson T, et al. Hoarding in children and adolescents with obsessive-compulsive disorder: prevalence, clinical correlates, and cognitive behavioral therapy outcome. Eur Child Adolesc Psychiatry 2019;28(8):1097–106.
104. Storch EA, Muroff J, Lewin AB, et al. Development and preliminary psychometric evaluation of the Children's Saving Inventory. Child Psychiatry Hum Dev 2011; 42(2):166–82.
105. Samuels JF, Bienvenu OJ, Grados MA, et al. Prevalence and correlates of hoarding behavior in a community-based sample. Behav Res Ther 2008; 46(7):836–44.
106. Diefenbach GJ, DiMauro J, Frost R, et al. Characteristics of hoarding in older adults. Am J Geriatr Psychiatry 2013;21(10):1043–7.
107. Dozier ME, Ayers CR. Validation of the Clutter Image Rating in older adults with hoarding disorder. Int Psychogeriatr 2015;27(5):769–76.
108. Dozier ME, Speed KJ, Davidson EJ, et al. The Association Between Sleep and Late Life Hoarding. Int J Aging Hum Dev 2021;93(4):931–42.
109. Howard I, Najmi S, Maddox M, et al. Hoarding in older adults. The oxford handbook of hoarding and acquiring. New York, NY: Oxford University Press; 2014.
110. Pittman JOE, Davidson EJ, Dozier ME, et al. Implementation and evaluation of a community-based treatment for late-life hoarding. Int Psychogeriatr 2021;33(9): 977–86.
111. Ayers CR, Davidson EJ, Dozier ME, et al. Cognitive rehabilitation and exposure/sorting therapy for late-life hoarding: effects on neuropsychological performance. J Gerontol B Psychol Sci Soc Sci 2020;75(6):1193–8.
112. Dozier ME, Wetherell JL, Amir N, et al. The association between age and experienced emotions in hoarding disorder. Clin Gerontol 2021;44(5):562–6.
113. Weiss ER, Landers A, Todman M, et al. Treatment outcomes in older adults with hoarding disorder: the impact of self-control, boredom and social support. Australas J Ageing 2020;39(4):375–80.
114. Kwok N, Bratiotis C, Luu M, et al. Examining the role of fire prevention on hoarding response teams: vancouver fire and rescue services as a case study. Fire Technology 2017;54(1):57–73.
115. Chasson GS, Carpenter A, Ewing J, et al. Empowering families to help a loved one with Hoarding Disorder: Pilot study of Family-As-Motivators training. Behav Res Ther 2014;63:9–16.
116. Neziroglu F, Upston M, Khemlani-Patel S. The psychological, relational and social impact in adult offspring of parents with hoarding disorder. Child Aust 2020; 45(3):153–8.
117. Drury H, Ajmi S, Fernández de la Cruz L, et al. Caregiver burden, family accommodation, health, and well-being in relatives of individuals with hoarding disorder. J Affect Disord 2014;159:7–14.

Body Dysmorphic Disorder

Amita Jassi, DClinPsy[a],*, Georgina Krebs, DClinPsy, Phd[a,b]

KEYWORDS

- Body dysmorphic disorder (BDD) • Cognitive behavior therapy (CBT)
- Selective serotonin reuptake inhibitors (SSRIs) • Cosmetic procedures
- Risk assessment

KEY POINTS

- BDD is a common and treatable condition, with evidence-based recommended treatments including cognitive behavior therapy (CBT) and serotonin reuptake inhibitor (SRI) medication.
- BDD is strikingly underdiagnosed, for a range of reasons including shame and embarrassment about disclosing appearance concerns, sufferers seeking cosmetic procedures instead of mental health support, and BDD being misdiagnosed as another condition (eg, social anxiety disorder or depression).
- A thorough and dynamic risk assessment is key, and it is important to assess whether they desire or have undertaken cosmetic procedures, including "DIY" procedures.
- Barriers to accessing CBT are being tackled with the development of Internet and app-based CBT, which show promising outcomes.

THE NATURE OF BODY DYSMORPHIC DISORDER

The cardinal feature of body dysmorphic disorder (BDD) is excessive and persistent preoccupation with perceived flaws in physical appearance[1,2] These perceived flaws are unobservable or appear very minimal to other people but are nevertheless a source of great distress for the BDD sufferer. The focus of preoccupation can vary greatly in BDD, but the most commonly reported appearance concerns relate to facial features, such as nose, eyes, teeth, skin, and hair.[3,4] Most individuals with BDD have worries about multiple features, although some of these may be more prominent than others. On the other hand, some individuals with BDD cannot pinpoint their concerns to *specific* aspects of their appearance, but instead describe *general* appearance worries, and may say that they look "ugly," "hideous," or even "abnormal."

[a] National & Specialist OCD, BDD, and Related Disorders Service, South London and Maudsley NHS Trust, London, SE5 8AZ, United Kingdom; [b] Department of Clinical, Educational and Health Psychology, University College London, 1-19 Torrington Place, London, WC1E 7HB, United Kingdom
* Corresponding author.
E-mail address: amita.jassi@slam.nhs.uk

Psychiatr Clin N Am 46 (2023) 197–209
https://doi.org/10.1016/j.psc.2022.10.005
0193-953X/23/© 2022 Elsevier Inc. All rights reserved.

In an attempt to cope with appearance concerns, BDD sufferers typically engage in a range of repetitive behaviors and mental acts, often aimed at checking, camouflaging, or correcting their perceived defects.[1,2] Checking behaviors may involve repeatedly looking in mirrors or other reflective surfaces, taking selfies, or physically touching the perceived flaw. Camouflaging can include concealing perceived flaws with excessive makeup or clothing (eg, covering hair with a hat) or using other body parts to hide perceived flaws (eg, holding a hand in front of mouth when talking to cover teeth). Attempts to correct perceived flaws can involve lengthy and costly grooming routines (eg, excessive use of skin and hair products), skin-picking, and seeking cosmetic treatments. In addition, avoidance is a common feature of BDD, which can range from subtle behaviors (eg, avoiding looking in reflective surfaces) to extreme and pervasive avoidance (eg, becoming housebound).

BDD typically develops during teenage years, with two-thirds of adults retrospectively reporting an onset during adolescence.[5] Without treatment, the disorder typically persists[6] and is associated with marked functional impairment across multiple domains. Among adults, BDD is associated with poor quality of life, high rates of occupational impairment, unemployment, and social isolation.[3] Similarly, among young people, BDD results in reduced academic performance, dropping out of school, and social withdrawal.[4] BDD often co-occurs with other psychiatric disorders, such as depression, social anxiety disorder, obsessive-compulsive disorder (OCD), and eating disorders.[4,7] BDD is also associated with concerningly high rates of suicidality; it is estimated that 1 in 4 individuals with BDD attempt suicide.[8]

A striking characteristic of BDD is that many, although not all, sufferers have poor insight.[3,4] That is, they do not recognize that their appearance concerns are excessive and are convinced that there is a physical problem with their appearance. There has been some debate about whether this feature of BDD should be viewed as a delusionality or lack of insight,[9] with the latter conceptualization being reflected in the current diagnostic symptoms, in which insight is a specifier for BDD.[1,2] Importantly, an individual's level of BDD insight is not static, and can vary greatly over short time intervals[10] and improve with treatment.[11]

Prevalence

BDD has an estimated point prevalence of approximately 2% in population-based samples of adults and young people.[12] Not surprisingly, BDD is substantially more common in certain settings, including psychiatric clinics and cosmetic surgery settings.[12] For example, it has been estimated that approximately 1 in 5 people who seek rhinoplasty meet diagnostic criteria for BDD,[12] highlighting the importance of screening for BDD in such settings.

Among young people, BDD has been found to be more common in girls than boys, but the sex difference seems to reduce in adulthood, where there is only a slight female preponderance.[12,13] This finding raises the possibility that BDD may emerge later in men than in women. The features of BDD are broadly similar in males and females. However, males are more likely to experience concerns about muscularity than females (referred to as muscle dysmorphia).[4,14] It has also been reported that males are more likely to be preoccupied with their genitals and thinning hair, whereas females are more likely to be preoccupied with hips, breasts, legs and excessive body hair.[15]

Little is known about whether the prevalence and phenomenology of BDD varies across countries and ethnic and/or cultural groups. Most community-based prevalence studies have been conducted within Europe and North America, but BDD has been reported across the world, including in Africa, Asia, and South America. Existing studies not only suggest that the prevalence and core features of BDD are similar across countries[16] but also highlight some potential differences. For example, a survey study conducted in the United States among adults with probable BDD found that Asian participants were more likely to report concerns about straight hair and dark skin, whereas White participants were more likely to report body shape concerns (eg, stomach, hips, buttocks).[17] Thus, it has been suggested that individuals from ethnic minority groups who develop BDD may be more likely to be concerned about body parts that are characteristic of their ethnic background, and differentiate them from the ethnic majority group.[17]

Assessment

BDD can often be overlooked or misdiagnosed in routine clinical practice[18,19]; this in part can be due to similarities with a range of other conditions. **Table 1** summarizes disorders in which differential diagnosis challenges often arise, highlighting similarities and important differences with BDD.

Studies have indicated that BDD is rarely spontaneously disclosed in routine clinical assessments.[18,20–23] However, if sufferers are explicitly asked about appearance concerns, they often disclose their symptoms.[24] For example, a single screening item assessing worries about appearance, as used in the BDD section of the Development and Well-Being Assessment,[25] was found to correctly identify 97% of young people with BDD.[26] Beyond screening, the Body Dysmorphic Disorder Yale-Brown Obsessive-Compulsive Scale (BDD-Y-BOCS)[27] is the gold-standard clinician administered measure of BDD severity. This measure has good psychometric properties in both the adult[28,29] and adolescent versions.[30] For young people, it is helpful to have other informants, such as parents, to help assess BDD, especially because young people have poorer insight into their BDD.[3]

Risk is a common characteristic of BDD and often brings sufferers to the attention of mental services. It is therefore important to conduct a thorough and dynamic risk assessment, with regular reviews. An assessment of suicidality and self-harm is vital given that around 25% of sufferers attempt to end their lives,[8] 80% have suicidal ideation,[8,24] and 50% self-harm.[4] In addition, given nearly half of sufferers report substance misuse,[18] this is also important to assess.

A unique feature of the BDD risk profile is seeking cosmetic procedures; it is estimated that up to 75% of individuals with BDD seek cosmetic procedures, including surgical interventions, in an attempt to "fix" their perceived defects.[31] The available evidence indicates that BDD symptoms do not improve following cosmetic interventions, and such procedures result in dissatisfaction, disappointment, and a deterioration in mental health.[31] Thus, cosmetic procedures are not recommended in individuals with BDD. In some instances, often when individuals are unable to access the cosmetic procedures that they desire through services, they attempt "DIY" surgery, such as bleaching their own skin or injecting saline solution into their lips,[32] which is clearly associated with substantial physical, as well as psychological, risk. In addition, approximately a third of BDD sufferers pick their skin in an attempt to improve its appearance,[33] and use instruments such as needles, razors, and knives to correct their perceived flaw. These repetitive behaviors could cause physical health consequences such as infections and damage to appearance, which could fuel distress. Therefore, it is important to consider the impact of repetitive behaviors in a risk assessment.

Treatment

The recommended evidence-based treatments for BDD are cognitive behavior therapy (CBT) and selective serotonin reuptake inhibitor (SSRI) medication.[34] CBT for

Table 1
Common differential diagnoses in body dysmorphic disorder

	Similarity to BDD	Key Differentiating Features
OCD	Repetitive behaviors, eg, grooming rituals, checking	BDD rituals are driven by attempts to correct perceived flaws in appearance. OCD rituals can be driven by a range of obsessions (eg, contamination, "just right," or need for symmetry)
Excoriation disorder	Repetitive skin picking	BDD skin picking is undertaken to fix a perceived appearance flaw in one's skin. Skin picking in excoriation disorder is typically described as being purely habitual or providing general tension relief
Trichotillomania	Repetitive hair pulling	In BDD sufferers may pluck or pull facial or body hair to improve appearance. Hair pulling in trichotillomania is typically described as being purely habitual or providing general tension relief
Eating disorders	Distressing preoccupation with body image	In eating disorders, the focus of appearance concern is shape and weight, and sufferers engage in eating behaviors and exercise to lose weight
Social anxiety disorder	Distress and avoidance of social situations	In BDD social avoidance is driven by fear of negative judgment about perceived appearance flaws. In social anxiety disorder this is driven by fear of doing or saying something embarrassing
Depression	Can involve feelings of ugliness and low self-esteem	In depression, appearance concerns are not the *primary* preoccupation and they are not typically accompanied by repetitive behaviors (eg,

(continued on next page)

	Similarity to BDD	Key Differentiating Features
Table 1 *(continued)*		
		grooming, mirror checking).
Gender dysphoria	Preoccupation and distress associated with sex-signifying aspects of appearance	In gender dysphoria, appearance distress is focused specifically on sex signifiers (eg, breasts, penis) because they represent the gender they do not identify with, accompanied by distress of possessing other sex signifiers, eg, tone of voice, and a feeling of not being the gender they wish to be. In BDD appearance concerns can be focused on a range of areas, including sex signifiers, the distress is focused on their appearance rather than the gender they represent
Visible difference in appearance	Preoccupation and distress associated with appearance	In BDD, the perceived "flaw" in appearance is not noticeable, or appears as minor, to others, whereas in those with visible difference, this is seen by others and there may not be a mismatch in perceived and actual appearance

Adapted from Krebs G, Fernández de la Cruz L, Mataix-Cols D. Recent advances in understanding and managing body dysmorphic disorder. Evidence-Based Mental Health. 2017;20(3):71-75. https://doi.org/10.1136/eb-2017-102702.

BDD protocols typically involves 12 to 22 sessions[35–37] and generally entails the components summarized in **Table 2**.

Treatment of adults and young people is broadly similar; however, for young people CBT is developmentally tailored with an emphasis on behavioral components and inclusion of a parent/carer as co-therapist.[39]

Evidence for CBT for BDD is primarily centered on adults, with 10 randomized controlled trials (RCTs) conducted to date. Only 1 RCT of CBT for BDD has been conducted in young people.[40] Early trials compared CBT with a waitlist control[36,41–43] with more recent trials using credible psychological control treatments such as anxiety management[35] and supportive psychotherapy.[37,44] Harrison and colleagues (2016)[11] conducted a meta-analysis including RCTs up to 2015 ($k = 7$; $N = 299$) and found CBT to be superior to waitlist and control treatments in reducing BDD symptoms (Cohen's $d = 1.22$). In addition, significant improvement in depression and BDD-related insight was evident.[11]

To date, the most promising treatment outcomes come from the largest adult RCT (N = 120) in which patients were randomized to 22 sessions of CBT or supportive psychotherapy.[37] The CBT response rate (defined by a reduction on BDD Y-BOCS ≤30%) at posttreatment was 83% to 85% across 2 treatment sites, which is higher than previous trials, which included 8 to 16 sessions.[36,41,42] There was also a significant reduction in depression, and an improvement in BDD-related insight and functioning. In their trial, Wilhelm and colleagues[37] found that patients continued to make gains after sessions 12 and 16, which would have been the end of treatment point in other trials (eg, Refs.[35,40]). Evidence suggests that even if there is minimal reduction in BDD symptoms within the first 4 to 12 sessions, patients can respond to a 24-session package of treatment.[45] Treatment of young people has improved with increasing number of sessions, with response rate of 40% to a 14-session package of CBT[40] to 79% to an extended 20-session package.[39] Taken together, these studies suggest that patients with BDD may benefit from longer treatment protocols.

Durability of outcomes has been found with treatment gains being maintained in follow-up of between 2 and 12 months and some further improvements in BDD symptoms, depression, and functioning.[37,39,44,46] Several studies have examined predictors and moderators of treatment outcomes. The most replicated finding is that higher baseline BDD symptom severity[6,39,47] is associated with less improvement in BDD symptoms. Some studies have also found higher motivation to change, greater treatment expectations, greater treatment credibility, expectation of improvement, better insight, shorter duration of BDD, and lower levels of depression to predict better outcomes,[6,47–49] although findings have been inconsistent.

There is no consensus yet on the active ingredients for effective CBT. Wilhelm and colleagues (2019)[37] found no significant differences in outcomes between supportive psychotherapy and CBT in 1 of their 2 treatment sites, potentially indicating that certain nonspecific therapy factors are associated with improvements in BDD (eg, feeling understood).[37] A recent study examining mechanisms of improvement in CBT for BDD found that within-subject cognitive (eg, negative beliefs about the importance of appearance) and behavioral (eg, checking, grooming, and avoidance) factors mediated treatment outcomes. This finding reinforces the importance of addressing beliefs about appearance (eg, "If my appearance is defective, I am worthless") and repetitive behaviors in CBT for BDD.[50]

In keeping with the current evidence base, clinical guidelines recommend SSRIs for the treatment of BDD, particularly among individuals with more severe impairment and/or those who decline CBT. Ideally, SSRIs should be offered in combination with CBT[34] but are effective as a standalone intervention.[3] A range of SSRIs have been used in the treatment of BDD, including fluoxetine[51] fluvoxamine,[52] citalopram,[53] and escitalopram,[54] as well as non-SSRIs such as clomipramine.[55] The bulk of the evidence for the efficacy of these pharmacologic treatments for BDD comes from open trials, and only 4 RCTs have been conducted.[51,54–56] Encouragingly, these RCTs have found SSRIs to be associated with response rates ranging from 53% to 70% among adults with BDD,[51,55] but they have also highlighted a need to remain on SSRIs medication for relatively long periods to reduce the likelihood of relapse occurring.[54]

Formal dose-finding studies have yet to be conducted in BDD, but the available evidence and expert clinical opinion indicates that BDD typically requires relatively high doses of SSRIs; higher than those required to treat depression.[57] At present, it is unclear whether certain SSRIs are more effective than others in the treatment of BDD, and further research is needed to compare efficacy. There is also a need to further evaluate pharmacologic augmentation strategies for patients with BDD who do not respond to initial trials of SSRIs. Clinical guidelines suggest that SSRI augmentation

Table 2
Overview of cognitive behavior therapy for body dysmorphic disorder

Treatment Component	Overview
Psychoeducation	Education on BDD, anxiety, and other emotions related to BDD (eg, shame, disgust).
Formulation and goal setting	Develop a shared psychological formulation considering how early experiences may have informed beliefs about appearance and how these feed into a cycle of thoughts, behaviors, and feelings, which maintain the problem. Processes such as selective attention, perceptual distortions, and self-focused attention are discussed in relation to how they contribute to BDD cycle. Patients are asked to consider this as an alternative formulation for their difficulties, that is, psychological vs physical problem. Treatment goals that are specific, measurable, achievable, relevant, and time bound are discussed
ERP	This is a key element of therapy whereby patients are supported to be exposed to feared and avoided situations while resisting the urge to engage in repetitive or safety behaviors; this can be guided by a hierarchy, and it is completed both in session and for homework to maximize the benefits. The goal of ERP is to learn to tolerate the distress and experience distress habituation
Behavioral experiments	Similar to ERP, however, the aim is to gather evidence for and against their beliefs about appearance
Evaluating thoughts	Patients learn to identify, track, and label maladaptive thoughts about appearance and are supported to look for patterns of cognitive errors, eg, mind reading, all or nothing. Using Socratic questioning, therapists ask them to consider evidence for and against beliefs and consider a more balanced view. Behavioral experiments can be used to gather evidence as part of this process
Mirror retraining	The goal of mirror retraining is 2-fold: one is to look at the body as a whole rather than focus in on perceived flaws and second, for the patient to be able to objectively describe their body without judgment. Patients are asked to stand in front of a full-length mirror to look at their entire body and are asked to describe it from head to toe in detail, using objective and nonjudgmental language (eg, "I have two eyes, they are 6 cm long and 4 cm wide, they are brown and I have black eyelashes").
Attention retraining	Like mirror retraining, the aim is to shift perspective from a narrow view to the bigger picture. For example, when engaging in ERP or

(*continued on next page*)

Table 2 *(continued)*	
Treatment Component	**Overview**
	behavioral experiments, it is helpful for patients to learn to focus externally by processing the 5 senses (eg, things they can see, hear, smell, taste, and feel); this can reduce self-focused attention, which allows them to take in external information and for distress to habituate
Habit reversal therapy (optional)	When patients engage in skin picking or hair pulling, habit reversal techniques may help to augment ERP, especially to manage strong urges
Motivational interviewing (optional)	This technique may be used before you start treatment or can be used at various points of treatment when patients are struggling to engage in CBT, especially due to poor insight and often wanting cosmetic procedures instead. Miller and Rollnick's (2012)[38] motivational interviewing techniques can be helpful.

Abbreviation: ERP, exposure and response prevention.

with an atypical antipsychotic can be beneficial,[34] but this is largely based on clinical experience as opposed to empirical evidence. Last, there have been no SSRI trials among young people with BDD, although clinical observational studies have highlighted the potential benefit of pharmacologic treatments in this population.[39]

Barriers to Access

BDD is strikingly underdiagnosed and undertreated. For example, previous survey studies conducted in Germany indicate that only 15% to 23% of adult BDD sufferers had received an accurate diagnosis.[58,59] Furthermore, a survey study conducted in the United States found that only 17% of adults with BDD had received CBT, and 34% had been prescribed an SSRI medication.[60] These findings are concerning, not least because BDD typically has a chronic course if left untreated[6,61] and causes profound impairment for the individual as well as potentially high costs for health care systems.

Understanding barriers to diagnosis and treatment are crucial to improve health care provision for BDD. Such barriers are likely to be multifaceted, encompassing characteristics related to the BDD sufferer (eg, shame, lack of insight), broader cultural and societal issues (eg, stigma), and constraints within health care settings (eg, lack of expertise and resources for accurate diagnostic assessment and treatment).

Undoubtably one of the main barriers to accessing CBT for BDD is the lack of trained therapists, and costs associated with the treatment.[44,62] In recent years, efforts have been made to address these obstacles by developing digitalized CBT for BDD programs, which combine self-help components with therapist support. For example, a therapist-assisted online CBT for BDD program has been developed and evaluated in an RCT, and shown to be effective relative to supportive therapy.[44] In this trial, therapists were clinical psychology students with no prior experience of BDD, and the average therapist time per patient per week was 13 minutes, highlighting the potential scalability of the program. More recently, an app-based CBT for BDD program has been developed and shown to be effective relative to waitlist control in an RCT.[63] In this trial, patients were supported by a bachelor's-level coach, as opposed to a trained clinician, which again demonstrates the scalability of this approach.

FUTURE DIRECTIONS

Research and understanding of BDD continues to develop but is still lagging compared with other related conditions such as OCD, despite the similar prevalence and morbidity. Further research is needed to better understand the mechanisms underpinning the development of BDD, which may inform early detection as well as prevention and/or early intervention strategies. In addition, predictors of treatment response and mechanisms of change is an important area for future research, because these remain poorly understood[6,39,47–49,64,65]; this may lead to a move toward an understanding of what works for whom and the development of individualized and tailored multimodal treatment packages. Research into low-intensity modes of delivery of CBT for BDD aims to increase access to effective treatments. Such low-intensity CBT-based programs may be best used as part of a stepped-care approach, with more severe or complex presentations requiring higher-intensity therapy. Nevertheless, the challenge to support sufferers to access mental health services remains, highlighting the importance of efforts to increase awareness of BDD in the wider community and in settings in which BDD sufferers are likely to present, such as cosmetic clinics.

DISCLOSURE

The authors have no conflicts of interest to disclose.

REFERENCES

1. American Psychiatric Association. The Diagnostic and Statistical Manual of Mental Disorders: DSM 5. Washington, DC: American Psychiatric Association; 2013.
2. World Health Organization. The ICD-11 classification of mental and behavioural disorders: clinical descriptions and diagnostic guidelines. World Health Organization; 2018.
3. Phillips KA, Didie ER, Menard W, et al. Clinical features of body dysmorphic disorder in adolescents and adults. Psychiatry Res 2006;141(3):305–14.
4. Rautio D, Jassi A, Krebs G, et al. Clinical characteristics of 172 children and adolescents with body dysmorphic disorder. Eur Child Adolesc Psychiatry 2020;1–12. https://doi.org/10.1007/s00787-020-01677-3.
5. Bjornsson AS, Didie ER, Grant J, et al. Age at onset and clinical correlates in body dysmorphic disorder. Compr Psychiatry 2013;54(7):893–903. https://doi.org/10.1016/j.comppsych.2013.03.019.
6. Phillips KA, Menard W, Quinn E, et al. A 4-year prospective observational follow-up study of course and predictors of course in body dysmorphic disorder. Psychol Med 2013;43(5):1109–17. https://doi.org/10.1017/s0033291712001730.
7. Gunstad J, Phillips KA. Axis I comorbidity in body dysmorphic disorder. Compr Psychiatry 2003;44(4):270–6. https://doi.org/10.1016/S0010-440X(03)00088-9.

8. Angelakis I, Gooding PA, Panagioti M. Suicidality in body dysmorphic disorder (BDD): A systematic review with meta-analysis. Clin Psychol Rev 2016;49: 55–66. https://doi.org/10.1016/j.cpr.2016.08.002.

9. Toh WL, Castle DJ, Mountjoy RL, et al. Insight in body dysmorphic disorder (BDD) relative to obsessive-compulsive disorder (OCD) and psychotic disorders: Revisiting this issue in light of DSM-5. Compr Psychiatry 2017;77:100–8. https://doi.org/10.1016/j.comppsych.2017.06.004.

10. Schulte J, Dietel FA, Wilhelm S, et al. Temporal dynamics of insight in body dysmorphic disorder: An ecological momentary assessment study. J Abnorm Psychol 2021;130(4):365. https://doi.org/10.1037/abn0000673.

11. Harrison A, Fernández de la Cruz L, Enander J, et al. Cognitive-behavioral therapy for body dysmorphic disorder: A systematic review and meta-analysis of randomized controlled trials. Clin Psychol Rev 2016;48:43–51. https://doi.org/10.1016/j.cpr.2016.05.007.

12. Veale D, Gledhill LJ, Christodoulou P, et al. Body dysmorphic disorder in different settings: A systematic review and estimated weighted prevalence. Body Image 2016;18:168–86. https://doi.org/10.1016/j.bodyim.2016.07.003.

13. Enander J, Ivanov VZ, Mataix-Cols D, et al. Prevalence and heritability of body dysmorphic symptoms in adolescents and young adults: a population-based nationwide twin study. Psychol Med 2018;48(16):2740–7. https://doi.org/10.1017/S0033291718000375.

14. Tod D, Edwards C, Cranswick I. Muscle dysmorphia: current insights. Psychol Res Behav Manag 2016;9:179. https://doi.org/10.2147/PRBM.S97404.

15. Phillips KA, Wilhelm S, Koran LM, et al. Body dysmorphic disorder: some key issues for DSM-V. Depress Anxiety 2010;27(6):573–91. https://doi.org/10.1002/da.20709.

16. Bohne A, Keuthen NJ, Wilhelm S, et al. Prevalence of symptoms of body dysmorphic disorder and its correlates: a cross-cultural comparison. Psychosomatics 2002;43(6):486–90. https://doi.org/10.1176/appi.psy.43.6.486.

17. Marques L, LeBlanc N, Weingarden H, et al. Body dysmorphic symptoms: Phenomenology and ethnicity. Body Image 2011;8(2):163–7. https://doi.org/10.1016/j.bodyim.2010.12.006.

18. Grant JE, Kim SW, Crow SJ. Prevalence and clinical features of body dysmorphic disorder in adolescent and adult psychiatric inpatients. J Clin Psychiatry 2001; 62(7):517–22. https://doi.org/10.4088/jcp.v62n07a03.

19. Krebs G, Fernández de la Cruz L, Mataix-Cols D. Recent advances in understanding and managing body dysmorphic disorder. Evidence-Based Ment Health 2017;20(3):71–5. https://doi.org/10.1136/eb-2017-102702.

20. Conroy M, Menard W, Fleming-Ives K, et al. Prevalence and clinical characteristics of body dysmorphic disorder in an adult inpatient setting. Gen Hosp Psychiatry 2008;30(1):67–72. https://doi.org/10.1016/j.genhosppsych.2007.09.004.

21. Dyl J, Kittler J, Phillips KA, et al. Body dysmorphic disorder and other clinically significant body image concerns in adolescent psychiatric inpatients: prevalence and clinical characteristics. Child Psychiatry Hum Dev 2006;36(4):369–82. https://doi.org/10.1007/s10578-006-0008-7.

22. Veale D, Akyüz EU, Hodsoll J. Prevalence of body dysmorphic disorder on a psychiatric inpatient ward and the value of a screening question. Psychiatry Res 2015;230(2):383–6. https://doi.org/10.1016/j.psychres.2015.09.023.

23. Schneider SC, Storch EA. Improving the detection of body dysmorphic disorder in clinical practice. J Cogn Psychotherapy 2017;31(4):230–41. https://doi.org/10.1891/0889-8391.31.4.230.

24. Phillips KA. The broken mirror: understanding and treating body dysmorphic disorder. USA: Oxford University Press; 2005.

25. Goodman R, Ford T, Richards H, et al. The Development and Well-Being Assessment: description and initial validation of an integrated assessment of child and adolescent psychopathology. J Child Psychol Psychiatry 2000;41(5):645–55. https://doi.org/10.1111/j.1469-7610.2000.tb02345.x.

26. Buckley V, Krebs G, Bowyer L, et al. Innovations in Practice: Body dysmorphic disorder in youth - using the Development and Well-Being Assessment as a tool to improve detection in routine clinical practice. Child Adolesc Ment Health 2018;23(3):291–4. https://doi.org/10.1111/camh.12268.

27. Phillips KA, Hollander E, Rasmussen SA, et al. A severity rating scale for body dysmorphic disorder: development, reliability, and validity of a modified version of the Yale-Brown Obsessive Compulsive Scale. Psychopharmacol Bull 1997; 33(1):17–22.

28. Phillips KA, Hart AS, Mendard W. Psychometric evaluation of the Yale-Brown obsessive-compulsive scale modified for body dysmorphic disorder (BDD-YBOCS). J Clin Psychiatry 2001;62(2):87. https://doi.org/10.4088/jcp.v62n0203.

29. Phillips KA, Hart AS, Menard W. Psychometric evaluation of the Yale–Brown Obsessive-Compulsive Scale Modified for Body Dysmorphic Disorder (BDD-YBOCS). J Obsessive-Compulsive Relat Disord 2014;3(3):205–8. https://doi.org/10.1016/j.jocrd.2014.04.004.

30. Monzani B, Fallah D, Rautio D, et al. Psychometric Evaluation of the Yale-Brown Obsessive-Compulsive Scale Modified for Body Dysmorphic Disorder for Adolescents (BDD-YBOCS-A). Child Psychiatry Hum Dev 2022. https://doi.org/10.1007/s10578-022-01376-x.

31. Bowyer L, Krebs G, Mataix-Cols D, et al. A critical review of cosmetic treatment outcomes in body dysmorphic disorder. Body Image 2016;19:1–8. https://doi.org/10.1016/j.bodyim.2016.07.001.

32. Veale D. Outcome of cosmetic surgery and 'DIY' surgery in patients with body dysmorphic disorder. Psychiatr Bull 2000;24:218–20. https://doi.org/10.1192/pb.24.6.218.

33. Grant JE, Menard W, Phillips KA. Pathological skin picking in individuals with body dysmorphic disorder. Gen Hosp Psychiatry 2006;28(6):487–93. https://doi.org/10.1016/j.genhosppsych.2006.08.009.

34. National Institute for Health and Clinical Excellence. Obsessive-compulsive disorder: Core interventions in the treatment of obsessive-compulsive disorder and body dysmorphic disorder. UK: National Institute for Health and Clinical Excellence; 2005.

35. Veale D, Anson M, Miles S, et al. Efficacy of cognitive behaviour therapy versus anxiety management for body dysmorphic disorder: a randomised controlled trial. Psychother Psychosom 2014;83(6):341–53. https://doi.org/10.1159/000360740.

36. Wilhelm S, Phillips KA, Didie E, et al. Modular cognitive-behavioral therapy for body dysmorphic disorder: a randomized controlled trial. Behav Ther 2014; 45(3):314–27. https://doi.org/10.1016/j.beth.2013.12.007.

37. Wilhelm S, Phillips KA, Greenberg JL, et al. Efficacy and Posttreatment Effects of Therapist-Delivered Cognitive Behavioral Therapy vs Supportive Psychotherapy for Adults With Body Dysmorphic Disorder: A Randomized Clinical Trial. JAMA Psychiatry Apr 1 2019;76(4):363–73. https://doi.org/10.1001/jamapsychiatry.2018.4156.

38. Miller WR, Rollnick S. Motivational interviewing: helping people change. Guildford press; 2012.

39. Rautio D, Gumpert M, Jassi A, et al. Effectiveness of multimodal treatment for young people with body dysmorphic disorder in two specialist clinics. Behav Ther 2022. https://doi.org/10.1016/j.beth.2022.04.010.

40. Mataix-Cols D, Fernández de la Cruz L, Isomura K, et al. A Pilot Randomized Controlled Trial of Cognitive-Behavioral Therapy for Adolescents With Body Dysmorphic Disorder. J Am Acad Child Adolesc Psychiatry 2015;54(11):895–904. https://doi.org/10.1016/j.jaac.2015.08.011.

41. Rosen JC, Reiter J, Orosan P. Cognitive-behavioral body image therapy for body dysmorphic disorder. J Consult Clin Psychol 1995;63(2):263–9. https://doi.org/10.1037//0022-006x.63.2.263.

42. Veale D, Gournay K, Dryden W, et al. Body dysmorphic disorder: a cognitive behavioural model and pilot randomised controlled trial. Behav Res Ther 1996;34(9):717–29. https://doi.org/10.1016/0005-7967(96)00025-3.

43. Rabiei M, Mulkens S, Kalantari M, et al. Metacognitive therapy for body dysmorphic disorder patients in Iran: acceptability and proof of concept. J Behav Ther Exp Psychiatry 2012;43(2):724–9. https://doi.org/10.1016/j.jbtep.2011.09.013.

44. Enander J, Andersson E, Mataix-Cols D, et al. Therapist guided internet based cognitive behavioural therapy for body dysmorphic disorder: single blind randomised controlled trial. Br Med J 2016;352:i241. https://doi.org/10.1136/bmj.i241.

45. Greenberg JL, Jacobson NC, Hoeppner SS, et al. Early response to cognitive behavioral therapy for body dysmorphic disorder as a predictor of outcomes. J Psychiatr Res 2022;152:7–13. https://doi.org/10.1016/j.jpsychires.2022.06.001.

46. Krebs G, Fernández de la Cruz L, Monzani B, et al. Long-Term Outcomes of Cognitive-Behavioral Therapy for Adolescent Body Dysmorphic Disorder. Behav Ther 2017;48(4):462–73. https://doi.org/10.1016/j.beth.2017.01.001.

47. Flygare O, Enander J, Andersson E, et al. Predictors of remission from body dysmorphic disorder after internet-delivered cognitive behavior therapy: a machine learning approach. BMC Psychiatry May 19 2020;20(1):247. https://doi.org/10.1186/s12888-020-02655-4.

48. Phillips KA, Greenberg JL, Hoeppner SS, et al. Predictors and moderators of symptom change during cognitive-behavioral therapy or supportive psychotherapy for body dysmorphic disorder. J Affect Disord 2021;287:34–40. https://doi.org/10.1016/j.jad.2021.03.011.

49. Greenberg JL, Phillips KA, Steketee G, et al. Predictors of Response to Cognitive-Behavioral Therapy for Body Dysmorphic Disorder. Behav Ther 2019;50(4):839–49. https://doi.org/10.1016/j.beth.2018.12.008.

50. Fang A, Steketee G, Keshaviah A, et al. Mechanisms of Change in Cognitive Behavioral Therapy for Body Dysmorphic Disorder. Cogn Ther Res 2020;44. https://doi.org/10.1007/s10608-020-10080-w.

51. Phillips KA, Albertini RS, Rasmussen SA. A randomized placebo-controlled trial of fluoxetine in body dysmorphic disorder. Arch Gen Psychiatry 2002;59(4):381–8. https://doi.org/10.1001/archpsyc.59.4.381.

52. Phillips KA, Dwight MM, McElroy SL. Efficacy and safety of fluvoxamine in body dysmorphic disorder. J Clin Psychiatry 1998;59(4):165–71. https://doi.org/10.4088/jcp.v59n0404.

53. Phillips KA, Najjar F. An open-label study of citalopram in body dysmorphic disorder. J Clin Psychiatry 2003;64(6):715–20. https://doi.org/10.4088/jcp.v64n0615.

54. Phillips KA, Keshaviah A, Dougherty DD, et al. Pharmacotherapy Relapse Prevention in Body Dysmorphic Disorder: A Double-Blind, Placebo-Controlled Trial. Am J Psychiatry 2016;173(9):887–95. https://doi.org/10.1176/appi.ajp.2016. 15091243.

55. Hollander E, Allen A, Kwon J, et al. Clomipramine vs desipramine crossover trial in body dysmorphic disorder: selective efficacy of a serotonin reuptake inhibitor in imagined ugliness. Arch Gen Psychiatry 1999;56(11):1033–9. https://doi.org/ 10.1001/archpsyc.56.11.1033.

56. Phillips KA. Placebo-Controlled Study of Pimozide Augmentation of Fluoxetine in Body Dysmorphic Disorder. Am J Psychiatry 2005;162(2):377–9. https://doi.org/ 10.1176/appi.ajp.162.2.377.

57. Phillips KA. Handbook on obsessive compulsive and related disorders. American Psychiatric Association; 2015.

58. Buhlmann U. Treatment barriers for individuals with body dysmorphic disorder: an internet survey. J nervous Ment Dis 2011;199(4):268–71. https://doi.org/10. 1097/NMD.0b013e31821245ce.

59. Schulte J, Schulz C, Wilhelm S, et al. Treatment utilization and treatment barriers in individuals with body dysmorphic disorder. BMC Psychiatry 2020;20(1):1–11. https://doi.org/10.1186/s12888-020-02489-0.

60. Marques L, Weingarden HM, LeBlanc NJ, et al. Treatment utilization and barriers to treatment engagement among people with body dysmorphic symptoms. J Psychosom Res 2011;70(3):286–93. https://doi.org/10.1016/j.jpsychores.2010. 10.002.

61. Phillips KA, Menard W, Pagano ME, et al. Delusional versus nondelusional body dysmorphic disorder: Clinical features and course of illness. J Psychiatr Res 2006;40(2):95–104. https://doi.org/10.1016/j.jpsychires.2005.08.005.

62. Marques L, LeBlanc NJ, Weingarden HM, et al. Barriers to treatment and service utilization in an internet sample of individuals with obsessive-compulsive symptoms. Depress Anxiety 2010;27(5):470–5. https://doi.org/10.1002/da.20694.

63. Wilhelm S, Weingarden H, Greenberg JL, et al. Efficacy of App-Based Cognitive Behavioral Therapy for Body Dysmorphic Disorder with Coach Support: Initial Randomized Controlled Clinical Trial. Psychother Psychosom 2022;91(4): 267–75. https://doi.org/10.1159/000524628.

64. Fang A, Porth R, Phillips KA, et al. Personality as a Predictor of Treatment Response to Escitalopram in Adults With Body Dysmorphic Disorder. J Psychiatr Pract 2019;25(5):347–57. https://doi.org/10.1097/pra. 0000000000000415.

65. Curtiss JE, Bernstein EE, Wilhelm S, et al. Predictors of pharmacotherapy outcomes for body dysmorphic disorder: a machine learning approach. Psychol Med 2022;1–11. https://doi.org/10.1017/s0033291721005390.

Moving?

Make sure your subscription moves with you!

To notify us of your new address, find your **Clinics Account Number** (located on your mailing label above your name), and contact customer service at:

Email: journalscustomerservice-usa@elsevier.com

800-654-2452 (subscribers in the U.S. & Canada)
314-447-8871 (subscribers outside of the U.S. & Canada)

Fax number: 314-447-8029

Elsevier Health Sciences Division
Subscription Customer Service
3251 Riverport Lane
Maryland Heights, MO 63043

*To ensure uninterrupted delivery of your subscription, please notify us at least 4 weeks in advance of move.

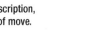

Printed and bound by CPI Group (UK) Ltd, Croydon, CR0 4YY

03/10/2024

01040470-0004